SLAM
Street-Level Airway Management

SLAM® Rescue Airway Flowchart

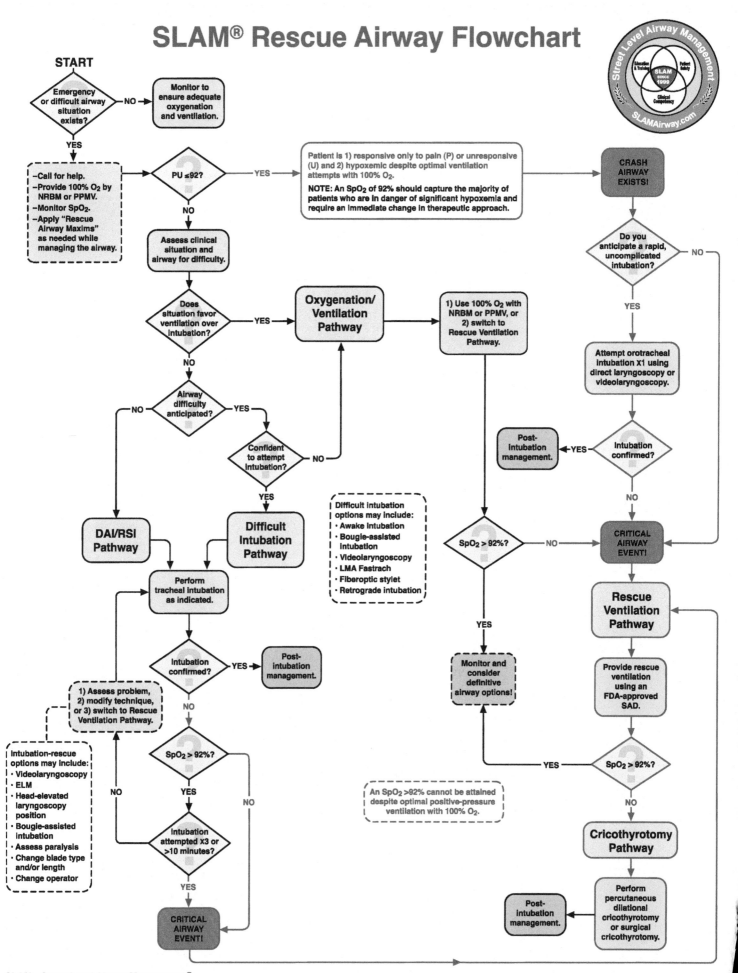

Color and Line Key

- [ ] Pathway headings are gray.
- ◇ Decision points are yellow with a question mark.
- [ ] Action blocks are aqua.
- [ ] Explanatory blocks are white.
- [ ] Critical blocks, borders, and lines are red: Treatment delays can lead to serious morbidity or mortality.
- [ ] Safe blocks are green: Definitive airway is established or oxygenation is attained and maintained using a ventilation technique.

Consideration borders and lines are dashed: Factors to consider include airway difficulty, clinical setting, clinical situation, provider skill, equipment/device availability, provider privileges, medical direction, and protocols/standing orders.

Abbreviations/Definitions

- **BAAM:** Beck Airway-Airflow Monitor (a.k.a. Beck whistle).
- **CMVCI:** Cannot mask ventilate–cannot intubate.
- **Cormack & Lehane laryngoscopic grades of the airway:** Grade 1—full view of the glottis from anterior to posterior commissure; grade 2—partial view of the glottis; grade 3—epiglottis only (3a—epiglottis can be lifted, 3b—epiglottis cannot be lifted from the posterior pharyngeal wall [may decrease success of bougie-assisted and fiberoptic intubation]); grade 4—soft tissue only, no visible laryngeal anatomy.
- **Crash airway:** Describes patients who have severe acute respiratory failure and typically 1) exhibit reduced responsiveness or are unresponsive; 2) have a respiratory rate of <10 or >30 breaths per minute; and 3) have severely depleted oxygen levels. Such patients are usually close to death and require either rapid tracheal intubation or immediate rescue ventilation.
- **Critical airway event:** Indicated by 1) any CMVCI situation; 2) three or more failed intubation attempts or attempted intubation for >10 minutes by an experienced laryngoscopist; or 3) sustained hypoxemia that is refractory to positive-pressure ventilation with 100% O_2.
- **DAI:** Drug-assisted intubation, with or without muscle relaxants.
- **Definitive airway:** Orotracheal tube, nasotracheal tube, or surgical airway.
- **Difficult intubation:** When multiple laryngoscopies, maneuvers, and/or blades are needed by an experienced practitioner.
- **Difficult/inadequate mask ventilation:** Inability of an experienced practitioner to prevent or reverse signs of inadequate ventilation with one- or two-person positive-pressure mask ventilation, using an oropharyngeal or nasopharyngeal airway (or both) and 100% O_2.
- **ELM:** External laryngeal manipulation to improve the laryngoscopic view.
- **Failed intubation:** Failure to intubate the trachea after multiple attempts, with or without hypoxemia.
- **Head-elevated laryngoscopy position:** Use of blankets, pillows, or a wedge pillow to raise the upper back and shoulders to improve the laryngoscopic view in large-framed and/or obese patients.
- **ILMA:** Intubating laryngeal mask airway or LMA Fastrach.
- **LMA:** Laryngeal mask airway (LMA Classic, LMA Fastrach, LMA Flexible, LMA ProSeal, LMA Supreme, LMA Unique, LMA CTrach).
- **MIAS:** Manual in-line axial stabilization to protect the c-spine.
- **NRBM:** Nonrebreathing mask.
- **PPMV:** Positive-pressure mask ventilation.
- **PU ≤92:** (From Mason's PU-92 Concept.) With the AVPU system (A = alert; V = responds to voice; P = responds only to pain; U = unresponsive), patients with "P" or "U" assessments have Glasgow Coma Scale scores of 9 or less. Hypoxemia exists with SpO_2 levels of 92% or less (generally allows for ±2% accuracy of pulse oximeters). If a "P" or "U" assessment and hypoxemia occur simultaneously (i.e., PU ≤92) despite optimal attempts at oxygenation using positive-pressure mask ventilation and 100% O_2, then a crash airway exists.
- **Rescue ventilation:** Administration of 100% O_2 and positive-pressure ventilation (preferably via an FDA-approved supraglottic airway device) to treat a critical airway event.
- **RSI:** Rapid sequence intubation. Relative indications are 1) head trauma with need for airway control and ventilation (e.g., Glasgow Coma Scale score ≤9); 2) uncooperative or combative patient with compromised airway; 3) uncontrolled seizure activity requiring airway control; 4) depressed level of consciousness in trauma patient; and 5) risk of pulmonary aspiration (e.g., full stomach).
- **SAD:** Supraglottic airway device.
- **SLAM:** Street Level Airway Management is an instructional system for rescuing the emergency and difficult airway (www.slamairway.com).
- **SpO_2:** Oxygen saturation as measured by a pulse oximeter.
- **Tracheal intubation:** Indications include 1) airway protection and risk of aspiration; 2) definitive maintenance of airway patency; 3) head injury and Glasgow Coma Scale score ≤9; 4) mechanical ventilation and respiratory failure; 5) emergency surgery and requirement for general anesthesia; 6) application of advanced cardiac life support and drug administration; 7) maintenance of oxygenation or positive end-expiratory pressure; 8) pulmonary toilet.

SLAM (Street Level Airway Management) Rescue Airway Maxims

1. **Call for help early. Maintain a portable emergency airway kit** with adjuncts that help to remedy difficult intubation, provide oxygenation/ventilation and rescue ventilation, facilitate cricothyrotomy, and confirm tracheal intubation. **Patients suffer death and disability from failure to oxygenate and failure to ventilate,** not failure to intubate.

2. **Emergency airway situation (e.g., acute respiratory failure, airway obstruction, CO poisoning, CPR, critical airway event, drug-induced coma, respiratory arrest, tension pneumothorax, traumatic airway disruption): The simple recognition that a patient needs a definitive airway** does not mean that the patient should receive a definitive airway if the provider is not skilled in establishing one. **Never exceed your ability,** experience, or scope of practice. **Consider naloxone or dextrose** to treat drug-induced coma. **Patients with a clenched jaw** will require paralysis and/or sedation in order to facilitate access to the oropharynx. In the absence of RSI drugs, insert one or two soft nasopharyngeal airways to optimize oxygenation.

3. **Oxygenation/ventilation: Provide 100% O_2 by nonrebreathing mask or positive-pressure mask ventilation (± chin lift/head tilt or jaw thrust with oral/nasal airway as tolerated). If tension pneumothorax exists,** decompress immediately. **Monitor SpO_2** (carbon monoxide toxicity will falsely elevate SpO_2). When a standard pulse oximeter probe fails to register a reading due to low perfusion, apply a probe to a different site or use Masimo SET technology. Hypoxemia is difficult to diagnose clinically, so make every attempt to use pulse oximetry or obtain a blood gas reading.

4. **Airway assessment: Perform a 6-D airway assessment** for potential signs of difficulty (e.g., evaluate for Disproportion, Distortion, Decreased range of motion, Decreased thyromental distance, Decreased interincisor gap, and Dental overbite). The potential for difficulty is proportional to the number of D signs. When no airway difficulty is predicted, unexpected difficulty managing the airway may still arise.

5. **C-spine protection: Use MIAS** in suspected or evident c-spine injury during all airway maneuvers and when c-spine collar is not in place. **Do not assess neck range of motion.** Any intubation technique is acceptable as long as MIAS is employed.

6. **Aspiration prophylaxis: Provide available aspiration prophylaxis,** e.g., cricoid pressure, particulate-free antacid, and metoclopramide, to help prevent silent aspiration or passive regurgitation. The aspiration prophylaxis afforded by double-lumen supraglottic airways (e.g., Combitube or EasyTube) is comparable to that of a tracheal tube. Supraglottic airways should generally protect against aspiration better than PPMV. Direct laryngoscopy and tracheal intubation without neuromuscular blockers has a higher documented incidence of aspiration than RSI with neuromuscular blockers.

7. **Tracheal intubation:** Use only methods with which you are trained and skilled. **Intubation attempts should generally be limited** to <10 minutes or ≤3 times by an experienced practitioner. Employ intubation-rescue techniques between attempts (to decrease the occurrence of trauma, bleeding, and edema in the airway, which can impair mask ventilation or subsequent intubation attempts and possibly cause a CMVCI situation). **Intubation-rescue techniques include** bougie-assisted intubation; ELM; head-elevated laryngoscopy position; assessing and/or improving neuromuscular blockade; and changing blade type (straight vs. curved) or blade length. **Difficult intubation options include but are not limited to** use of 1) intubation-rescue techniques, 2) blind nasotracheal intubation, 3) LMA Fastrach ± spontaneous ventilation/(± BAAM, 4) optical stylet, and 5) a video laryngoscope. Combined use of the head-elevated laryngoscopy position, ELM, and bougie introducer can facilitate intubation in patients with limited range of motion due to c-spine precautions (MIAS), morbid obesity, and other causes of Cormack & Lehane grade 3 or 4 laryngoscopic views. **A definitive airway is always best;** however, rescue ventilation can provide interim improvement in oxygenation and ventilation until a definitive airway is established.

8. **Confirmation of tracheal intubation: Always confirm and document intubation** using an evidence-based method (capnography, esophageal detector device, or videolaryngoscopy) in conjunction with auscultation over the mid-axillary lines and abdomen. Use capnography in patients with a perfusing cardiac rhythm. Use an esophageal detector device in patients with a nonperfusing cardiac rhythm.

9. **Rescue ventilation: Provide rescue ventilation using an FDA-approved supraglottic airway device** in the presence of a critical airway event. Supraglottic airway devices can only assist with a supraglottic (above the glottis) obstruction. If rescue ventilation fails, the final option is cricothyrotomy. Glottic or subglottic obstructions require intervention using either a tracheal tube or cricothyrotomy.

10. **Traumatized or burn airway: Avoid blind intubation techniques** in the presence of laryngotracheal trauma. Avoid neuromuscular blockers in blunt neck trauma to prevent potential airway collapse. Up to 6% of patients with blunt airway trauma may have coexisting c-spine injuries. Use only a tracheal tube to maintain patency of a surgical airway for acute burn and inhalation injuries and thus prevent subsequent edema of the anterior neck tissues from engulfing the surgical airway.

SLAM® Rescue Airway Flowchart

- **The advice featured in this flowchart should be overridden when medical direction, clinical experience, the clinical situation, and/or local protocols dictate.**
- **This flowchart is intended for use in adult patients and should only be used by advanced airway practitioners who at a minimum are competent in the use of airway management drugs, direct laryngoscopy, tracheal intubation, rescue ventilation techniques, and cricothyrotomy.**
- **A thorough understanding of the flowchart is necessary prior to its use. Algorithms by their very nature cannot be all-encompassing and need to be interpreted, modified, and applied according to individual patient assessment and good clinical judgment.**

SLAM
Street-Level Airway Management

James Michael Rich

EMETH PRESS
www.emethpress.com

SLAM, Street-Level Airway Management

First Printing by Pearson Prentice Hall 2007

Library of Congress Cataloging-in-Publication Data

Rich, James Michael, author.
  SLAM : street-level airway management / James Michael Rich.
      p. ; cm.
  Street-level airway management
  Includes bibliographical references and index.
  Originally published: Upper Saddle River, N.J. : Pearson/Prentice Hall, c2008.
  ISBN 978-1-60947-085-2 (alk. paper)
  I. Title. II. Title: Street-level airway management.
  [DNLM: 1. Airway Obstruction—therapy. 2. Airway Obstruction—prevention & control. 3. Emergency
Treatment—methods. 4. Intubation, Intratracheal—instrumentation. 5. Intubation, Intratracheal—methods.
6. Respiration, Artificial—methods. WF 145]
  RM388
  615.8'36—dc23
            2014041216

To my wife Alice, the love of my life
and constant companion through thick and thin.

Contents

Chapter **12**

Cricothyrotomy   213

Chapter **13**

The Traumatized Airway   237

Chapter **14**

The Cervical-Spine-Injured Patient   247

Chapter **15**

Burns and Inhalation Injuries   259

Preface

Introduction: The SLAM Concept

Street Level Airway Management (SLAM) and the SLAM Concept involve that overlapping area of clinical practice where practitioners of Prehospital Care, Emergency Medicine and Anesthesiology perform emergency airway management. Several years ago, I developed an airway training program for respiratory care practitioners at a hospital where I was practicing. While doing research for this course and simultaneously working on a manuscript I was preparing on airway management, I began thinking about the concept of street-level airway management (SLAM). I realized that the vast majority of airway management I had provided during my previous two decades in anesthesia could have been applied in or out of the operating room or hospital. With certain exceptions, SLAM principles can generally be applied to any arena in which airway management is performed.

The SLAM concept first and foremost involves having a plan of care. I offer one plan around which this book is written: the SLAM Universal Adult Airway Flowchart (see inside front cover). This is a universal flowchart that can be used by practitioners in different disciplines, such as emergency medicine, prehospital care, and anesthesiology, to navigate through the pitfalls of emergency airway management. The concept also includes clinical options that can be applied in order to avoid the "law of insanity." The law of insanity is defined as doing the same thing again and again while expecting a different result. Not all options work for all situations, and when an option or technique fails, it should be augmented or replaced by another technique to improve the likelihood of success.

The SLAM concept includes pre-use inspection of airway equipment, airway assessment and evaluation, denitrogenation (preoxygenation), primary ventilation and oxygenation, airway control, application of cricoid pressure for aspiration prophylaxis, availability and rational use of airway adjuncts, cervical-spine immobilization (when indicated), safe tracheal intubation and extubation, rescue ventilation and cricothyrotomy. Obviously some situations limit application of advanced airway techniques (i.e., flexible fiberoptic intubation) in the prehospital area, while basic techniques, like optimal patient positioning, optimal external laryngeal manipulation, head-elevated laryngoscopy position (HELP), and the use of bougie-assisted intubation, should be applied in all locations.

At the heart of SLAM is the overarching principle that background knowledge and preparation in both basic and advanced airway management techniques can be applied to nearly all emergency and rescue airway situations, regardless of location. As we know from experience, an airway emergency may arise when least expected. At the moment an airway problem arises, one must be able to assess and effectively remedy the situation using the means at his or her disposal. Successfully overcoming airway emergencies requires knowledge of both basic and advanced airway techniques and adjuncts. For effective airway management, these techniques and adjuncts must be understood and available in all practice locations.

Emergency and rescue airway techniques are central to the SLAM concept. Adjuncts such as the Combitube and laryngeal mask airway can be used effectively in or out of the hospital; however, without thorough knowledge of these adjuncts, benefit from their application remains limited. With the current national emphasis on field rapid-sequence tracheal intubation, it is imperative that these devices be understood and made available due to the temporizing benefits they offer as evidence-based rescue ventilation devices.

Finally, at its most fundamental level, SLAM is about practitioners and health care organizations being willing to invest time, effort, and resources in both acquiring and teaching the skills necessary to help patients avoid airway misadventures. Ready availability and application of multidisciplinary instruction in airway management is needed for the prehospital, hospital, and office/clinic areas. Available areas and resources should be utilized for this endeavor, to include but not necessarily be limited to physician/nurse anesthesia, surgery, medicine, pulmonary care, paramedicine, flight nurse training, and sedation nursing in realistic environments using simulators or cadavers. Periodicals, books, conferences, workshops, and the Internet can provide current updates in airway management. Instruction and application of this knowledge can facilitate effective airway management when an airway emergency arises by having a knowledgeable practitioner do all that is humanly possible to ensure the continuance of life that we all hold so dear.

That airway education program eventually led to the development of the SLAM Advanced Airway Provider Course and the SLAM Express 1-Day Advanced Airway Workshop. I hope that this book, in conjunction with these and other courses, will assist you in the practice of emergency airway management in your particular specialty.

JAMES MICHAEL RICH, CRNA, MA
SLAM Airway Training Institute
www.SLAMAirway.com

Acknowledgements

The author wishes to acknowledge the following:

* Especially grateful to the Lord for my life, family, friends, and colleagues.
* My mother and father for a lifetime of love and encouragement.
* My dear friend and colleague Dr. Michael Frass, MD, of the University of Vienna, in Vienna, Austria who has been a constant source of encouragement and support.
* My friend, colleague and benefactor, Michael A.E. Ramsay, MD, FRCA of the Department of Anesthesiology and Pain Management at Baylor University Medical Center in Dallas, Texas for his direction and encouragement in spurring me on and singularly enabling me to stay on track. A man to which I owe so much but am able to repay so little.
* My friend and colleague, Dr. Andrew M. Mason, MB BS MRCS LRCP, of the Suffolk Accident Rescue Service, Ipswich, United Kingdom for generously sharing his time and talents in collaborating on the SLAM Universal Adult Airway Flowchart, the many readings of this manuscript and the furtherance of the SLAM concept.
* My friend and colleague, William "Gene" Gandy, JD, LP, and my many EMS friends and colleagues without which SLAM would not have continued as it has.
* All the contributors of this work who added greatly to its depth, breadth, and currency.
* Dr. Adolph "Buddy" Gieseke, Dr. Chris Grande, and the International Trauma Anesthesia and Critical Care Society who early on facilitated the educational mission of SLAM.
* Carson Harrod, PhD, of the Baylor Institute of Research in Dallas, Texas for his editorial assistance in the preparation of this manuscript.
* The many nurse anesthetists, anesthesiologists, and anesthesia technicians who have taught me so much over the past 28 years.
* The thousands of students and attendees at SLAM Workshops that I have had the privilege of teaching, who in reality have given far more to me than I have given to them.

Reviewers

Bryan E. Bledsoe, D.O., F. A., C.E.P., EMT-P
Emergency Physician
Midlothian, Texas
and
Adjunct Associate Professor of Emergency Medicine
The George Washington University Medical Center
Washington, DC

Timothy P. Duncan, RN CCRN CEN CFRN EMTP
Flight Nurse/St. Vincent Mercy Medical Center Life Flight
Toledo, OH

Randal Gray, MA Ed., NREMT-P
Director, Office of EMS
University of Alabama at Birmingham

Russell Griffin, NR/CC-P
EMS Captain
McKinney Fire/EMS
McKinney, Texas

Sean Kivlehan, EMT-P
New York-Presbyterian Hospital
New York, NY

Justin Klis, NREMT-P
EMS Coordinator/Instructor
Mount Pleasant Fire Dept.
Racine, WI

Joseph J. Mistovich, M.Ed, NREMT-P
Chair and Professor
Department of Health Professions
Youngstown State University
Youngstown, Ohio

Brian Petrone PA-C, EMT-P
Burlington, Massachusetts

Susie Vigh, BSRRT, NREMT-P, EMSI
EMT Program Instructor
Polaris Career Center
Middleburg Hts, OH

Matthew Zavarella, RN, NREMT-P, MS, SRNA, CFRN, CCRN, CEN
Flight Nurse STAT MedEvac
Pittsburgh, PA

Contributors

Brett D. Arnoldo, MD
Assistant Professor, Surgery
University of Texas Southwestern Medical School
Dallas, TX

George Beck, MD
Anesthesiologist
Lubbock, TX

Tareg Bey, MD, FACEP, ABMT, DEAA
Clinical Professor of Emergency Medicine
Director, International Emergency Medicine
Department of Emergency Medicine
University of California, Irvine
UCI Medical Center
Orange, CA

Janice A. Follmer, CRNA
Summit Anesthesia
Summit Medical Center
Frisco, CO

Michael Frakes, RN, APRN, CCNS, CFRN
Senior Flight Nurse
Clinical Practice and Research Coordinator
Life Star/Hartford Hospital
Hartford, CT

Michael Frass, MD
Professor of Medicine, Intensive Care Unit
Department of Internal Medicine I
Medical University of Vienna
Vienna, Austria

William E. Gandy, JD, LP
EMS Educator and Consultant
Tucson, AZ

Dr. Med. Harald V. Genzwuerker
Clinic of Anaesthesiology and Intensive Care Medicine
University Hospital Mannheim
Mannheim, Germany

Abid U. Ghafoor, MD
Assistant Professor of Anesthesiology
University of Arkansas for Medical Sciences
Staff Anesthesiologist
Arkansas Children's Hospital
Little Rock, AR

Carson Harrod, PhD
Senior Research Associate for Scientific Communication
Baylor Research Institute
Dallas, TX
Founder & Senior Editor
Scientific & Professional Editors
Murphy, TX

John L. Hunt, MD
Co-Director, Burn Unit, Parkland Memorial Hospital
Professor, Department of Surgery
UT Southwestern Medical Center
Dallas, TX

Peter Krafft, MD
Professor, Department of Anesthesiology and General Intensive Care
Medical University of Vienna
Vienna, Austria

Timothy W. Martin, MD, MBA
Professor of Anesthesiology
Vice Chair for Education and Administration
Department of Anesthesiology
UAMS College of Medicine
Chief, Division of Pediatric Anesthesiology
Arkansas Children's Hospital
Little Rock, AR

Andrew M. Mason, MB BS MRCS LRCP
Immediate Care Physician
Suffolk Accident Rescue Service
Ipswich, UK

Alexandre F. Migala, DO
Emergency Medicine Physician
Dallas, TX

W. Patrick Monaghan, CLS, SBB, PhD
Professor, College of Medicine
Anesthesiology Department
University of Florida, Shands,
Jacksonville, FL

Dave Nigel Nanan, MD
Anesthesiologist
Pembroke Pines, FL

Edgar J. Pierre MD
Asst. Professor of Anesthesiology, Surgery and Critical Care
University of Miami Ryder Trauma Center
Miami, FL

Gary Purdue, MD
Co-Director, Burn Unit, Parkland Memorial Hospital
Professor, Department of Surgery
UT Southwestern Medical Center
Dallas, TX

Michael A.E. Ramsay, MD, FRCA
Chief of Service
Department of Anesthesiology and Pain Management
Baylor University Medical Center
Dallas, TX

James Michael Rich, CRNA, MA
Nurse Anesthetist — Northstar Anesthesia, P.A.
Department of Anesthesiology and Pain Management
Baylor University Medical Center
Dallas, TX

Adjunct Faculty
Emergency Medicine Education Program
School of Allied Health Sciences
University of Texas Southwestern Medical Center at Dallas
Dallas, TX

Executive Director
The SLAM Airway Training Institute &
The SLAM Society
3526 Lakeview Parkway, Suite B238
Rowlett, TX 75088
Email: jamesrich.crna@gmail.com

Micha Y. Shamir, MD
Attending Anesthesiologist
Head, Resuscitation School and Service
Department of Anesthesiology and Critical Care Medicine
Hadassah – Hebrew University Medical Center
Hebrew University Medical School
Jerusalem, Israel

Charles E. Smith, MD, FRCPC
Professor of Anesthesia
Director, Cardiothoracic Anesthesia
MetroHealth Medical Center
Case Western Reserve University School of Medicine
Cleveland, OH

Darko Vodopich, MD
Department of Anesthesia
Kaiser Permanente
Walnut Creek Medical Center
Walnut Creek, CA

CHAPTER 1

SLAM Universal
Adult Airway Flowchart

James Michael Rich

Chapter Objectives

After reading this chapter, you should be able to:

- State the goals and functions of the SLAM Universal Adult Airway Flowchart (SUAAF).

- Describe ways of providing primary oxygen and ventilation.

- Define an emergency airway situation.

- Define the limits on attempts to perform intubation.

- Describe the methods of managing rescue ventilation.

- Describe evidence-based techniques for confirming tracheal tube placement.

- Describe Mason's PU-92 concept.

- List the limitations on the SUAAF.

- List the recommended content of an emergency airway kit.

CASE Study

Flight paramedic Mike Jacobs, NREMT-P, and flight nurse Cindy Reyes, RN, arrive on Flight-1 at the scene of an accident involving an SUV. The firefighter paramedics report that the driver of the SUV hit a patch of ice, lost control of the vehicle, and hit a guard rail. He was not wearing a seatbelt and he was ejected from his vehicle.

The firefighter paramedics describe the patient's condition as hypotensive and tachycardic. They have applied a rigid c-spine collar, inserted an oropharyngeal airway, and are administering oxygen by nonrebreathing mask at 15 liters per minute. An IV bolus of 250 mL of Ringer's lactate is infused and restores a radial pulse. However, the patient's breathing is rapid and shallow, and his SpO_2 reading is only 90%, despite oxygen therapy. The patient has a GCS of 5, equating to a P grading on the AVPU scale. A rapid 6-D airway assessment is performed.

The paramedics decide to undertake rapid sequence intubation (RSI) in order to secure the patient's airway and improve oxygenation and ventilation. The RSI drugs are drawn up and labeled, and the intubation equipment is checked and readied. The anterior portion of the c-spine collar is removed while manual in-line axial stabilization (MIAS) is continually applied.

After receiving lidocaine 100 mg, the patient is given etomidate 14 mg and succinylcholine 120 mg while Sellick's maneuver is performed. In an attempt to raise the SpO_2, the patient is gently ventilated by positive pressure mask ventilation while cricoid pressure is maintained. Within 45 seconds, the SpO_2 has improved to 96%.

On the first laryngoscopy attempt using a 3 Macintosh laryngoscope blade, only the tip of the epiglottis is visible, and the patient's SpO_2 drops to 90%. Laryngoscopy is halted, and the patient is given positive pressure mask ventilation with 100% oxygen. The MIAS and Sellick's maneuver are continued without interruption. The SpO_2 rises to 96% once again.

On the second laryngoscopy attempt, a bougie introducer is inserted just posterior to the tip of the epiglottis. As the bougie is advanced, the laryngoscopist feels tracheal clicking. A tracheal tube is then railroaded over the bougie, the tracheal tube cuff is inflated, and position is confirmed using a portable handheld capnograph and chest auscultation.

At this point Sellick's maneuver is released, and the anterior portion of the c-spine collar is reattached. The tracheal tube is secured with a commercial tube holder, and the patient is ventilated by bag-valve device. Ventilation and oxygenation are monitored continuously using the capnograph and pulse oximeter as part of the postintubation management process.

The patient is transported to a Level I trauma center where he undergoes an exploratory laparotomy resulting in a splenectomy. He also undergoes evacuation of a subdural hematoma and open reduction and internal fixation of a right femur fracture. He makes a good recovery without incident in the surgical intensive care unit and is discharged from the hospital 10 days later with no neurological deficit.

Introduction

Street Level Airway Management® (SLAM®) is an instructional system for teaching emergency airway management to multidisciplinary groups of practitioners who practice from street level through all areas of the hospital. The prehospital area (i.e., the street level) is the most challenging area for emergency airway management because of the uncontrolled clinical situations that are prone to occur there. The two key aspects of the SLAM system are the SLAM Concept and the SLAM Universal Adult Airway Flowchart[1] (SUAAF) (see the inside front cover of this book). A major goal of these two entities is to increase patient safety by improving practitioner skill in emergency and difficult airway management.

KEY TERMS

BURP, p. 14	gum-elastic bougie, p. 7	6-D method, p. 6
crash airway, p. 9	HELP, p. 14	SLAM concept, p. 2
critical airway event, p. 8	interincisor gap, p. 6	SSAAA, p. 5
ELM, p. 14	Mason's PU-92 concept, p. 10	thyromental distance, p. 6

Overview of the SLAM Universal Adult Airway Flowchart

SLAM concept
The idea that most airway techniques used in anesthesiology can be applied from the prehospital environment through all areas of the hospital.

The SLAM Universal Adult Airway Flowchart (SUAAF) is based on the **SLAM concept**,[2] which maintains that most airway techniques used in anesthesiology can be generally applied to other locations where emergency airway management is performed—from the street level[3,4] through all areas within the hospital.[5] Problems encountered during emergency airway management, regardless of the clinical situation,[6-12] are often multivariate. In addition to basic training and advanced skill acquisition, successful airway management requires familiarity, availability, and application of decision-making strategies,[13-19] airway drugs,[7,8,11] adjunctive airway devices,[11,20-23] equipment for tracheal intubation,[24-28] and monitoring of lung ventilation.[17,27,29,30]

A number of airway management flowcharts have been published in recent years (Table 1-1). Most of these flowcharts are intended for physicians and are hospital-based.[13,14,16,19]

Table 1-1 Comparisons of Airway Management Algorithms/Flowcharts[25]

	Target Group	Target Location	Advocates Airway Evaluation?	Offers Intubation-Rescue Techniques?	Presents Rescue Ventilation Techniques?	Presents Information on Aspiration Prophylaxis?	Advocates Evidenced-Based Techniques for Confirmation of Tracheal Intubation?
ASA Difficult Airway Algorithm[13]	Anesthesiologists and those supervised by them	Anesthetizing locations	Yes: 11-step preoperative assessment plan	No	Yes	No	Yes: capnography or esophageal detector device
ERC Flowchart for Advanced Management of the Airway and Ventilation[14]	Physicians	Prehospital and hospital locations	No	No	Yes	No	No
SLAM Universal Adult Airway Flowchart[32]	Advanced airway practitioners: nurses, physicians, paramedics, and others	Prehospital and non–operating room hospital locations	Yes: quick 4-step assessment	Yes	Yes	Yes: cricoid pressure, nonparticulate antacid, and metoclopramide	Yes: capnography or esophageal detector device
Algorithms of R.M. Wallis[19]	Emergency medical physicians	Emergency Department	Yes	Yes	Yes	Yes: cricoid pressure	No
DAS guidelines for management of the unanticipated difficult intubation[16]	Anesthesiologists	Anesthetizing locations for adult nonobstetrical patients	No	Yes	Yes	Yes	No

ASA = American Society of Anesthesiologists

ERC = The European Resuscitation Council

DAS = Difficult Airway Society (modified from reference)[25]

Emergency airway management in closed spaces. The victim is trapped in a vehicle and in need of rapid oxygenation and ventilation. After preoxygenation, induction, and intravenous sedation, a Combitube was inserted and ventilation provided until the victim was extricated from the vehicle.
(Courtesy of Dr. Peer G. Knacke)

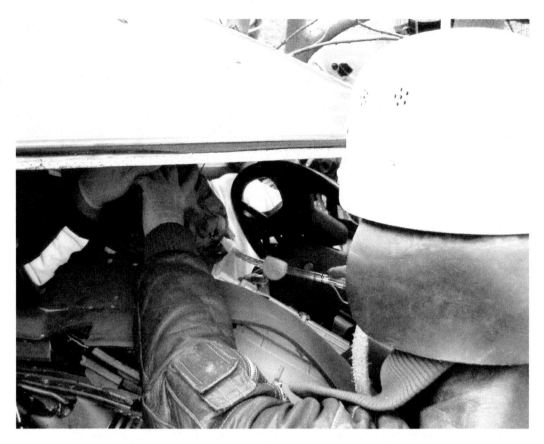

However, an emergency airway situation can occur anywhere across the spectrum of health care.[3-6,22,23,31,32] Whether the provider is a physician, nurse, or paramedic, he or she is responsible for provision of safe and effective airway management. The patient requires a patent airway along with effective oxygenation and ventilation. Therefore, the SUAAF does not differentiate between practitioners in its approach to airway management training because providers at all levels can encounter airway pitfalls. In reality, those having the least access to clinical training for airway management (e.g., paramedics) frequently encounter the most complicated emergency airway situations.[22] Entrapment, closed-space rescue, airway and multiple trauma secondary to motor-vehicle collisions create tremendous challenges for prehospital paramedic rescuers (Figure 1-1).[3,4,31]

PEARLS   A difficult airway situation can occur without warning and regardless of the practitioner's experience or scope of practice.

It is reported that death or brain damage occurred in approximately 85% of 522 anesthesia-related airway closed liability claims that were analyzed through 1985.[9] The findings of the closed malpractice liability claims on adverse respiratory events that were published by the American Society of Anesthesiologists[5,9] and the American Association of Nurse Anesthetists[33,34] document the need for additional comprehensive proficiency in airway management. Inadequate ventilation, unrecognized esophageal intubation, and difficult intubation accounted for approximately 75% of the adverse respiratory events that were reported.[9] Improvements in monitoring within the operating room have decreased the first two mechanisms of injury in anesthesiology.[22] However, reports of airway injury, inadequate ventilation, unrecognized esophageal intubation, and other complications of airway management continue to be reported.[6,8,12]

ON TARGET

The SUAAF should be overridden when medical direction, clinical experience, the clinical situation, and/or local protocols dictate. One algorithm cannot fit all situations. Good clinical judgment must always be exercised.

The **SUAAF** is intended, at a minimum, to assist in preventing these types of airway complications through a comprehensive system that alerts practitioners to dangerous airway pitfalls that can occur during airway management. While other algorithms target a particular group of practitioners (e.g., anesthesiologists or emergency physicians),[14,16,19,35] the SUAAF was developed for application by a wide variety of airway practitioners, especially paramedics and prehospital advanced airway practitioners. During development, the SUAAF was presented in various formats at several educational conferences,[18,36-41] and it received the award for best scientific exhibit for clinical application at the 57th Postgraduate Assembly of the New York State Society of Anesthesiologists in December 2003.[42]

The SUAAF was originally introduced as The SLAM Emergency Airway Flowchart.[25] However, the title was changed to reflect its universal application with regard to the site of airway injury (e.g., prehospital or hospital) the clinical situation (emergency or difficult), as well as the type of advanced airway practitioner (physician versus nonphysician). The flowchart is designed to assist advanced airway practitioners in the acquisition of critical decision-making skills and the improvement of patient care with regard to emergency airway management.

SUAAF fills a dual role by focusing on the prevention and management of difficult airway situations through practical methods to rectify failed intubation, while simultaneously providing emergency airway practitioners with clinical guidance on deciding when (1) tracheal intubation is appropriate, (2) to stop attempting tracheal intubation, and (3) to undertake rescue ventilation (Chapter 8). It provides clear and comprehensive strategies for treating emergency airway situations, especially those occurring in the prehospital[3,4,6,17,31,43] and non–operating room[5] hospital environments. It stresses prevention, rapid recognition, and treatment of critical airway events, while assisting practitioners in developing critical decision-making skills in emergency airway management.

The overall intent of the SUAAF is to foster improvement in patient safety with regard to emergency and difficult airway management.[22,23] However, it is limited to use by advanced airway practitioners who are trained in oxygenation and ventilation techniques (Chapter 3), direct laryngoscopy and tracheal intubation (Chapter 4), application of evidence-based techniques to confirm tracheal intubation and monitor oxygenation and ventilation (Chapter 5), the administration of drugs for airway rapid sequence intubation (RSI) (Chapter 7), rescue ventilation techniques (Chapter 8),[22] difficult-airway intubation techniques (Chapter 9), and cricothyrotomy (Chapter 12).[44,45]

Airway management is performed in various clinical settings and by different types of practitioners possessing different levels of training and experience.[3,4,6,8,22,23,46-48] The location of care can affect the clinical situation by creating difficulty in what might otherwise be an uncomplicated airway management encounter (e.g., prehospital confined-space rescue).[3,4,49] A recent report reveals that the timing and location of airway management in the hospital can have a direct effect on patient outcome; that is, the severity of injury can increase and survivability can decrease the greater the distance that the incident occurs from the operating room area.[5] No such reports exist for the prehospital environment, but it can be assumed from this report that lack of preparation in basic training, skill maintenance, and logistics may have a detrimental effect on provision of airway management.

Airway Assessment and Evaluation

Tracheal intubation is not always achievable, and airway difficulty is not always predictable.[11] Additionally, difficult laryngoscopy is reported to occur in up to 6% of laryngoscopies in anesthesia.[11] Difficult laryngoscopy created by the need for a neutral head position (e.g., unstable cervical-spine precautions) occurs with an incidence as high as 42%.[50] Paramedics are exposed to this situation more than any other advanced airway practitioner.

Therefore, the SUAAF does not differentiate between physician and nonphysician. For this reason, the SUAAF promotes the practice of assessing the airway whenever feasible and prior to implementation of airway management. Beyond patient factors that create difficulty, paramedics are exposed to clinical situations that can increase difficulty, such as entrapment and closed-space rescue. For this reason, paramedics must always consider the impact of the scene and its potential effect on the management of the airway.

Always assess the airway first. Recognizing a difficult airway before you begin to manage it can help prevent or decrease the incidence of a difficult laryngoscopy and failed intubation. One way to recognize a potentially difficult airway is to use the 6-D method. It was developed by the author[51] from a previously described method of airway assessment.[52] It examines the airway for six signs that can be associated with difficult intubation:

- Distortion of the airway.
- Disproportion.
- Decreased **thyromental distance.**
- Decreased **interincisor gap.**
- Decreased range of motion.
- Dental overbite.

This rapid method of airway assessment[51-55] helps practitioners remember to assess for signs that can be associated with a difficult intubation. The potential for difficult intubation is generally proportional to the number of signs observed. However, no method of airway assessment is infallible and may produce either false-negative or false-positive signs of difficult intubation. (More about the **6-D** method will be offered in Chapter 2.)

Provision of Emergency Airway Management in the Prehospital Area and Remote Hospital Locations

Prior planning can prevent poor outcomes during airway rescue. Two prerequisites to safe delivery of airway care include availability of well-trained personnel and provision of an appropriately stocked airway kit. Ready availability of appropriate items for emergency airway management will assist in prevention of complications and improvement of patient outcome in remote locations. Maintaining a prepared kit that can be carried to remote locations is recommended (Figure 1-2).

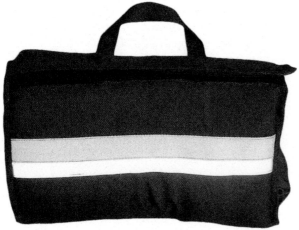

Photo credit: SunMed Medical Solutions

(a)

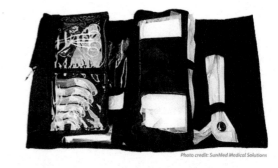

Photo credit: SunMed Medical Solutions

(b)

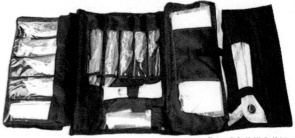

Photo credit: SunMed Medical Solutions

(c)

FIGURE 1-2
An example of a commercially available emergency airway kit (Sun-Med, Largo, FL, Airwaystore.com) for both primary ventilation, orotracheal intubation, and nasotracheal intubation. This kit rolls up for easy storage.
(Courtesy of Sun-Med USA, Largo, FL)

Always maintain and carry a prepared kit containing everything you will need to handle an airway emergency.

Portable airway kits should be ready for use and available to treat adverse respiratory events at all times. At a minimum, these kits should contain appropriate airway drugs (Chapter 6), conventional tracheal intubation equipment (Chapter 4), devices to treat difficult intubation (Chapter 9), evidence-based devices to confirm tracheal intubation (Chapter 5), and devices for rescue ventilation (Chapter 8) (Table 1-2). These kits should either be exchanged

---

Table 1-2   Recommended Contents for the Portable Emergency Airway Kit[25]

1. Tracheal intubation components
   a. Beck airway airflow monitor (BAAM whistle)[56]
   b. Blades: straight (#1, #2, #3, and #4) and curved (#1, #2, #3 and #4)
   c. Drugs
      i. Atropine or glycopyrrolate
      ii. Midazolam
      iii. Etomidate
      iv. 2% lidocaine jelly
      v. 4% topical lidocaine
      vi. Oxymetazoline nasal spray
      vii. Rocuronium
      viii. Succinylcholine
      ix. Vecuronium
   d. Exam gloves
   e. Flexible bougie introducer/stylet (e.g., **gum-elastic bougie**)
   f. K-Y jelly
   g. Laryngoscope handle (2)
   h. Magill forceps
   i. Malleable stylet
   j. Syringes and needles
   k. Tape, trach-tape, or Thomas tube holder to secure tracheal tube or laryngeal mask airway
   l. Tracheal tubes (sizes pediatric through adult)
   m. Tracheal tube exchange catheter (e.g., Cook exchange catheter)

2. Ventilation devices and adjuncts
   a. Combitube SA (37 F)
   b. Laryngeal mask airway (#1, #2, #3, #4, and #5)
   c. Oropharyngeal airways (pediatric through adult)
   d. Nasopharyngeal airways (all sizes)
   e. Ventilation bag with various face masks

3. Devices to confirm tracheal intubation
   a. Portable carbon dioxide detector (electronic or colorimetric)
   b. Esophageal detector device (e.g., self-inflating bulb)
   c. Stethoscope

4. Infection control product
   a. Decontamination wipes
   b. Exam gloves
   c. Biohazard bag

---

gum-elastic bougie
A long flexible "stylet" that is placed in the trachea as a guide for the ET tube. It is useful when a good view of the cords is impossible, but the epiglottis or posterior arytenoids can be identified.

Modified from Rich J, Mason A, Ramsay M. The SLAM emergency airway flowchart: a new guide for advanced airway practitioners. *AANA J.* 2004; 72: 431–439.

for a new one after use or immediately restocked. A color-coded breakaway lock can be used to indicate that the kit has been restocked and is ready for use.

Using the SLAM Universal Adult Airway Flowchart

Note that the advice featured in the SUAAF should be overridden when medical direction, clinical experience, the clinical situation, and/or local protocols dictate. It is also important to understand that algorithms cannot, by their very nature, be all-encompassing; they must be interpreted, modified, and applied according to individual patient assessment and good clinical judgment.

The SUAAF has been designed with instructional blocks of various shapes and colors. Each color and shape denotes important emergency airway management considerations such as clinical pathways, clinical situations, and clinical questions. When using the flowchart, the goal should be to arrive at a green rectangular block, indicating that tracheal intubation has been confirmed (Chapter 5), or that rescue ventilation has been applied effectively (Chapter 8). Treatment pathways are indicated by gray blocks. The five treatment pathways are:

- Oxygenation/ventilation.
- Rapid sequence intubation.
- Difficult intubation.
- Rescue ventilation.
- Cricothyrotomy.

Each pathway poses clinical questions contained in yellow diamond-shaped decision blocks, which are designed to assist the practitioner in making clinical decisions. Each decision contains a clinical question with a yes or no reply. Depending on the answer, care is either continued on the treatment pathway currently being used, or care is switched to an alternate treatment pathway.

Green indicates a safe block, and red indicates a critical block or pathway. Safe blocks show that a definitive airway (i.e., orotracheal tube, nasotracheal tube, or surgical airway) has been established or that oxygenation and ventilation has been achieved using a rescue ventilation technique or cricothyrotomy. Arriving at a red block indicates that a critical airway situation exists, demanding either rapid intubation or effective rescue ventilation. Delayed or inadequate management of red-block situations can lead to serious morbidity or mortality.

Blue blocks are action blocks that direct the practitioner to proceed with a particular intervention or action. Dashed lines or borders indicate that a further clinical consideration is required. Explanatory notes are indicated by white blocks.

The Rescue Ventilation Pathway, Mason's PU-92 Concept, and the Cricothyrotomy Pathway

The SUAAF brings a new term to airway management: **critical airway event.** It summarizes dangerous airway conditions that could lead to death or disability if allowed to continue without intervention and that are generally reversible using rescue ventilation.[5,9,22] A critical airway event is indicated by:

- Any cannot-mask-ventilate/cannot-intubate (CMVCI) situation.
- Three or more failed intubation attempts or attempting intubation for longer than 10 minutes (by an experienced practitioner).
- Sustained hypoxemia that is refractory to positive pressure ventilation with 100% oxygen.[25]

critical airway event
Any cannot-mask-ventilate/cannot-intubate situation, three or more failed intubation attempts or attempting intubation for longer than 10 minutes (by an experienced practitioner), or sustained hypoxemia that is refractory to positive pressure ventilation with 100% oxygen.

Table 1-3 *Adjunctive Supraglottic Airway Ventilation Devices*[1,22,59]

Device	AHA/ILCOR* Classification	Manufacturer
AMBU laryngeal mask	Not yet rated	AMBU, Glen Burnie, MD
Cobra PLA	Not yet rated	Engineered Medical Systems, Indianapolis, IN
Combitube	Class II-a[†]	Tyco-Healthcare-Nellcor, Pleasanton, CA
EasyTube	Not yet rated	Rusch, Research Triangle Park, NC
Intubating laryngeal airway	Not yet rated	Mercury Medical, Clearwater, FL
King laryngeal tube	Not yet rated	King Systems, Noblesville, IN
Laryngoseal laryngeal mask	Not yet rated	Tyco-Healthcare-Nellcor, Pleasanton, CA
LMA-Classic	Class II-a[†]	LMA North America, San Diego, CA
LMA-Fastrach	Not yet rated	LMA North America, San Diego, CA

*AHA/ILCOR stands for American Heart Association/International Liaison Committee on Resuscitation. Devices are classified at the AHA/ILCOR conferences that occur every five years. Classification is based on review and discussion of research articles and case reports from the peer-reviewed literature. Many new supraglottic airway devices have been introduced since the 2000 conference was held. However, the 2005 conference did not expand the range of such devices awarded Class IIa status beyond the existing Combitube and LMA.

[†]Class IIa status denotes a therapeutic option for which the weight of evidence is in favor of its usefulness and efficacy.

Used by permission from Rich J. Recognition and management of the difficult airway with special emphasis on the Intubating LMA-Fastrach/whistle technique: a brief review with case reports. BUMC Proceedings 2005; 18: 220–227.

ON TARGET As with all supraglottic airway devices, the Combitube and LMA offer no assistance in overcoming a glottic or subglottic obstruction. These types of obstructions require a tracheal tube or cricothyrotomy.[29] If rescue ventilation fails, the final option is to undertake a cricothyrotomy (Chapter 12).[44,45]

ON TARGET Oxygenation and ventilation are emphasized over intubation because patients suffer brain death or die from failure to ventilate and oxygenate, not failure to intubate!

crash airway
A patient with a Glascow Coma Scale (GCS) score of 9 or less, or an AVPU score of "P" or "U", an oxygen saturation of less than or equal to 92%, a respiratory rate of less than 10 or greater than 30 breaths per minute, and who has not responded to basic methods of ventilation.

Regardless of why laryngoscopy is difficult or why failed intubation occurs, the situation can usually be temporized using rescue ventilation.[1,22,25,57,58] Rescue ventilation involves using 100% oxygen and positive pressure ventilation, ideally by way of a Class IIa adjunctive airway device, such as a Combitube or laryngeal mask airway (LMA), to resolve a critical airway event.[22,59,60] (Class IIa designates a therapeutic option for which the weight of evidence is in favor of its usefulness and efficacy.[61])

Rescue ventilation is indicated for rapid treatment of a critical airway event.[1,25] Newer supraglottic adjunctive airway devices (Table 1-3) are proving effective for rescue ventilation[57] and may receive a Class IIa designation for rescue ventilation in the foreseeable future. However, the esophageal tracheal Combitube (ETC) and LMA (Figure 1-3) are currently the only alternative airway devices with a Class IIa designation (Table 1-3) from the American Heart Association and the International Liaison Committee on Resuscitation[22] and therefore are preferentially recommended for treatment of critical airway events.[11,13,14,19,22,23,29,32,58]

The SUAAF assists in rapid recognition and treatment of a patient with a **crash airway** (Table 1-4). Walls[19] originally described the crash airway[13,21,26,38,48] to categorize patients with acute respiratory failure who are unconscious, apneic, or having agonal respirations; arrested or near death; and anticipated to be unresponsive to (i.e., tolerant of) laryngoscopy.

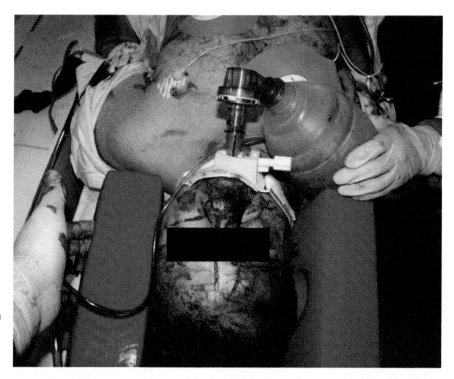

Mason's PU-92 concept
A simple scheme to identify patients requiring immediate intubation or rescue ventilation using pulse oximetry and the AVPU scale.

Rapid recognition of a crash airway can be accomplished by the use of **Mason's PU-92 concept,** a simple scheme for the identification of patients requiring either immediate intubation or rescue ventilation (Figure 1-4).[17] Look at the SUAAF at the beginning of your book. Mason's PU-92 concept appears in the second yellow decision diamond from the flowchart's starting point.[25]

Mason's PU-92 concept combines an assessment of the level of responsiveness using the AVPU scale (A = alert, V = responds to voice, P = responds only to pain, U = unresponsive) in combination with the patient's SpO_2 level.[17,62] Those who are either responsive only to pain (P) or are unresponsive (U) and have a simultaneous SpO_2 reading of 92% or less are classified as crash-airway patients, requiring immediate tracheal intubation or rescue ventilation.[17,25] A score of P or U corresponds to a Glasgow Coma Scale score of <9.[62]

The "92" in Mason's PU-92 concept refers to the threshold for hypoxemia using a pulse oximeter. A study of the oxyhemoglobin dissociation curve shows that the hypoxemia

Patients who simultaneously exhibit the following triad of signs should be considered to have a crash airway:

- Significantly reduced responsiveness (having a Glasgow Coma Scale score of 9 or less).
- Significantly depleted oxygen levels[†] (having an SaO_2 level of 90% or less).
- A respiratory rate of <10 or >30 breaths per minute,[17,22] the hypoxemia having been unresponsive to basic methods to improve oxygenation (e.g., positioning and clearing of the airway and use of a nonrebreathing mask or bag-valve-mask ventilation together with high-flow oxygen therapy).

*Use of this revised model for the crash airway should ensure that trauma patients who might benefit from immediate airway intervention are not overlooked in the prehospital phase of treatment.

†Early oxygenation by way of a secure airway is of vital importance for patients who have sustained serious brain injuries because the combination of hypoxemia and hypercarbia is potentially lethal in patients who already have a primary cerebral insult.

Used by permission from Rich J, Mason A, Ramsay M. The SLAM emergency airway flowchart: a new guide for advanced airway practitioners. AANA J. 2004; 72: 431–439.

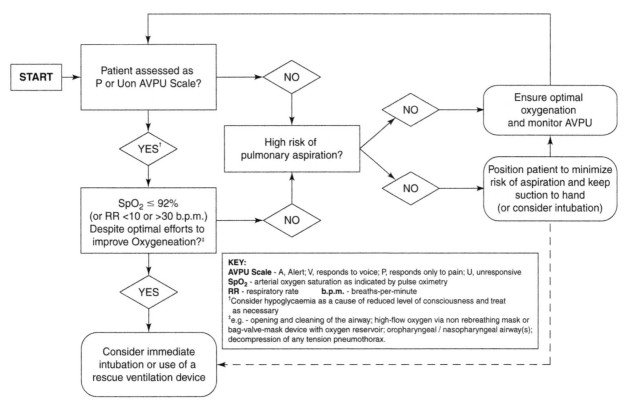

FIGURE 1-4

Mason's PU-92 concept is a simple scheme to identify patients requiring immediate intubation or rescue ventilation. (Courtesy of Dr. Andrew M. Mason)

threshold is reached when the SaO_2 value falls to 90% (Figure 1-5). However, an SaO_2 reading (arterial oxygen saturation) requires arterial blood sampling, which is not feasible in most emergency situations where rescuers will be relying on readings from a pulse oximeter displaying SpO_2 values. SpO_2 readings are simply estimates of the arterial oxygen saturation level generated from algorithms. The majority of pulse oximeters have a tolerance of $\pm 2\%$ accuracy.[30] So to ensure that the great majority of patients who are truly hypoxemic will be captured, Mason's scheme uses an SpO_2 threshold of 92%.

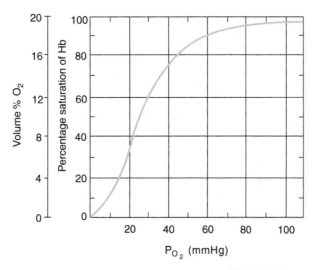

FIGURE 1-5

Oxyhemoglobin-dissociation curve.

The benefits of Mason's PU-92 concept stem from its straightforward structure consisting of just two components that are quick and simple to administer (an AVPU grading and an SpO_2 reading). Previously, practitioners have lacked a simple, practical method of identifying a critical airway situation despite the fact that persistent hypoxemia and a Glasgow Coma Scale (GCS) score of less than 9 are both widely accepted indications for emergency intubation.

Oxygenation/Ventilation Pathway

A "no" answer to the PU≤92 question indicates that the patient does not require immediate intubation or rescue ventilation. In these circumstances, simple methods can be used to open the airway and provide adequate oxygenation, such as a jaw-thrust maneuver in conjunction with a nonrebreathing oxygen mask in those who are breathing spontaneously or bag-valve-mask ventilation with an oropharyngeal (O/P) or nasopharyngeal (N/P) airway in those who require ventilatory support.

At an early stage, the SUAAF directs the operator to assess the airway for difficulty (Table 1-1) in an attempt to determine whether the patient should be treated using the RSI pathway, the difficult intubation pathway, or the oxygenation/ventilation pathway. A host of adjunctive supraglottic airway devices can be used for primary ventilation (Table 1-3). (See the SUAAF on the inside front cover of the book.[3,4,23,49]) The main goal is to ensure that the patient is well oxygenated and ventilated until a definitive airway can be established.

Difficult Intubation Pathway

Difficult intubation continues to be a source of disability and death during emergency airway management.[8,9,11,12] Therefore, the SUAAF goes beyond some algorithms[13,14] by recommending additional techniques for treating difficult intubation (Table 1-5)[63] and application of intubation-rescue techniques (Table 1-6).[4,29,63-67] Use of these techniques can attenuate difficult intubation and may diminish the airway trauma that has been reported to cause death or disability.[9,12,29] A recent report indicates that regular practice along with the use of a practical algorithm is the key to success in overcoming difficult airway situations.[68] The choice of a difficult-airway intubation technique depends on the clinical situation and the practitioner's familiarity and skill in using any particular device. Not every difficult-airway technique must be learned or mastered, but practitioners should be familiar with more than one technique to increase the likelihood of success.[51]

Rapid Sequence Intubation Pathway

The rapid sequence intubation (RSI) pathway is recommended for use only in patients meeting the criteria for RSI.[48] The SUAAF recommends techniques that promote aspiration prophylaxsis (Chapter 7).[29,48,69] Both the RSI and difficult tracheal intubation pathway use a common format to direct the practitioner to do the following:

- Confirm intubation using an evidence-based method, that is, carbon dioxide detection in the presence of a perfusing cardiac rhythm, and an esophageal detector device (EDD) in the presence of a nonperfusing cardiac rhythm.[70]

Table 1-5 Techniques for Difficult Tracheal Intubation[51]

Difficult-Airway Intubation Technique	Considerations and Requirements
Awake laryngoscopic intubation[71]	Judicious intravenous sedation[72] Topical anesthesia[72] Gentle use of the laryngoscope
Awake blind nasotracheal intubation[56]	Judicious intravenous sedation[72] Topical anesthesia[72] Spontaneous ventilation Vasoconstrictor[72] Patil intubation guide or Beck airway airflow monitor[56]
Intubating laryngeal mask airway in the awake patient	Judicious intravenous sedation[72] Topical anesthesia[72] Chandy maneuver[73] Spontaneous ventilation Patil intubation guide or Beck airway airflow monitor
Intubating laryngeal mask airway in the apneic patient[73]	Chandy maneuver[73] Positive pressure ventilation
Retrograde intubation[72]	"Can-mask-ventilate/cannot-intubate" situation Parker endotracheal tube Direct laryngoscopy
Indirect rigid fiberoptic laryngoscopy[74]	Upsher, Wu, or Bullard laryngoscope[74]
Flexible fiberoptic laryngoscopy[75]	General anesthesia Judicious intravenous sedation[72] Topical anesthesia[72] Spontaneous ventilation[75]
Lightwand intubation[74]	Should not be used in patients with pharyngeal masses or anatomic abnormalities of the upper airway[74]
Videolaryngoscopic devices[76]	GlideScope[76]
Malleable fiberoptic stylet	Shikani seeing stylet[77] Direct laryngoscopy

Used by permission from Rich J. Recognition and management of the difficult airway with special emphasis on the Intubating LMA-Fastrach/whistle technique: a brief review with case reports. BUMC Proceedings 2005; 18: 220–227.

- Generally limit intubation attempts to less than 10 minutes or no more than three attempts (by an experienced laryngoscopist).
- Assess the reason for the failed intubation and modify the intubation technique on the next attempt using an intubation-rescue technique (Table 1-6).[32,63,64]
- Attempt to maintain an SpO_2 >92% between failed intubation attempts.

It is not intended that the practitioner should abandon intubation or proceed with rescue ventilation merely because the oxygen saturation has dropped briefly to ≤92%, providing that adequate oxygenation can be reestablished quickly using positive pressure ventilation with 100% oxygen. However, leaving an intubation pathway and proceeding with rescue ventilation is essential when there is sustained hypoxemia that is refractory to optimal ventilation attempts using 100% oxygen. Alternatively, the rescuer can choose to

Table 1-6 Intubation Rescue Techniques[51]

- External laryngeal manipulation (**ELM**) on the thyroid cartilage[78]
- Backward, upward, rightward pressure (**BURP**) on the thyroid cartilage[79]
- Lever-tip (McCoy-type) laryngoscope[50]
- Head-elevated laryngoscopy position (**HELP**)[32,64]
- Assessing for proper degree of muscle paralysis[78]
- Changing the blade length (e.g., #2 Miller to #3 Miller)[78]
- Changing the blade type (e.g., curved to straight)[78]
- Changing the operator (one with more experience or better access)
- Bougie-assisted intubation (e.g., gum-elastic bougie)[80]
- Combined use of a lever-tip laryngoscope and bougie introducer for patients requiring cervical-spine precautions or a neutral head position[50]

Used by permission from Rich J. Recognition and management of the difficult airway with special emphasis on the Intubating LMA-Fastrach/whistle technique: a brief review with case reports. BUMC Proceedings 2005; 18: 220–227.

switch early to the rescue ventilation pathway if intubation is judged not feasible after just one or two failed attempts. On the other hand, if there is a persistent failure to intubate or sustained hypoxemia cannot be readily corrected, the practitioner should proceed directly with rescue ventilation.[22] As mentioned previously, if rescue ventilation fails, the final option is to perform a cricothyrotomy.[44,45] Throughout the SUAAF, oxygenation and ventilation are emphasized over intubation because patients suffer brain death or die from failure to ventilate and oxygenate rather than failure to intubate.[6,9,47,81]

Confirmation of Tracheal Intubation and Monitoring of Lung Ventilation

ON TARGET Clinical signs such as bilateral breath sounds, lack of gastric insufflation over the epigastrium, compliance of the BVM, and fogging of the tracheal tube are unreliable signs for confirmation of tube placement. It is necessary to use a carbon dioxide detector; an esophageal detector device (EDD); or, best of all, waveform capnography to confirm tube placement in a patient with a perfusing cardiac rhythm or an EDD in the patient with a nonperfusing cardiac rhythm.

The SUAAF stresses evidence-based confirmation of tracheal intubation and monitoring of lung ventilation (Table 1-7).[82] The use of routine clinical signs (e.g., chest movement with bilateral breath sounds, lack of gastric insufflation over the epigastrium, movement or adequate compliance of the reservoir bag, and fogging of the endotracheal tube) for confirmation of tracheal intubation by themselves are unreliable and not failsafe.[82-84] At a minimum, confirmation should include bilateral chest auscultation over the four thoracic quadrants, along the midaxillary lines, and over the epigastrium in combination with an appropriate evidence-based near-failsafe device (carbon dioxide detector or EDD).[70,82]

If the patient has a perfusing cardiac rhythm, capnometry (either electronic or colorimetric) can be used to confirm tracheal intubation. If the patient has a nonperfusing rhythm (e.g., ventricular fibrillation, asystole, or pulseless electrical activity), confirmation should be accomplished using an EDD such as a self-inflating bulb (Chapter 5). Auscultation of bilateral breath sounds helps ensure midtracheal placement of the distal tip of the tracheal tube in order to prevent unilateral lung ventilation and possible aspiration of the unprotected lung.[1,22,23,25,82]

Postintubation management of the patient should not proceed without first confirming that a definitive airway has been securely placed. If tracheal intubation is not possible, lung ventilation (using bag-valve-mask ventilation or an adjunctive supraglottic airway device) should be monitored using a carbon dioxide detector, and oxygenation should be monitored using a pulse oximeter.

Table 1-7 Confirmation of Tracheal Intubation[25,70,82]

Non-Failsafe Methods

- Auscultated breath sounds over chest
- No breath sounds auscultated over abdomen
- No gastric distention
- Chest rise and fall
- Intercostal spaces flare out with inspiration
- Large spontaneous exhaled tidal volume
- Tracheal tube fogging (− with inspiration and + with expiration)
- Air heard exiting the tracheal tube when chest is compressed
- Reservoir bag has appropriate compliance
- Reciprocating pulsed pressures between ETT pilot balloon and suprasternal notch when suprasternal notch is compressed

Near-Failsafe Methods

- Carbon dioxide detectors and esophageal detector devices (EDD)
- The choice of portable carbon dioxide detectors includes:
  —Disposable qualitative colorimetric carbon dioxide detectors
  —Portable qualitative nonwaveform electronic carbon dioxide detectors
  —Portable quantitative electronic waveform carbon dioxide devices
- The EDD and carbon dioxide detector are considered to be *near–failsafe* because either occasionally can produce false-positive or false-negative readings.[82,85,86]
- Disposable qualitative colorimetric carbon dioxide detectors

- Portable electronic qualitative nonwaveform CO_2 detector
  —Provides a qualitative range of CO_2 (e.g., 30–50 mm HG) via a lighted LED readout rather than an actual CO_2 reading
  —Includes apnea alarm

- Portable electronic quantitative waveform CO_2 detector
  —Provides a quantitative reading of CO_2 in mm Hg.
  —Provides a capnographic CO_2 waveform
  —Includes apnea alarm

Non-Failsafe: Recommendations, Benefits, Hazards

- Non-failsafe methods should be used only in conjunction with other evidence-based methods.
- Use of only non-failsafe methods has resulted in death and brain death secondary to the occurrence of undetected esophageal intubation.[6,9,82-84]

Near-Failsafe: Recommendations, Benefits, Hazards

- Near-failsafe devices are evidence-based and are recommended for confirmation of tracheal intubation.[82]
- Use of a near-failsafe device should also include auscultation over the midaxillary lines and epigastrium to help ensure the presence of bilateral lung ventilation.
- Choice of carbon dioxide detector versus EDD is based on the patient's cardiac perfusion status.[70]
  —Perfusing cardiac rhythm—CO_2 detector[70]
  —Nonperfusing cardiac rhythm—EDD[70]
- Use of CO_2 detectors also permits monitoring of lung ventilation.[22]

- Colorimetric CO_2 detectors are adequate for both confirming tracheal intubation and monitoring lung ventilation during postintubation management. However, they are not durable and can stop working after an indeterminate period of time.[22]
- Use carbon dioxide detection in patients with a perfusing cardiac rhythm.[70]

- Adequate for both confirming tracheal intubation and monitoring lung ventilation during postintubation management.[22,23,70,82]
- No capnographic waveform is displayed, which does not allow for the use of other capnographic-waveform benefits (e.g., lower airway obstruction).

- Best for confirmation of tracheal intubation and monitoring of lung ventilation in the presence of a perfusing cardiac rhythm because:
  —Gives CO_2 reading in mm Hg
  —Has the benefit of a capnographic waveform

(continued)

Table 1-7 *Confirmation of Tracheal Intubation[25,70,82] (continued)*

Near-Failsafe Methods	Near-Failsafe: Recommendations, Benefits, Hazards

• Esophageal detector device (EDD)
  —Self-inflating bulb (SIB)
  —Syringe-type EDD
	• EDD is adequate for detecting esophageal intubation but occurrence false positives and false negatives must be understood.[22,82,85-88]
	• Use an EDD (e.g., self-inflating bulb) in patients with a nonperfusing cardiac rhythm (e.g., CPR; severe traumatic hemorrhage). EDD may also be used in patients with a tension pneumothorax.[22,23,70,82]
	• Self-inflating bulb (SIB) primarily assesses ETC location within the esophagus or the trachea

Failsafe Methods	**Failsafe: Recommendations, Benefits, Hazards**
• Recognition of supraglottic anatomy around the endotracheal tube during a second laryngoscopic look (e.g., epiglottis, arytenoids, vocal cords)	Recommended in the absence of CO_2 or if EDD is indeterminate or not available[82]
• Recognition of subglottic anatomy using flexible fiberoptic bronchoscope within the endotracheal tube (e.g., tracheal rings, carina, right and left mainstem bronchi)	Recommended during flexible fiberoptic intubation and can confirm any intubation if it is immediately available[82]

Used by permission. James Michael Rich, CRNA–SLAM Airway Training Institute, www.airwayeducation.com.

Summary

The SUAAF promotes the use of evidence-based methods throughout the emergency airway management process. A careful and methodical assessment of the airway is recommended to alert practitioners to the possibility of a potential difficult intubation allowing them to:

- Attempt intubation using a difficult-airway intubation technique from the outset.
- Proceed using a standard direct laryngoscopy technique while simultaneously preparing for an intubation-rescue technique (Chapters 4 and 7).
- Apply an adjunctive ventilation technique (Table 1-4) (Chapters 3 and 8) when intubation or ventilation proves to be difficult.

The use of intubation rescue techniques,[32,51,63,64] difficult intubation techniques,[51] and rescue ventilation techniques (SUAAF)[22,57,58,89-92] (e.g., administration of 100% oxygen and positive pressure ventilation, preferably by way of a Class IIa alternative airway device such as a Combitube or LMA)[25,59,61] to treat a critical airway event are central to the SUAAF.

PEDIATRIC NOTES

The SUAAF is suitable for use with adult patients only.

The main limitations of the SUAAF are that it is suitable for use only with adult patients and by advanced airway practitioners who are trained in the use of anesthetic drugs and neuromuscular blocking agents to facilitate intubation, direct laryngoscopy, tracheal intubation, rescue ventilation techniques, and cricothyrotomy. The SUAAF also depends heavily on an assessment of the SpO_2. If this information is not available, rescuers should proceed using their best judgment concerning the likely level of oxygenation. However, because hypoxemia is so difficult to diagnose clinically,[93] every effort should be made to obtain a pulse oximeter reading. In situations where an SpO_2 reading is lacking, a respiratory rate of <10 or >30 breaths per minute could be an indication that a crash-airway situation exists. Use of the SUAAF may decrease the incidence of difficult intubation and/or help prevent airway trauma, which has been reported to cause death or disability.[9,12]

The SUAAF assists both in the teaching and learning of emergency airway management and is intended to improve patient care. The SLAM concept holds that the emergency airway can occur anywhere across the spectrum of health care.[3-6,22,23,31] It also maintains that most airway techniques used in anesthesiology can be applied by advanced airway practitioners working at the street level[3,4] and throughout the hospital.[5] However, the advice featured in the SUAAF should always be overridden when medical direction, clinical experience, the clinical situation, and/or local protocols dictate. It is also important to understand that algorithms cannot, by their very nature, be all-encompassing and must be interpreted, modified, and applied according to individual patient assessment and good clinical judgment.

REVIEW QUESTIONS

1. Describe the ways of providing primary oxygenation and ventilation.

2. What are the number of intubation attempts generally limited to 3 or less?

3. List three simple methods for rescuing failed intubation.

4. Describe the evidence-based techniques for confirming tracheal tube placement.

5. When should rescue ventilation using a Combitube or laryngeal mask airway be employed?

6. Describe how does Mason's PU-92 concept functions?

7. What are the limitations of the SUAAF?

CHAPTER 2

Airway Anatomy and Assessment

Andrew M. Mason
James Michael Rich

After reading this chapter, you should be able to:

- Identify the structures and functions of the human airway.
- Assess the respiratory status of a patient.
- Describe techniques for difficult tracheal intubation.
- Describe the Cormack and Lehane grading system.

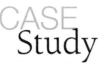

CASE Study _____

Medic 42 responds to a motor-vehicle crash on the interstate. The highway patrol on scene has reported a two-car collision with one trapped female in critical condition. When the paramedics arrive, they find fire department personnel removing the roof of a small passenger car that has sustained major frontal damage with significant intrusion into the passenger compartment. One of the fire crew is already positioned inside the vehicle, supporting the patient's head and neck in neutral alignment from behind.

The patient is of college age. She is sitting in the driver's seat, wearing a seatbelt. The steering wheel and curtain airbags have deployed. The patient is only responding to painful stimuli with groans. Her pupils are of equal size and are responding normally to light, but her radial pulse is weak and rapid with a rate of 130 beats per minute. Respirations are noted to be shallow with a rate of 35 breaths per minute. Pulse oximetry reveals an SpO_2 reading of 85%.

A paramedic inserts an oropharyngeal airway, which is tolerated without gagging, and oxygen is administered via nonrebreathing mask at a rate of 15 liters per minute. A rigid cervical collar is then applied, after which an IV line is established and a 250 ml bolus of Ringer's lactate is infused.

When the patient is extricated from the vehicle, she is secured to a long spine board. Despite oxygen therapy, the SpO_2 readings do not rise above 88%, which means the patient meets the criteria for the establishment of a definitive airway. The paramedics prepare the equipment for intubation and perform a 6-D airway assessment. There is no disproportion or distortion of her anatomical features. She is wearing a cervical collar, so there is a decrease in the available range of movement. She is noted to have a small dental overbite with a decrease in her interincisor gap, but there is no decrease in the thyromental distance.

A decision is made to attempt rapid sequence intubation (RSI). The anterior portion of the c-spine collar is removed while manual in-line axial stabilization (MIAS) is applied continuously. Sellick's maneuver is performed while the medications are administered and is maintained both during preoxygenation with a bag-valve-mask device and throughout the subsequent intubation procedure. In anticipation of a difficult intubation, a bougie introducer is utilized together with size 3 Macintosh blade. The arytenoid cartilages are visualized, and the bougie introducer is inserted anterior to these structures in the midline. As the bougie is advanced, tracheal clicking is felt, and a tracheal tube is railroaded over the bougie into the airway. Positive pressure ventilation is then initiated.

Decreased breath sounds are found on the right side of the chest, and the endotracheal tube is noted to be inserted to a depth of 25 cm. The tube is repositioned to 21 cm at the interincisor gap, and there is a return of equal bilateral breath sounds with no sounds heard over the epigastric area. The endotracheal tube is secured, and the cervical collar is repositioned. An $ETCO_2$ monitor shows correct tube placement, and SpO_2 readings rise steadily to 99%.

Hand ventilation is continued to maintain good oxygenation while keeping the $ETCO_2$ values between 30 and 35 mmHg. IV fluid is administered as necessary to maintain a palpable radial pulse. The patient is transported to the local trauma center without further incident.

Introduction

To understand and assess the respiratory status of the patient, it is important that all practitioners who perform airway management have a working knowledge of both airway anatomy and respiratory physiology. This chapter focuses on airway anatomy and assessment of the airway for difficulty.

KEY TERMS

Cormack and Lehane grading, p. 27

Sellick's maneuver, p. 25

Airway Anatomy

The respiratory tract (Figure 2-1) begins at the nose and mouth and ends in over 300 million tiny air sacs called alveoli (singular, alveolus) that are situated in the lungs. The adult larynx lies at the level of the fourth, fifth, and sixth cervical vertebrae and is continuous with the pharynx above and the trachea below (Figure 2-2). The larynx (or voice box) (Figure 2-3) is composed of three paired and three unpaired structures made from cartilage. The three small paired cartilages are the cuneiform, corniculate, and arytenoid cartilages. The three larger unpaired cartilages are the epiglottal, thyroid, and cricoid cartilages.

All of those cartilages are held together in a cylindrical shape by various ligaments to produce a dynamic structure that protects the trachea and distal air passages from the entry of food, drink, and other foreign substances, while allowing the intake of air and expulsion of exhaled gases.

The larynx is also the organ of phonation, generating the sounds necessary for speech. The sounds produced by vocal-cord vibration are then modified by the articulatory actions of the rest of the vocal apparatus, including the tongue.

It is important that advanced airway practitioners are totally familiar with the appearance of the larynx as seen during direct laryngoscopy (Figure 2-3) as well as with laryngeal anatomy.

Airway Anatomy of the Anterior Neck

Thyroid Cartilage

The thyroid cartilage (Figure 2-3) is the largest of the nine cartilages that make up the skeleton of the human larynx. It consists of two plates called the laminae, the anterior borders of

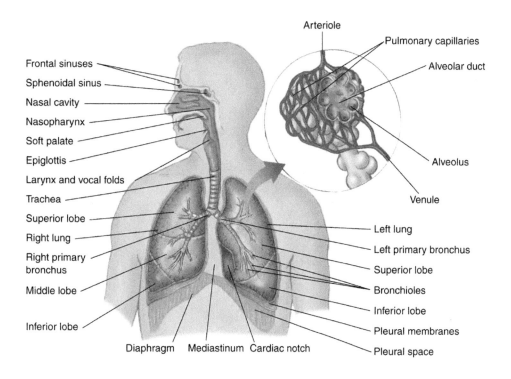

Frontal sinuses
Sphenoidal sinus
Nasal cavity
Nasopharynx
Soft palate
Epiglottis
Larynx and vocal folds
Trachea
Superior lobe
Right lung
Right primary bronchus
Middle lobe
Inferior lobe
Diaphragm   Mediastinum   Cardiac notch

Arteriole
Pulmonary capillaries
Alveolar duct
Alveolus
Venule

Left lung
Left primary bronchus
Superior lobe
Bronchioles
Inferior lobe
Pleural membranes
Pleural space

FIGURE 2-1
Overview of the upper and lower airways.

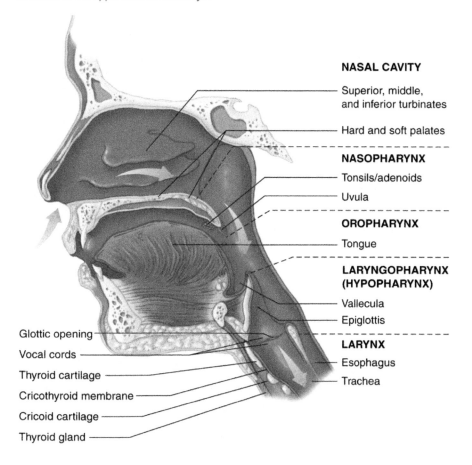

NASAL CAVITY
Superior, middle, and inferior turbinates
Hard and soft palates

NASOPHARYNX
Tonsils/adenoids
Uvula

OROPHARYNX
Tongue

LARYNGOPHARYNX (HYPOPHARYNX)
Vallecula
Epiglottis

Glottic opening
Vocal cords
Thyroid cartilage
Cricothyroid membrane
Cricoid cartilage
Thyroid gland

LARYNX
Esophagus
Trachea

FIGURE 2-2
Anatomy of the upper airway.

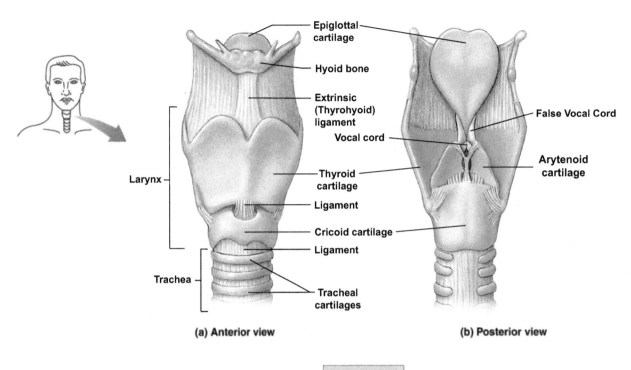

(a) Anterior view   (b) Posterior view

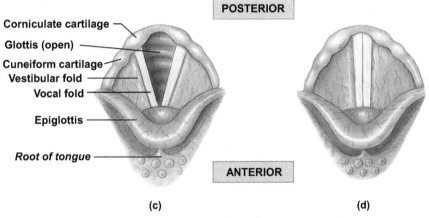

POSTERIOR

Corniculate cartilage
Glottis (open)
Cuneiform cartilage
Vestibular fold
Vocal fold
Epiglottis
Root of tongue

ANTERIOR

(c)   (d)

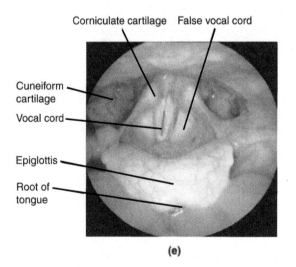

Corniculate cartilage   False vocal cord

Cuneiform cartilage
Vocal cord
Epiglottis
Root of tongue

(e)

FIGURE 2-3

Anatomy of the vocal cords: (a) anterior view of the larynx, (b) posterior view of the larynx, (c) superior view of the larynx with the glottis open and (d) with the glottis closed, and (e) fiberoptic view with the glottis closed.

which are fused together in the midline of the neck. The laminae meet at an acute angle anteriorly forming a distinct ridge, the upper portion of which is called the laryngeal prominence, or Adam's apple. After puberty, this prominence is much more distinct in men than in women.

Posteriorly, the thyroid cartilage has two striking horns above and below on either side. Above, the cartilage is suspended from the hyoid bone by the thyrohyoid membrane, the central portion of which is thickened anteriorly to form the thyrohyoid ligament. In the midline below, the thyroid cartilage is attached to the cricoid cartilage by a narrow fibrous band called the cricothyroid ligament.

At the upper aspect of the laryngeal prominence is the superior thyroid notch.[1] The ability to identify and manipulate this notch is important for anyone attempting to perform external laryngeal manipulation (ELM), a maneuver that can greatly improve the laryngeal view during laryngoscopy.[2] When the glottic structures cannot be viewed or are barely visible during direct laryngoscopy, pressure applied to the laryngeal prominence using the BURP maneuver, which is backward, upward, rightward pressure, or pressure directed backward (B) against the cervical vertebrae and upward (U) as far as possible and slightly laterally to the patient's right (R) side. This maneuver can bring vocal cords that are otherwise invisible into the full view of the laryngoscopist.[3]

The ability to identify the small gap between the thyroid and cricoid cartilages by palpation is essential to knowing where emergency access to the airway can be gained below the level of the vocal cords (e.g., when undertaking a cricothyrotomy). A clear knowledge of this laryngeal landmark is also important when administering local anesthetic blocks to the airway or attempting retrograde wire-guided intubation of the trachea.

Cricoid Cartilage

The cricoid cartilage is smaller than the thyroid cartilage, but it is thicker and stronger. It lies at the most inferior aspect of the larynx (Figure 2-3). Its shape has been compared to that of a signet ring, with a narrow anterior arch and a much wider posterior quadrate lamina.[1] At the junction of the lamina and arch on either side is a small round facet that articulates with the inferior horn of the thyroid cartilage. The cricoid cartilage is the only continuous ring of cartilage within the airway. Just below it lies the trachea, with its incomplete C-shaped cartilaginous rings.

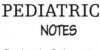

PEDIATRIC
NOTES

The level of the cricoid cartilage represents the narrowest portion of the funnel-shaped pediatric larynx; whereas, in adults, the narrowest portion of the more cylindrical larynx is at the level of the glottis.

The arytenoid cartilages (Figure 2-3) are two pyramidal structures that sit on top of the cricoid lamina. The base of each of these pyramids articulates with a sloping oval facet on the upper outer border of the cricoid lamina. At the tip of each arytenoid sits a small cone of elastic cartilage called the corniculate cartilage. Two further elongated pieces of elastic cartilage lie within the folds of mucous membrane (aryepiglottic folds) and curve from the apex of the arytenoid cartilages round to each side of the base of the epiglottis. Called the cuneiform cartilages (of Wrisberg), they are visible to the laryngoscopist, together with the corniculate cartilages, as small oval swellings within the aryepiglottic folds on each side. These are key laryngeal landmarks on laryngoscopy because they lie immediately behind and lateral to the glottic opening.

The arytenoids are surprisingly mobile structures, their anterolateral surfaces serving as the posterior attachment for the vocal cords. Anteriorly, the vocal cords are attached to the back of the angle of the thyroid cartilage either side of the midline and immediately below the attachment of the epiglottis. With their apices curved backward and toward the medial, rotation of the arytenoids on their vertical axes causes the glottic opening to widen or narrow. Opening

FIGURE 2-4
The hypoepiglottic ligament, epiglottis, and other laryngeal cartilages.
(Courtesy of JM Rich, CRNA)

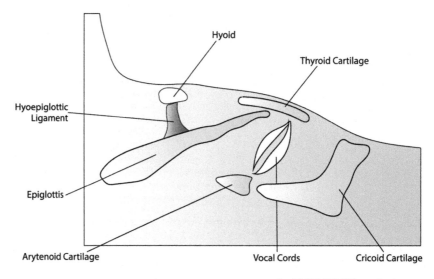

Copyright 2015-J. Rich, CRNA-www.slamairway.com

and closing of the glottis is further achieved as the bases of the arytenoids glide up and down the articular facets on the shoulders of the cricoid lamina in synchrony with the rotary motion.

Epiglottis

The epiglottis is a thin tongue-shaped sheet of fibrocartilage. It is the last of the nine cartilages that make up the larynx (Figure 2-3). It gains attachment by its narrow stalklike base to the inner surface of the angle of the thyroid laminae just below the superior thyroid notch. Close to its point of attachment on its anterior surface, an elastic ligament (the hyoepiglottic ligament) connects it to the hyoid bone above (Figure 2-4). The broad, rounded, free end of the epiglottis projects obliquely upward behind the root of the tongue from where, upon swallowing, it folds backward and downward to direct food and drink posteriorly into the esophagus and away from the glottic opening.

Between the base of the tongue and the root of the epiglottis is a blind recess called the vallecula into which the tip of the curved (Macintosh) blade of a laryngoscope can be inserted (Figure 2-5). With the blade tip placed here, lifting the handle of the laryngoscope

Indirect Glottic Exposure

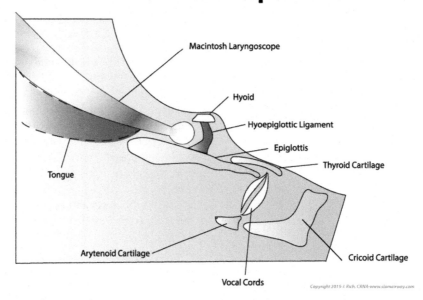

FIGURE 2-5
Upon entering the vallecula, the tip of the Macintosh blade stretches the hypoepiglottic ligament, which indirectly lifts the epiglottis and exposes the laryngeal inlet.
(Courtesy of JM Rich, CRNA)

Copyright 2015-J. Rich, CRNA-www.slamairway.com

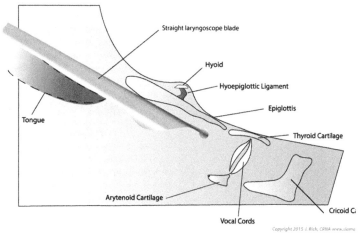

FIGURE 2-6
The straight blade is brought into contact with the posterior surface of the epiglottis in order to directly lift the epiglottis and expose the laryngeal inlet. (Courtesy of JM Rich, CRNA)

lifts both the tongue and epiglottis and opens up a view of the laryngeal inlet to the laryngoscopist. The epiglottis is sometimes clearly visible behind the back of the tongue, especially in children and, in the days before immunization against Hib (Haemophilus influenzae type B), it was frequently prone to sudden attacks of inflammation, sometimes resulting in life-threatening restriction of the child's airway (i.e., epiglottitis).

Between the base of the epiglottis and the root of the tongue lies a groove called the epiglottic vallecula. This is the structure into which the tip of the blade of a Macintosh laryngoscope is inserted to lift the epiglottis indirectly and reveal the laryngeal inlet (Figure 2-5). Alternatively, a straight Miller blade can be applied against the posterior surface of the epiglottis to lift it directly (Figure 2-6).

The ability to identify the cricoid cartilage by external palpation is important in airway management for two reasons. First, applying pressure to the anterior arch of the cricoid cartilage causes its posterior laminar surface to press against, flatten, and finally occlude the esophagus, which lies directly behind it. Cricoid pressure has become a standard part of rapid sequence intubation and is known as **Sellick's maneuver,** named after the British anesthetist, Brian Arthur Sellick.[4] It is widely believed to aid in the prevention of silent regurgitation of gastric contents into the lungs during airway management, although there is little hard evidence of its effectiveness in the medical literature.[5]

The second important reason for being able to identify the junction of the cricoid and thyroid cartilages is to locate the cricothyroid membrane. This is the structure through which percutaneous or surgical entrance to the larynx is obtained for emergency airway access, as well as for administration of local anesthetics to produce topical anesthesia below the level of the vocal cords. The cricothyroid membrane is situated in the small mid-line depression that lies between the cricoid and thyroid cartilages anteriorly.

Trachea

The trachea (windpipe) extends from immediately below the cricoid cartilage at the level of the sixth cervical vertebra to the upper border of the fifth thoracic vertebra, where it divides into the two primary bronchi, one for each lung (Figure 2-7). In adults, it measures about 11 cm in length and has a diameter of between 2 and 2.5 cm. It is larger in men than in women.

The trachea is a tubular structure that is not quite cylindrical because it is flattened posteriorly. It consists of incomplete rings of cartilage stacked one on top of another. Hyaline cartilage makes up about two-thirds of each ring anteriorly, but it is absent behind where the tube is completed by fibrous tissue and involuntary muscle fibers. Each ring is firmly bound to its neighbor by fibrous tissue, and the inner aspect of the trachea is lined with a mucous membrane having a surface of ciliated epithelium.

Sellick's maneuver
The application of pressure on the cricoid cartilage to occlude the esophagus and prevent silent regurgitation of gastric contents.

ON TARGET Mucus secreted by the ciliated epithelium helps to trap small inhaled particles and organisms. The cilia then beat these materials back in the direction of the oropharynx, a process assisted by coughing. Any loss of cilia (as occurs in smokers) or any interference with the normal coughing process (such as with painful rib fractures or a drug overdose) can lead to a dangerous accumulation of mucus and debris within the lower air passages.

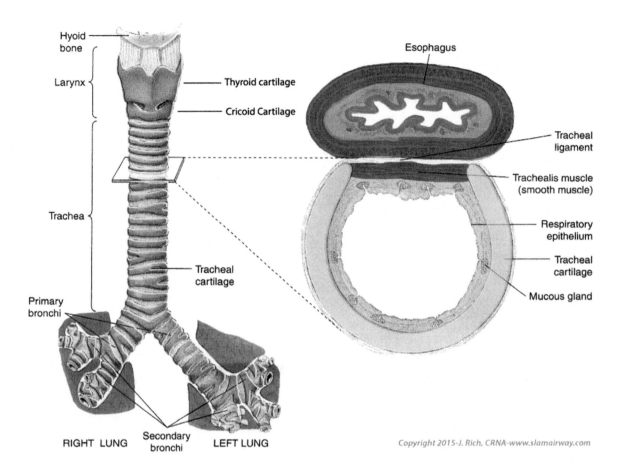

Labels on figure:
- Hyoid bone
- Larynx
- Thyroid cartilage
- Cricoid Cartilage
- Esophagus
- Tracheal ligament
- Trachealis muscle (smooth muscle)
- Respiratory epithelium
- Tracheal cartilage
- Mucous gland
- Trachea
- Tracheal cartilage
- Primary bronchi
- Secondary bronchi
- RIGHT LUNG
- LEFT LUNG

FIGURE 2-7

Anatomy of the trachea: (a) anterior view showing the plane of section for (b) a cross-sectional view of the trachea and esophagus.

PEARLS When a gum-elastic bougie is inserted through the glottic opening into the trachea, a characteristic vibration is felt as the bougie is advanced and its tip bumps over the tracheal rings (i.e., tracheal clicking). This is not felt if the bougie is mistakenly inserted into the esophagus, which sits immediately behind the trachea.

ON TARGET Listening for equal air entry into both lungs is an essential part of a postintubation check.

The cartilages of the trachea vary from 16 to 20 in number because two or more often unite, either partially or totally. They are highly elastic in children but tend to become calcified and more rigid with advancing age.

The trachea divides distally into the two primary bronchi. The right primary bronchus is shorter, about 2.5 cm in length. It follows a more vertical path than the left, entering the right lung almost opposite the fifth thoracic vertebra. The left primary bronchus is smaller in caliber but longer than the right, being nearly 5 cm long. It enters the root of the left lung opposite the sixth thoracic vertebra. The larger diameter of the right main bronchus coupled with its straighter path explains why foreign bodies tend to enter on this side. For the same reason, a tracheal tube inserted too far will preferentially enter the right primary bronchus.

Nerve Supply to the Larynx

The larynx is innervated by the laryngeal nerves, which are branches of the tenth cranial (vagus) nerve. As it descends to the larynx, the superior laryngeal nerve divides into two main branches, which are the internal and external laryngeal nerves. The internal laryngeal nerve provides sensation to the mucous membrane above the vocal cords. The external laryngeal nerve provides motor innervation to the cricothyroid muscle.

The recurrent laryngeal nerve provides sensation to the upper trachea and mucous membrane of the larynx below the vocal cords, as well as motor innervation to all intrinsic muscles of the larynx (apart from the cricothyroid muscle). The term *recurrent* is used because this branch of the vagus nerve first descends into the thorax before returning to the neck. It takes a slightly different route on each side and can be prone to injury anywhere along its tortuous course. Division of a recurrent laryngeal nerve (e.g., during surgery to the thyroid gland) results in complete paralysis of the vocal cord on that side. The motor supply to the various extrinsic muscles of the larynx is by way of the fifth, seventh, and twelfth cranial nerves.

Laryngoscopic Anatomy of the Airway

The laryngeal inlet (Figures 2-2 and 2-3) is the opening between the supraglottic area of the pharynx above and the sub- or infraglottic portion of the larynx below. Its borders are formed by the curved free edge of the epiglottis anteriorly, and the aryepiglottic folds laterally, which curve around to meet at the interarytenoid notch posteriorly.

Posteriolaterally, the tiny cuneiform cartilages sit at the four o'clock and eight o'clock positions within the aryepiglottic folds. The corniculate cartilages, which cap the apices of the arytenoid cartilages, rest side by side and close to the six o'clock position of the laryngeal inlet. Because of their location, these three paired cartilages are sometimes referred to collectively as the posterior cartilages. The interarytenoid notch is an important landmark for the laryngoscopist because it separates the laryngeal inlet anteriorly from the esophagus posteriorly.[6]

The floor of the laryngeal inlet consists of a space called the glottic inlet, which is bounded by the true vocal cords and, further laterally, the folds of tissue referred to as the false vocal cords, or vestibular folds. The tracheal tube is inserted through the glottic inlet to protect the airway and maintain its patency during airway management.

The pyriform fossae are those small recesses on either side of the larynx bounded by the aryepiglottic fold medially and by the thyroid cartilage and thyrohyoid membrane laterally. They are considered to be part of the hypopharynx.

Laryngeal Grades of the Airway Seen During Direct Laryngoscopy

Cormack and Lehane grading

A useful method for grading the laryngeal view of the airway as seen with the laryngoscope and estimating the difficulty of the intubation.

Direct laryngoscopy will produce one of four possible views of the airway. These four views were originally defined by Cormack and Lehane (Table 2-1)[7] and are called **Cormack and Lehane grading** (Figure 2-8). Understanding the laryngeal grades and their significance to tracheal intubation is essential to a practical understanding of direct laryngoscopy and airway management.

The desired view of the airway is to see the entire laryngeal inlet from the anterior to the posterior commissure, or at least enough of the glottic opening to be able to pass a tracheal tube with confidence. After obtaining the best laryngeal view possible, the laryngoscopist will see one of the four laryngeal grades.[7] The Cormack and Lehane grading is an important tool to document and communicate the laryngoscopic view for future interventions.

Table 2-1 Cormack and Lehane Laryngeal Grades of the Airway[7]

Laryngeal Grade	Visualized Oral Anatomy	Potential Intubation Implications
1	Visualization of the entire glottic opening from the anterior to posterior commissure	Should facilitate an easy intubation
2	Visualization of just the posterior portion of glottis	Normally not difficult to pass a styleted endotracheal tube through the laryngeal aperture
3a*	Visualization of the epiglottis only (epiglottis can be lifted using a laryngoscope blade)	Intubation is difficult but possible using a bougie introducer or flexible fiberoptic scope
3b*	Visualization of the epiglottis only (but epiglottis cannot be lifted from the posterior pharynx using a laryngoscope blade)	Intubation can be difficult because insertion of a bougie introducer (e.g., gum-elastic bougie) may be impeded, which can directly affect the successful use of a bougie introducer or a flexible fiberoptic scope
4*	Only soft tissue is viewed, with no identifiable airway anatomy	Difficult intubation, requiring advanced techniques to intubate the trachea

For additional information on grades 1, 2, and 4, see reference 8.

For additional information on grade 3, see reference 9.

*Tracheal intubation normally requires an advanced airway technique other than direct laryngoscopy. Modified from reference 10.

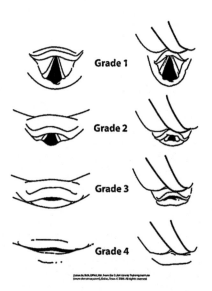

FIGURE 2-8
The Cormack and Lehane grading system of glottic exposure classifies the optimal laryngeal view obtainable with laryngoscopy.
(Courtesy of JM Rich, CRNA)

Cormack and Lehane Laryngeal Grades

Airway Assessment

The aim of airway assessment is to help anticipate whether or not the laryngeal inlet will be visible using direct laryngoscopy.[11] Assessment of the airway is recommended to predict the presence of a difficult airway before embarking on airway management.[9,12-17]

Assess the airway before attempting intubation to help prevent and better prepare for a potentially difficult airway.

The Mallampati classification system (Table 2-2) (Figure 2-9) was one of the first methods implemented to predict difficult intubation. It was developed to correlate theoretically with Cormack and Lehane's grades (Figure 2-10). However, its reliability has been questioned[16] because it assesses for only one aspect of the airway for difficulty (i.e., intraoral disproportion).[17]

A comprehensive airway examination incorporates both quantitative and qualitative tests that, when used together, increase the probability of predicting difficult intubation.[11] One such method[10] is the 6-D Method of airway assessment (Table 2-3), which is based on some of Mallampati's ideas.[11] Airway examination is carried out by assessing for the presence of:

1. Distortion of the airway caused by trauma, scarring, or a medical condition (Table 2-2).
2. Disproportion using the Mallampati score (Table 2-3).
3. Decreased thyromental distance (Figure 2-11).

Table 2-2	Mallampati Airway Classification System	
Mallampati Class	Visualized Intraoral Anatomy	Implications
I	Uvula, faucial pillars, and soft palate	Generally associated with an easy intubation
II	Faucial pillars, soft palate	Generally associated with an easy intubation
III	Only soft palate	Potential for intubation difficulty
IV	Only hard palate	Potential for intubation difficulty

Based on references 11, 17–19.

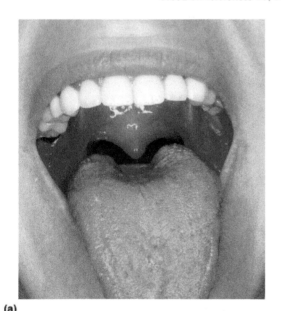

(a)

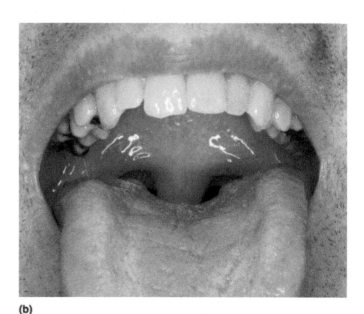

(b)

FIGURE 2-9

The Mallampati classification compares tongue size to the oropharyngeal space (i.e., disproportion). The patient must fully open the mouth and extend the tongue so that the test can be performed correctly.
a. Mallampati I: Soft palate, fauces, uvula, and anterior and posterior pillars. This is generally associated with an easy intubation.
b. Mallampati II: Soft palate, faucial pillars, and uvula. Generally associated with an easy intubation.

Airway Anatomy and Assessment 29

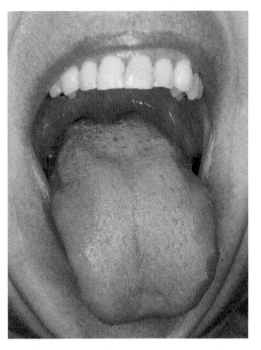 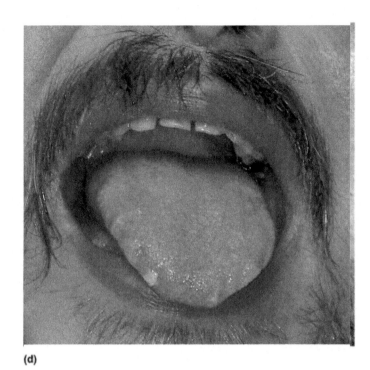

(c)   **(d)**

FIGURE 2-9
(continued)

c. Mallampati III: Only soft palate, base of uvula is seen.

d. Mallampati IV: Soft palate is not visible at all; only the hard palate is visible. Potential for intubation difficulty exists.

(Courtesy of JM Rich, CRNA)

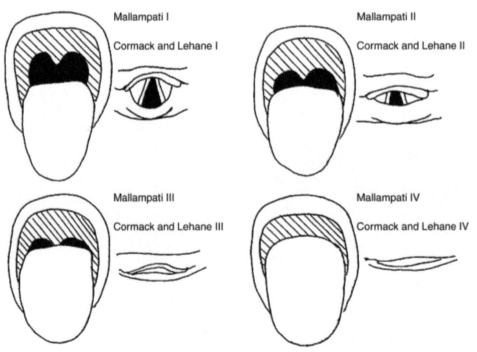

FIGURE 2-10
Postulated correlation of Mallampati with Cormack and Lehane. It was originally postulated that the Mallampati classification correlated with the Cormack and Lehane grades. However, the causes of a decreased laryngeal view are multivariate, which may or may not be affected by the level of disproportion.

(Courtesy of Dr. Harald V. Genzwuerker, MD)

Table 2-3 The 6-D Method of Airway Assessment

Difficult Signs	Description	Findings Reported to Be Associated with Difficulty	Acceptable Findings Not Usually Associated with Difficulty
Distortion	Airway swelling	May be difficult to assess	Midline trachea
	Airway trauma (blunt or penetrating)	Blunt or penetrating airway trauma	No contractures of the neck
	Tissue consolidation (e.g., secondary to radiation)	Tracheal deviation	No surgical airway scar
	Neck mass	Neck asymmetry	Mobile laryngeal anatomy
	Neck hematoma	Voice changes	Easily palpated thyroid cartilage
	Neck abscess	Subcutaneous emphysema (crepitus)	Easily palpated cricoid cartilage
	Arthritic changes in the joints of the neck	Laryngeal immobility	
	Previous surgical airway	Nonpalpable thyroid cartilage	
		Nonpalpable cricoid cartilage	
Disproportion	Increased size of tongue in relation to pharyngeal size	Mallampati class III or IV	Mallampati class I or II
Decreased thyromental distance	Anterior larynx and decreased mandibular space	Thyromental distance <7 cm (<3 finger breadths), measured from the superior aspect of the thyroid cartilage to the tip of the chin	Thyromental distance ≥7 cm (approximately 3 finger breadths)
	Information about the amount of space available for laryngoscopic retraction		No receding chin
		Receding chin	
Decreased interincisor gap	Reduced mouth opening	Distance between upper and lower incisors (i.e., interincisor gap <4 cm [<2 finger breadths])	Interincisor gap ≥4 cm (approximately 2 finger breadths)
	Related to decreased range of motion of the temporomandibular joints, or to the presence of long teeth, or a combination of the two	Mandibular condyle fracture	
		Rigid cervical-spine collar	
Decreased range of motion in any or all of the joints of the airway (i.e., atlanto-occipital joint, temporomandibular joints, cervical spine)	Limited head extension	Head extension <35°	Head extension ≥35° of atlanto-occipital extension
	Atlanto-occipital range of motion is critical for assuming the sniffing position secondary to arthritis, diabetes, or other diseases	Neck flexion <35°	Cervical-spine flexion ≥35°
		Short, thick neck	Long, thin neck
		Cervical-spine collar or cervical-spine immobilization	No cervical-spine collar or cervical-spine immobilization
	Previous neck radiation and/or radical surgery		
	Neck contractures secondary to burns or trauma		
Dental overbite	Large angled teeth disrupting the alignment of the airway axes and possibly decreasing the interincisor distance	Dental overbite	No dental overbite

Disproportion of tongue size to pharyngeal size is assessed by the Mallampati classification system. Distortion assessment comprises visual assessment of the airway for swelling and trauma. Decreased thyromental distance and decreased intercisor gap are measured using the first three fingers of the hand.

Based on references 11, 13, 15, 17, and 19. Modified with permission from reference 10.

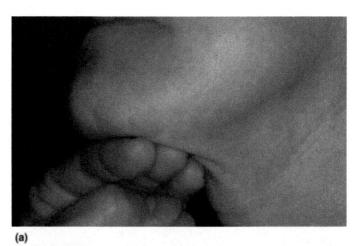

(a)

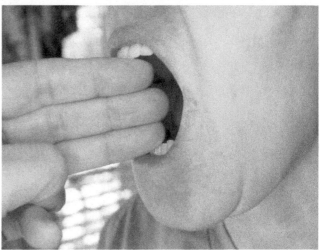

(b)

FIGURE 2-11
(a) Measuring the thyromental distance. (b) Measuring interincisor gap.

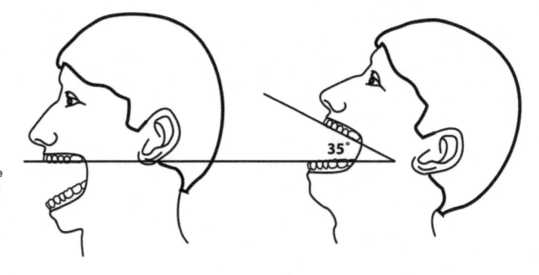

FIGURE 2-12
The range of motion of the atlanto-occipital joint can be measured by estimating the angle that is created by the change of position of the maxillary teeth when the neck is extended.

(Courtesy of JM Rich, CRNA)

4. Decreased interincisor gap (Figure 2-11).
5. Decreased range of motion of any of the joints in and around the airway (Figure 2-12).
6. Dental overbite (Figure 2-13).

The 6-D assessment method helps in remembering the six "D-is-for-difficulty" signs. The potential for a difficult intubation is generally related to the number of D signs that are present. However, regardless of the method of airway evaluation, it is important to under-

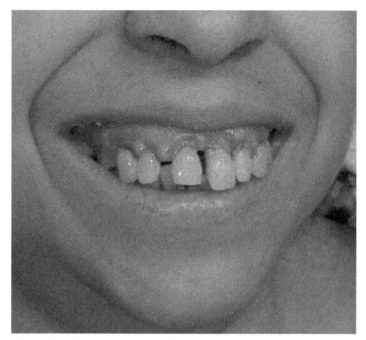

(a)

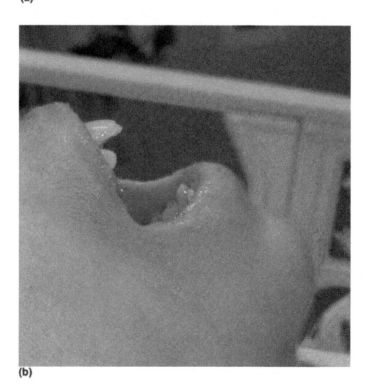

(b)

Table 2-4   Techniques for Difficult Tracheal Intubation[3,18,21-26]

Difficult-Airway Intubation Technique	Considerations/Requirements
Awake laryngoscopic intubation[27]	Judicious intravenous sedation[28]
	Topical anesthesia[28]
	Gentle use of the laryngoscope
Awake blind nasotracheal intubation[29]	Judicious intravenous sedation[28]
	Topical anesthesia[28]
	Spontaneous ventilation
	Vasoconstrictor[28]
	Patil intubation guide or Beck airway airflow monitor[29]
Intubating laryngeal mask airway in the awake patient	Judicious intravenous sedation[28]
	Topical anesthesia[28]
	Chandy maneuver[30]
	Spontaneous ventilation
	Patil intubation guide or Beck airway airflow monitor
	Dedicated tracheal tube (recommended)
Intubating laryngeal mask airway in the apneic patient	Chandy maneuver[30]
	Positive pressure ventilation
	Dedicated tracheal tube (recommended)
Retrograde intubation[31]	"Can-mask-ventilate/cannot-intubate" situation
	Parker endotracheal tube
	Direct laryngoscopy
Indirect rigid fiberoptic laryngoscopy[32]	Upsher, Wu, or Bullard laryngoscope[32]
Flexible fiberoptic laryngoscopy[33]	General anesthesia
	Judicious intravenous sedation[28]
	Topical anesthesia[28]
	Spontaneous ventilation[33]
Lightwand intubation[32]	Should not be used in patients with pharyngeal masses or anatomic abnormalities of the upper airway[32]
Videolaryngoscopic devices[34]	GlideScope®[34]
Malleable fiberoptic stylet	Shikani seeing stylet
	Direct laryngoscopy[35]

Modified by permission of reference 10.

stand that airway assessment is not infallible and can produce both false-negative and false-positive signs of difficult intubation. Nonetheless, airway examination is beneficial because it can alert practitioners to the presence of a potentially difficult intubation and allow them either to attempt intubation using a difficult-airway intubation technique from the outset (Table 2-4) or to proceed using a standard direct laryngoscopy technique while simultaneously being prepared to apply an intubation rescue technique or an adjunctive ventilation technique should intubation or ventilation prove to be difficult.

Intubation rescue techniques (Table 2-5) may assist with an anticipated or unanticipated difficult intubation. Intubation rescue is indicated following failed intubation, but the use of

Table 2-5 Intubation Rescue Techniques

- External laryngeal manipulation (ELM) on the thyroid cartilage[21]
- Backward upward rightward pressure (BURP) on the thyroid cartilage[3]
- Lever-tip (McCoy-type) laryngoscope[26]
- Head-elevated laryngoscopy position (HELP)[23,25]
- Assess for proper degree of muscle paralysis
- Changing the blade length (e.g., #2 Miller to #3 Miller)[18]
- Changing the blade type (e.g., curved to straight)[18]
- Changing the operator (one with more experience or better access)
- Bougie-assisted intubation (e.g., gum-elastic bougie)[22,32]
- Combined use of a lever-tip laryngoscope and bougie introducer for patients requiring cervical-spine precautions or the neutral head position[26]

Modified from reference 10.

direct laryngoscopy can continue provided that no more than three laryngoscopic attempts have been made, laryngoscopy has not been attempted for more than 10 minutes, and the patient's oxygen saturation as measured by pulse oximetry (SpO_2) can be maintained at greater than 92%. Otherwise, intubation attempts should be aborted and rescue ventilation using a Combitube or LMA should be instituted until a definitive airway can be safely inserted using a different technique.

 PEARLS The choice of a difficult-airway intubation technique depends on the clinical situation and the practitioner's familiarity and skill in using a particular device (Table 2-4). Not all techniques need to be learned or mastered, but it is best to have more than one technique available to increase the likelihood of success.

When a difficult airway is strongly suspected, it may be advantageous to secure the airway while the patient is awake,[2] unless there is a specific contraindication.[20,21] Of the various difficult-airway intubation techniques described in Table 2-4, most can be performed with the patient awake, although judicious sedation would be a minimum requirement.

Summary

The purpose of this chapter has been to provide the practitioner with clear information about the anatomy and assessment of the human airway to ensure the safest possible conclusion to any airway intervention. A sound knowledge of airway anatomy and the factors associated with difficulty should result in higher first-time success rates for intubation, early identification of the potentially difficult airway, and the selection of the best alternative technique in both anticipated and unanticipated difficult-intubation situations.

REVIEW QUESTIONS

1. Name two methods that may be used to manipulate the thyroid cartilage in order to improve the laryngeal view.

2. Where does the cricoid cartilage lie?

3. What are the narrowest portions of the pediatric larynx and the adult larynx?

4. Describe how bougie-assisted intubation can simplify a difficult intubation.

5. What does a Cormack and Lehane Grade 4 view indicate?

Oxygenation and Ventilation in Adults

Harald V. Genzwuerker
James Michael Rich
Andrew M. Mason

Chapter Objectives

After reading this chapter, you should be able to:

- Describe the mechanics, physiology, and processes of respiration.

- Identify complications of breathing.

- Discuss basic techniques of oxygenation and ventilation.

- Discuss advanced techniques of oxygenation and ventilation.

- Describe the devices used in basic and advanced airway management.

- Discuss the standard of care for airway management.

CASE Study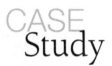

Medic 24 is dispatched to a pediatrician's office for a medical emergency. On arrival, crew members are directed to a side room to find most of the office staff crowded around a stretcher. The crew identify themselves as paramedics and ask who is in charge. Dr. Smith, the pediatrician, informs them that the patient, Johnny B., is a 15-year-old with a long history of asthma who presented with increased shortness of breath less than an hour earlier. The medical assistant who initially saw Johnny said that she did not hear any wheezes, so she put him in the side room to be seen in turn. When Dr. Smith entered the room, the patient was unresponsive, so staff started rescue breathing for Johnny and immediately called 911.

While the clinic staff members continue with resuscitation, the paramedics begin their assessment and attach their monitors. The patient is unresponsive to any stimulus. His airway is open with an oropharyngeal airway in place. The office staff members are ventilating with a pediatric bag-valve-mask device at a rate of 12 breaths per minute, but there is a large air leak coming from around the mask. There is very little rise and fall of the chest, but faint wheezes are audible on chest auscultation. The patient's radial pulse is strong, rapid, and regular. The monitors reveal sinus tachycardia with a heart rate of 130 beats per minute, a pulse oximetry reading of 72% with a waveform matching the pulse rate, and blood pressure of 98/50 mm Hg.

The paramedics start by switching to an adult bag-valve-mask device. They then ask a separate rescuer to help form a tight mask seal and instruct the staff members to squeeze the bag until the chest is seen to rise. It is then noticed that the oxygen reservoir bag is not filling. Further investigation reveals that the oxygen tank is empty.

After the paramedics attach their own oxygen tank, the bag fills rapidly. Reassessment shows that the patient is receiving adequate respiratory volumes, and there is satisfactory chest rise with no evidence of a tension pneumothorax. The pulse oximetry reading increases to 90%, but no further improvement can be obtained and the patient remains unconscious and unresponsive to any stimuli.

The paramedics prepare for intubation by checking their equipment. Direct laryngoscopy is performed without difficulty, and a cuffed endotracheal tube (ETT) is passed between the vocal cords. Correct placement of the ETT is confirmed by capnography and also by chest auscultation. They ventilate the patient at a rate of 16 breaths per minute. The end-tidal carbon dioxide (ETCO$_2$) reading is noted to be 58 mm Hg.

After the paramedics secure the patient to a stretcher, they begin transport to the hospital. En route they insert an orogastric tube and remove a large amount of air from the patient's stomach. They then administer a beta agonist using an in-line nebulizer and give the patient intravenous corticosteroids.

As the ambulance backs up to the emergency department, the patient begins to regain consciousness and starts following simple commands. Upon reexamination of the chest, wheezes are now more audible. The pulse oximeter shows a reading of 95%, and the ETCO$_2$ reading has fallen to 40 mm Hg.

Introduction

The process of respiration involves four integrated steps:

- Pulmonary ventilation, or breathing, involving the physical movement of air into and out of the lungs.
- Gas diffusion across the respiratory membrane, which separates alveolar air from the blood within the alveolar capillaries.
- Storage and transport of oxygen and carbon dioxide in the blood as these gases move between the alveolar capillaries and body tissues.
- Exchange of oxygen and carbon dioxide between the blood and the interstitial fluid in the tissues, with release of oxygen into the tissues and uptake of carbon dioxide into the blood for transport back to the lungs.

All living cells need energy for maintenance, growth, defense, and replication. Cells obtain this energy by harnessing certain foods as fuel. But energy production is also dependent on aerobic respiration, a process that consumes oxygen (O$_2$) and generates carbon dioxide (CO$_2$). This gaseous exchange takes place through the delicate membrane that lines the millions of tiny air sacs called *alveoli*, which are deep within the lungs. With about 400,000,000 alveoli distributed over a total surface area of 100 to 150 square meters, the respiratory system represents the largest interface that our body has with the outside world, larger even than the skin.

The goal of respiration is to expel excess carbon dioxide and replace it with a fresh supply of oxygen, thus preventing a build up of CO$_2$. Carbon dioxide dissolves in our body to form the weak acid, carbonic acid (CO$_2$ + H$_2$O $\rightleftharpoons$ H$_2$CO$_3$ $\rightleftharpoons$ H$^+$ + HCO$_3^-$), so respiration plays a vital role in regulating the acidity of the blood and body fluids. Although breathing is the obvious outward manifestation of this gaseous exchange process, normal respiration is also dependent upon a functioning circulatory system. In addition, the respiratory system plays a key role in the process of speech, using a series of specialized structures for phonation within the airway.

In fulfilling these important roles, the respiratory system presents a potential portal of entry into the body for viruses and bacteria as well as for inhaled foreign material. So the respiratory tract must also possess mechanisms for dealing with these challenges.

In this chapter, the mechanics of breathing, as well as the physiology of respiration in terms of gas transport and its exchange between the blood and tissues, will be considered. Discussion will also include the assessment of breathing and practical methods to provide oxygenation and ventilation from patients in the prehospital environment through all areas of the hospital.

Respiratory Physiology and Assessment

Control of Breathing

ON TARGET

The functions of the respiratory system are to:

- Move air to and from the gas-exchange surfaces of the lungs.
- Help control the pH (acidity/alkalinity) of the body fluids.
- Permit vocal communication.
- Provide specific defenses against the invasion of pathogens and other foreign material.

Hering-Breuer reflex

A reflex, initiated by stretch receptors in the airways and lungs, that causes inspiration to stop and thus prevents overinflation of the lungs.

The involuntary control of breathing is undertaken by specialized cells within the brainstem, which ensure the continuation of normal respiration during sleep (Figure 3-1). Various receptors play an important part in this process. Central chemoreceptors in the medulla of the brain detect a fall in pH caused by a rise in CO_2 levels in plasma and cerebral spinal fluid, triggering an increase in respiration. Peripheral chemoreceptors, located in special nodes within the aorta and common carotid artery (the so-called aortic and carotid bodies), mainly detect changes in the arterial oxygen concentration, but they also respond to changes in CO_2 and pH. Signals from these peripheral chemoreceptors are mediated by the ninth and tenth cranial nerves and are fed back to the respiratory center in the brain to stimulate respiration, particularly when there is a fall in the oxygen concentration in the blood.

Mechanoreceptors located in the airways and lung parenchyma initiate a variety of reflex responses. The **Hering-Breuer reflex** is initiated by stretch receptors that signal to terminate inspiration, thereby preventing overinflation of the lungs. Other receptors in the upper airway are responsible for sneezing, coughing, closure of the glottis (laryngospasm), and hiccups. Certain other reflexes, including the gasping response, are initiated via the spinal cord.

In addition to these involuntary mechanisms, breathing can also be controlled voluntarily to some degree, although voluntary breath-holding is always followed, after a varying period, by an irresistible desire to breathe again. Emotional state also has an effect on respiration, as does body temperature which is regulated by the hypothalamus.

The muscles that facilitate breathing are the intercostal muscles between the ribs and the diaphragm between the thoracic and abdominal cavities (Figure 3-2). The intercostal muscles are innervated via the ventral rami of the thoracic nerves (intercostal nerves), whereas the diaphragm is innervated by cervical nerve roots three, four, and five ("C3, 4, and 5 keep the diaphragm alive"). Therefore, after complete transection of the spinal cord in the lower cervical region, there will be immediate and complete paralysis of the intercostal muscles, but diaphragmatic contraction will be unaffected.

Mechanics of Breathing

Normal quiet breathing involves an active inspiratory phase and a passive expiratory phase. During inspiration, a flat sheet of muscle called the diaphragm, which separates the abdominal and thoracic cavities, descends, pulling the lungs downward. Simultaneous contraction

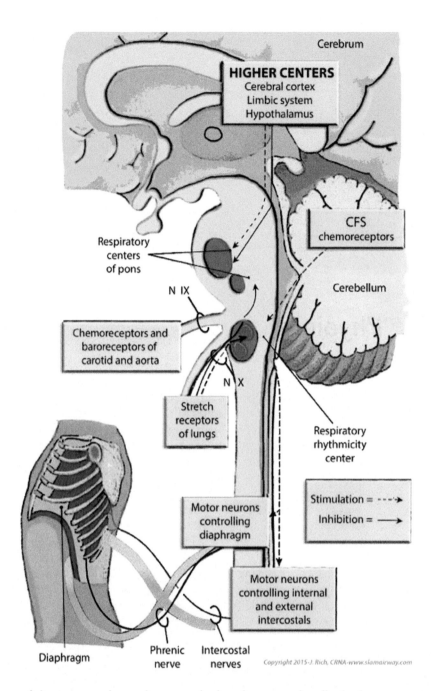

FIGURE 3-1
The control of respiration.

Diaphragm   Phrenic   Intercostal
             nerve   nerves

of the intercostal muscles expands the rib cage and pulls the lungs outward. These movements create a negative pressure within the thoracic cavity, and air is drawn into the lungs. The active inspiratory phase of quiet breathing (Figure 3-3) is followed by a passive expiratory phase in which the air is expelled purely by recoil of elastic tissues within the chest wall and lungs.

The proportion of lung expansion that comes from descent of the diaphragm (abdominal breathing) or expansion of the rib cage (thoracic breathing) varies among individuals, abdominal breathing often being more pronounced in men.

Central to any study of the mechanics of breathing is an understanding of lung volumes and capacities (Figure 3-4). When assessing respiratory movement, it is useful to expose both the chest and abdomen, and then to look along the line of the abdomen and chest from a position close to the patient's feet. From there it is often possible to spot small differences in the degree of expansion of the two sides of the chest (as can occur with a pneumothorax), which may be invisible from directly above the patient. Also, paradoxical respiration, in

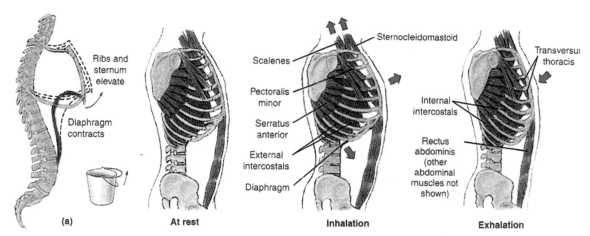

(a)   At rest   Inhalation   Exhalation

Labels in figure (a)–Inhalation/Exhalation:
- Ribs and sternum elevate
- Diaphragm contracts
- Sternocleidomastoid
- Scalenes
- Pectoralis minor
- Serratus anterior
- External intercostals
- Diaphragm
- Transversus thoracis
- Internal intercostals
- Rectus abdominis (other abdominal muscles not shown)

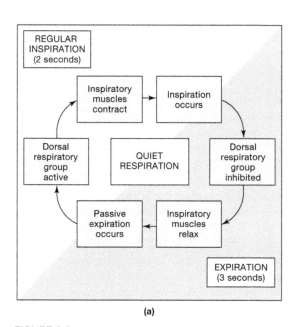

FIGURE 3-2

Pressure and volume relationships in the lungs. (a) Raising the curved handle of the bucket increases the amount of space between it and the bucket. Similarly, the volume of the thoracic cavity is increased when the ribs are elevated or the diaphragm is depressed when it contracts. (b) An anterior view at rest, with no air movement. (c) During inhalation, elevation of the rib cage and depression of the diaphragm increases the size of the thoracic cavity. Pressure decreases and air flows into the lungs. (d) Exhalation occurs when the rib cage returns to its original position or the diaphragm relaxes and the volume of the thoracic cavity decreases. Pressure rises, and air moves out of the lungs. Accessory muscles may assist such movements of the rib cage to increase the depth and rate of respiration.

Labels in figure (b)-(d):
- Pleural space
- Mediastinum
- Diaphragm

(b) Pressure outside and inside are equal, so no movement occurs
$P_o = P_i$

(c) Volume increases Pressure inside falls, and air flows in
$P_o > P_i$

(d) Volume decreases Pressure inside rises, so air flows out
$P_o < P_i$

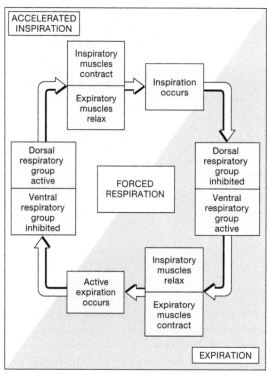

REGULAR INSPIRATION (2 seconds)

Inspiratory muscles contract → Inspiration occurs → Dorsal respiratory group inhibited → Inspiratory muscles relax → Passive expiration occurs → Dorsal respiratory group active →

QUIET RESPIRATION

EXPIRATION (3 seconds)

(a)

ACCELERATED INSPIRATION

Inspiratory muscles contract / Expiratory muscles relax → Inspiration occurs → Dorsal respiratory group inhibited / Ventral respiratory group active → Inspiratory muscles relax / Expiratory muscles contract → Active expiration occurs → Dorsal respiratory group active / Ventral respiratory group inhibited →

FORCED RESPIRATION

EXPIRATION

(b)

FIGURE 3-3

Basic regulatory patterns: (a) quiet respiration and (b) forced respiration.

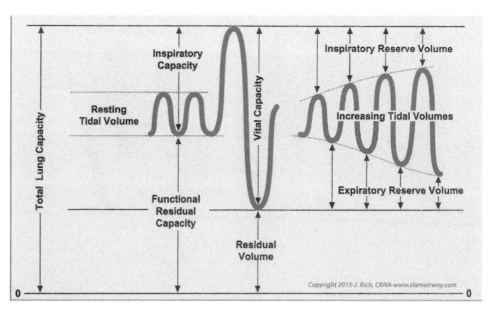

FIGURE 3-4

Lung volumes and capacities. Depending on prevailing circumstances, a normal respiratory rate lies somewhere in the range of 8 to 20 breaths per minute. In adults, the amount of air inspired or expired per breath, known as the resting tidal volume, is approximately 500 ml. The largest quantity of air that an individual can expel with a single breath following a maximal inspiration is called the vital capacity (VC), and it is around 3.2 liters in the female and 4.8 liters in the male. However, any condition that splints the diaphragm (e.g., obesity, pregnancy, and ascites) or restricts expansion of the chest wall (e.g., spinal kyphosis and ankylosing spondylitis) will, in turn, reduce the VC. The volume of air remaining in the lungs at the end of a resting expiration is known as the functional residual capacity (FRC). At the end of a forced expiration, the quantity of air remaining in the lungs is called the residual volume (RV). The difference between the FRC and the RV is known as the expiratory reserve volume (ERV). The maximum quantity of air that can be inhaled following a resting expiration is called the inspiratory capacity (IC). The difference between the IC and the resting tidal volume is known as the inspiratory reserve volume (IRV). Clearly, as tidal volumes increase, so the IRC and ERC decrease proportionally. The greatest volume of air that can be ventilated on command during a given interval (usually tested over a 15-second interval) is known as the maximum ventilatory volume (MVV) and is expressed in liters per minute. Young men can sometimes achieve MVV values approaching 170 L/min, but the levels are often much lower in females and in the elderly. The MVV is often profoundly reduced in patients with emphysema and those with obstructive pulmonary disease. (Redrawn by Dr. Andrew M. Mason after Pappenheimer Jr. et al. Fed Proc. 1950 Sep; 9(3):602)

which part of the chest wall is seen to inflate during expiration and deflate during inspiration, is often easier to appreciate from an oblique viewing angle, aiding in the diagnosis of a flail segment of chest wall.

During forceful breathing, the so-called accessory muscles of respiration are brought into play in order to increase the depth and frequency of respiration. The muscles of the abdominal wall, usually inactive during quiet breathing, are the most important muscles involved in forced expiration. When they contract, they increase the intra-abdominal pressure and force the diaphragm upward. At the same time, they pull the lower ribs downward and medially. Other muscles attached between the chest wall and head and neck, notably the sternomastoids and scalene muscles, become active with increased respiratory effort. Also, with the upper limbs fixed, the pectoral muscles, which attach between the chest wall and upper arms, can further assist in raising the chest wall. This is why patients in severe respiratory distress will often be seen leaning forward with their arms braced against fixed objects, such as their own knees or a wall or table. Inspiration can be further assisted by muscles that flare the nostrils.

Intercostal retractions are characterized by an inward movement of the intercostal muscles between the ribs as a result of high negative intrathoracic pressure. They are a sign of severe airway restriction and indicate respiratory distress. Retraction of soft tissue may

intercostal retractions
Inward movements of the muscles between the ribs. A sign of severe airway restriction and respiratory distress.

also be noticed in the suprasternal and supraclavicular regions. In neonates and young children, retraction of the sternum can also occur, but this is generally not seen in adults because their chest walls are much more bony and less pliable.

Breath Sounds

Breath sounds are examined by listening over the chest wall with a stethoscope, a procedure known as auscultation. Lung sounds are normally heard over all areas of the chest from above the clavicles to the bottom of the rib cage. Normal breath sounds have a soft, rustling quality and are termed **vesicular breath sounds.**

Abnormal breath sounds include rales, wheezes, and rhonchi. **Rales** (sometimes called crepitations) are tiny crackling, bubbling, or rattling noises within the lung and are sometimes further classified as being moist, dry, coarse, or fine. Wheezes are high-pitched, musical sounds found typically in asthmatics and are produced when turbulent air flows through narrowed air passages, particularly those smaller passages deep within the lung. Wheezing is mainly detected during expiration and may be loud enough to be heard without the aid of a stethoscope at some distance from the patient. **Rhonchi** are coarser sounds than wheezes and resemble soft snoring. They are produced when turbulent air passes through a restricted larger airway.

Auscultation may also reveal decreased or absent breath sounds, indicating a significant reduction of air flow to an area of lung. One type of breath sound audible without a stethoscope is **stridor,** a harsh vibrating noise caused by a high obstruction within the airway. It is usually louder during inhalation and can indicate an inhaled foreign body or some other restriction within the throat, larynx, or trachea. It should be regarded as a serious sign, especially in children, because their narrow upper airway is particularly prone to blockage.

Chest Percussion

In addition to auscultation, **percussion** over the chest wall can provide the practitioner with important information. Percussion is carried out by placing the palmar surface of the middle finger of the nondominant hand in isolation against the chest wall and tapping firmly over the middle phalanx, using the tip of the opposite middle finger. The degree of resonance of the underlying lung is assessed by listening and, to a lesser extent, by feeling vibrations from the chest wall.

Increased resonance upon percussion indicates hyperinflated lungs (emphysema) or the presence of air in a pleural cavity (pneumothorax). Decreased resonance suggests an underlying consolidation of lung tissue (e.g., pneumonia or tumor). A significant quantity of fluid within the pleural cavity (pleural effusion) gives a characteristic stony dullness at the base of one or both lungs.

Oxygen Transport

Oxygen saturation reflects the percentage of hemoglobin that is bound with oxygen, but it must be clearly understood that it is not the same as the pO_2, the partial pressure of oxygen dissolved in plasma. Under normal circumstances, 97% of the oxygen delivered to the tissues is carried by a specialized molecule within the red blood cells called **hemoglobin,** with just 3% being transported in simple solution.

Hemoglobin (Hb) is composed of four globin subunits, each consisting of a protein chain closely associated with a nonprotein heme group. The heme group contains one iron atom at the center of a porphyrin ring structure. The special way in which oxygen binds to hemoglobin results in the characteristic S-shaped sigmoidal oxygen dissociation curve (Figure 3-5). The shape of this curve enables hemoglobin to be highly saturated with oxygen

vesicular breath sounds
Normal breath sounds.

rales
Also called crepitations. Tiny crackling, bubbling, or rattling noises within the lungs that sound like hair being twisted together or salt being poured on a piece of paper.

rhonchi
Coarse sounds resembling soft snoring that come from the larger airways.

stridor
A harsh, vibrating noise caused by an obstruction high in the airway.

percussion
A tapping on the chest by placing one middle finger against the chest wall and tapping it with the tip of the other middle finger.

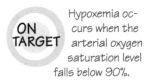

ON TARGET Hypoxemia occurs when the arterial oxygen saturation level falls below 90%.

hemoglobin
The oxygen-carrying, iron-containing compound of the blood. It is measured by weight per unit volume, such as 14.5 grams per deciliter, or 14.5 g/dl.

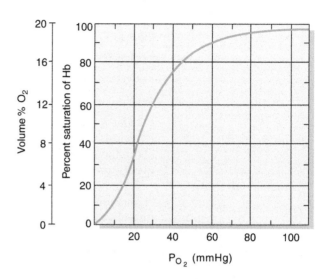

FIGURE 3-5
Oxyhemoglobin dissociation curve.

(usually more than 97%) when it leaves the lungs, yet able to unload large quantities of oxygen very rapidly into the tissues, where much lower oxygen tensions are encountered. Study of the S-shaped oxyhemoglobin dissociation curve shows that, as the partial pressure of oxygen increases, more and more molecules of oxygen combine with hemoglobin. Once fully saturated, the blood can only be made to carry more oxygen by increasing the hemoglobin concentration (e.g., by blood transfusion, erythropoietin [EPO] therapy) or by providing supplemental oxygen to increase the oxygen dissolved in plasma.

The hemoglobin molecule is around 90% saturated with oxygen at a paO_2 of 60 mm Hg. Above this level, increasingly greater rises in paO_2 are necessary to produce rises in percentage saturation as the molecule approaches full saturation. The more horizontal section of the curve is known as the flat-loading portion, and its presence ensures that the oxygen content of the blood remains reasonably steady, even with relatively large changes in paO_2. By contrast, the steep portion of the curve is known as the unloading portion, where small drops in paO_2 produce large falls in percentage saturation. This is the part of the curve that facilitates rapid unloading of oxygen in peripheral tissues where it is needed.

When hemoglobin is 100% saturated with oxygen, 100 ml of blood with a hemoglobin concentration of 15 g/dl can carry around 20 ml of oxygen. The bright-red compound that results is known as **oxyhemoglobin.** At rest, only around 25% of the oxygen carried is released into the tissues, rising to some 85% during strenuous exercise. The affinity that hemoglobin has for oxygen alters according to the chemical environment, an increased affinity resulting in a shift of the oxygen dissociation curve to the left and a decreased affinity shifting it to the right. Factors that decrease the oxygen affinity and allow greater quantities of oxygen to dissociate from the hemoglobin molecule include an increase in both temperature and the acidity of the blood (Figure 3-6).

As mentioned in the introduction to this chapter, carbon dioxide (CO_2) is a waste product of cellular metabolism that must be eliminated from the body (Figure 3-7). On its way back to the lungs for excretion, CO_2 binds to hemoglobin but at a different site than does oxygen. It also dissolves in the water of the plasma to form a weak acid (carbonic acid), a reaction that is catalyzed by an enzyme called *carbonic anhydrase*. Blood containing a higher level of CO_2 is therefore more acidic with a lower pH reading. Such conditions decrease the affinity that hemoglobin has for oxygen, thus promoting oxygen release to the tissues. This rightward shift in the oxyhemoglobin dissociation curve is known as the **Bohr effect.**

Conversely, when CO_2 is released from the pulmonary capillaries into the alveoli, the pH of the blood immediately rises, and the high affinity of haemoglobin for oxygen is re-

oxyhemoglobin

The compound that results from oxygen combining with hemoglobin.

ON TARGET Pulse oximeters cannot tell the difference between oxyhemoglobin and carboxyhemoglobin. Therefore, a person whose hemoglobin is heavily contaminated with carbon monoxide still shows a pulse oximetry reading of 100%.

Bohr effect

The effect of a rise in blood acidity on oxyhemoglobin, increasing its ability to release oxygen.

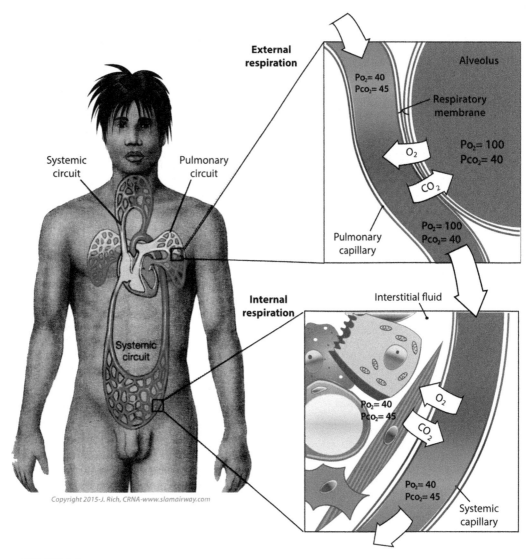

External
respiration

Alveolus

$P_{O_2}= 40$
$P_{CO_2}= 45$

Respiratory
membrane

O_2

$P_{O_2}= 100$
$P_{CO_2}= 40$

CO_2

Systemic
circuit

Pulmonary
circuit

Pulmonary
capillary

$P_{O_2}= 100$
$P_{CO_2}= 40$

Systemic
circuit

Internal
respiration

Interstitial fluid

$P_{O_2}= 40$
$P_{CO_2}= 45$

O_2

CO_2

$P_{O_2}= 40$
$P_{CO_2}= 45$

Systemic
capillary

Copyright 2015-J. Rich, CRNA-www.slamairway.com

FIGURE 3-6
An overview of respiration and respiratory processes.

stored. In this way the blood is rapidly recharged with oxygen in preparation for another cycle through the tissues.

Carboxyhemoglobin

The affinity of hemoglobin for the toxic gas carbon monoxide (CO) is around 200 times greater than its affinity for oxygen. Consequently, even small quantities of CO in inspired air can quickly tie up the hemoglobin in the bloodstream and block its ability to transport oxygen. When CO combines with hemoglobin it creates a relatively stable compound called **carboxyhemoglobin**, which has a bright cherry-red appearance. Once formed, and despite removal of a victim of poisoning to a CO-free environment, carboxyhemoglobin releases its CO back into the lungs only very slowly. In this way, atmospheric concentrations of CO as low as 0.1% can lead to unconsciousness and eventual death from hypoxemia because the brain is extremely sensitive to the lack of oxygen.

Carbon monoxide is created during incomplete combustion of hydrocarbon compounds and, in heavy smokers, as much as 20% of hemoglobin can be tied up in the carboxyhemaglobin form. Practitioners should be aware that pulse oximeters are unable to differentiate between oxyhemoglobin and carboxyhemoglobin, explaining why an SpO_2 reading is an unreliable guide to true oxygenation in cases of suspected CO poisoning.

carboxyhemoglobin
The compound that results from carbon monoxide combining with hemoglobin.

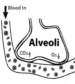 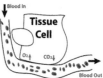

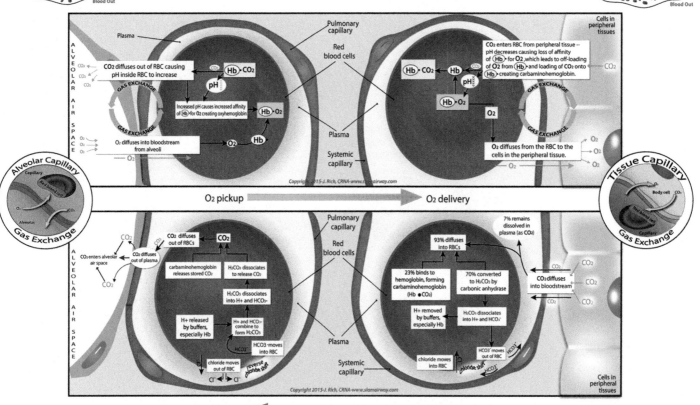

Gases in Alveolar Air

The pressure exerted by the atmosphere varies according to altitude, with the pressure falling the higher one climbs. At sea level the atmosphere exerts a force of 760 mm Hg, 101 kPa, or 15 psi—all equivalent to one atmosphere. Air is made up of a number of different gases, and the total air pressure is simply the sum of the pressures of its constituent parts.

Atmospheric air contains small quantities of carbon dioxide, argon, and helium, but 99% of dry atmospheric air is made up of nitrogen (78%) and oxygen (21%). The pressure that each gas exerts in any mixture of gases is known as its partial pressure, and gases tend to move from an area of high partial pressure to one where the partial pressure is lower. However, water vapor is another gaseous constituent of air, and its presence displaces the other gases to a varying degree, depending on the prevailing humidity.

Within the alveoli, where the air is fully saturated with water vapor and where there is a combination of inhaled fresh air and air for exhalation, the normal mixture consists of 75.1% nitrogen (N_2), 13.4% oxygen (O_2), 6.2% water vapor (H_2O), and 5.2% carbon dioxide (CO_2) (See Table 3-1). The shorthand symbol for the partial pressure of a gas is usually shown as a lowercase p followed by its chemical symbol (e.g., pO_2, pCO_2, pH_2O, pN_2).

Alveolar Gas Exchange

Blood returning via the pulmonary arteries to the lungs from the tissues has a low pO_2 of around 40 mm Hg. In the pulmonary capillaries, which surround alveoli, oxygen diffuses from the high partial pressure of 102 mm Hg to the lower pO_2 of 40 mm Hg found within the pulmonary capillaries. In a perfect lung, all alveoli would receive an equal share of alveolar ventilation and vascular perfusion, and the pO_2 of reoxygenated blood within the pul-

Table 3-1	Partial Pressures of Gases in Alveolar Air
Constituent Gas	**Partial Pressure (at Sea Level)**
Oxygen (O_2)	102 mm Hg
Carbon dioxide (CO_2)	40 mm Hg
Water vapor (H_2O)	47 mm Hg
Nitrogen (N_2)	571 mm Hg
	TOTAL: 760 mm Hg

ventilation/perfusion mismatch

A condition that occurs when some alveoli are overventilated and underperfused, and others are underventilated and overperfused, resulting in suboptimal oxygenation of the blood.

shunting

A condition that occurs when deoxygenated blood passes straight through unventilated sections of the lung without picking up oxygen or shedding carbon dioxide. This can happen when alveoli collapse (atelectasis) or pulmonary edema replaces the air in the alveoli.

ON TARGET When hemoglobin is 100% saturated with oxygen, 100 ml of blood with a hemoglobin concentration of 15 grams per deciliter can carry around 20 ml of oxygen. The bright red compound that results is known as oxyhemoglobin.

monary veins would reach that within the alveolus (paO_2). In such a model, ventilation and perfusion would be perfectly matched.

In diseased lungs, there may be marked differences between the ventilation and the perfusion of different areas of lung. Some alveoli are relatively overventilated, while others are relatively overperfused. Underventilated alveoli cannot oxygenate the blood to their maximum potential. Therefore, the oxygenated blood returning to the heart via the pulmonary veins, being of a mixture of pulmonary capillary blood from all alveoli, has a reduced pO_2 compared to the paO_2. This is termed a **ventilation/perfusion mismatch.**

Even normal lungs exhibit this to some degree because the upper zones tend to be relatively overventilated and the lower zones relatively overperfused and underventilated. The situation is worsened when so-called shunting takes place. **Shunting** occurs when deoxygenated blood passes straight through unventilated sections of lung with no opportunity to absorb O_2 or shed CO_2 as occurs in atelectasis (collapse of the alveoli) or pulmonary edema, where fluid in the alveoli has replaced the air.

Diffusion of oxygen into the blood is very rapid in normal lung tissue but, in cases of pulmonary fibrosis, the speed at which O_2 diffuses through the wall of the alveolus may be so slow that oxygenation is incomplete. Ventilation/perfusion mismatch, shunting, and slow diffusion can all contribute to lowering the pO_2 in the pulmonary capillaries compared to that of the alveoli, but blood vessels within the lung are capable of constricting and diverting blood flow from areas that are underventilated, thus reducing the impact of shunting.

Oxygen Deprivation

Hypoxemia occurs when the arterial oxygen saturation falls below 90%. Because of the sigmoidal shape of the oxyhemoglobin dissociation curve, each 100 ml of normal blood with a 90% saturation level still contains some 18 ml of oxygen, despite the fact that the partial pressure of oxygen in the arterial blood will have fallen from just over 100 to around 80 mm Hg. Thereafter, there are relatively large drops in SaO_2 for relative small falls in paO_2 as the patient enters the steep section of the oxyhemoglobin dissociation curve. Hypoxemic patients generally become confused and are often agitated or combative before losing consciousness. Such behavior should always alert the rescuer to the possibility of oxygen lack.

PEARLS Peripheral cyanosis is not a good indicator of hypoxia. Central cyanosis involving the lips, tongue, and truncal skin is a more ominous finding. The hypoxic patient becomes restless, agitated, and confused.

Cellular hypoxia occurs from either a decrease of oxygen delivery to the cell (e.g., decreased cardiac output) or the inability of the cell to use oxygen (e.g., cellular poisoning). There are four causes of cellular hypoxia: (1) hypoxemic hypoxia, (2) anemic hypoxia, (3) stagnant hypoxia, and (4) histotoxic hypoxia. The first three are caused by a decrease in oxygen delivery to the tissues. Hypoxic hypoxia is the most important cause of cellular hypoxia and can result from any one of the following: (1) apnea, (2) breathing a hypoxic gas mixture, (3) airway obstruction, or (4) a right-to-left shunt in the heart. This is the type of cellular hypoxia normally associated with difficult-airway management. Anemic hypoxia results from a decreased concentration of hemoglobin or a reduction in the number of erythrocytes (i.e. decreased **hematocrit**). It is usually not critical because the heart compensates for it by increasing cardiac output, thus increasing blood flow to the tissues. Stagnant hypoxia can occur either globally on a large scale (e.g., congestive heart failure) or regionally on a smaller scale (arterial blockage from a thrombus). The ashen gray color of a patient experiencing a myocardial infarction is caused by stagnant hypoxia secondary to a decrease in cardiac output. The fourth cause of cellular hypoxia, histotoxic hypoxia, occurs when there is an inability of the cells to take up or utilize oxygen from the bloodstream, despite physiologically normal delivery of oxygen to the cells and tissues. Histotoxic hypoxia occurs when tissues are affected by poisons such as alcohol, narcotics, and cyanide (which acts by inhibiting cytochrome oxidase), thus preventing them from utilizing oxygen. Carbon monoxide (CO) poisoning results in a mixed quasi-anemic hypoxia (as hemoglobin is progressively tied up as carboxyhemoglobin, becoming unavailable for oxygen transport) and a histotoxic hypoxia due to its direct effect upon cells. Carbon monoxide prevents electron transfer within mitochondrial cytochromes leading to depletion of ATP, lactic acidosis, and cell death. However, CO does not bind to cytochrome oxidase with the same affinity as oxygen, so significant intracellular hypoxia is necessary before such binding takes place and cell death results. This explains why some individuals recover completely from seemingly severe episodes of CO poisoning without sequelae, the presence of still sufficient quantities of oxygen in the bloodstream presumably inhibiting the histotoxic effect of CO at a cellular level.

Cyanosis is a blue or purplish tinge to the skin and mucous membranes. Before the advent of the pulse oximeter, the presence of cyanosis of the lips or fingernails was the only physical clue to the presence of hypoxemia in the prehospital setting. However, clinical assessment of hypoxemia is now known to be highly unreliable because the presence of cyanosis requires a concentration of at least 5 g/dl of reduced (deoxygenated) hemoglobin in the capillaries. With normal hemoglobin concentrations of 15 g/dl, patients do not accumulate such levels of reduced hemoglobin until the SaO_2 level falls to 85%. With hemoglobin levels of 9 g/dl, cyanosis is not evident until the SaO_2 reaches the highly dangerous level of 73%. Furthermore, in anemic individuals with hemoglobin concentrations of 8 g/dl and below, the patient could easily die from hypoxemia without cyanosis ever becoming evident. On the other hand, peripheral cyanosis of the extremities can occur in normal individuals without true hypoxemia being present. Certain silver salts and drugs such as amiodarone and chloroquine can impart a bluish tinge to the skin and mucous membranes called pseudocyanosis.

Finally, the ability of the observer to detect cyanosis depends on experience and good eyesight and can be adversely affected by the color balance of the ambient lighting and by dark skin pigmentation. For all these reasons, it is most important that hypoxemia is diagnosed, wherever possible, by the application of pulse oximeter probe, while remembering that carbon monoxide poisoning is likely to give a false-normal result.

Respiratory failure is complex and multifactorial in its etiology (Table 3-2). Paramedics and others working in the prehospital environment will encounter patients with respiratory failure stemming from both traumatic and medical causes. Depending on the status of the patient, anatomical variations, clinical situation, and the access to the patient's head, the best choice for oxygenation and ventilation must take into account the resources that are available along with the training and experience of the rescuer.

Used separately or in combination, four general options are available for achieving and maintaining adequate oxygenation in the high-risk emergency patient:

- Spontaneous ventilation by the patient (with or without supplemental oxygen and an N/P or O/P airway).
- Mask ventilation (assisted or controlled).

Table 3-2 Etiology of Respiratory Failure in Critically Ill Patients and Trauma Patients[4]

Airway Causes	Ventilatory Causes	Cardiovascular Causes	Other Causes
Foreign body	Pulmonary aspiration of gastric contents	Shock	Spinal-cord lesion
Soft-tissue obstruction	Hemothorax	Nonperfusing cardiac rhythm	Head injury
Airway edema	Pneumothorax	Myocardial trauma	Neck trauma
Airway hemorrhage	Pulmonary contusion	Pericardial tamponade	Poisoning/overdose
Laryngeal, tracheal, or bronchial injury	Pulmonary edema	Dissecting or ruptured aortic aneurysm	Preexisting medical condition (e.g., Guillain-Barré syndrome, tetanus)
Ligature or manual strangulation	Flail chest	Valvular heart disease	
Laryngospasm secondary to instrumentation or drowning	Inhalation of noxious gases	Pulmonary embolus	
	Depressurization of aircraft at high altitude		

- Placement of an endotracheal tube or supraglottic airway device.
- Creation of a surgical airway.

It is generally easier for patients to breathe spontaneously or to be manually ventilated if they are in the sniffing position, with the head slightly elevated, extension at the antlanto-occipital joint, and slight flexion of the cervical spine.[1,2] Care should always be exercised when injury to the cervical spine is suspected, but opening the airway to ensure adequate oxygenation must take priority if the alternative is hypoxemia.

Advanced techniques such as the use of supraglottic airways or endotracheal intubation require training in elective situations to allow a realistic chance of success in the emergency setting. When simple measures to improve oxygenation fail, then supraglottic devices can provide both oxygenation and ventilation without the need for endotracheal intubation. Their ease of use, coupled with the fact that they can be inserted blindly into the airway, make them particularly suitable for prehospital use (e.g., closed-space airway management of a casualty victim trapped in a vehicle).[3]

Spontaneous Versus Assisted/Controlled Ventilation

The reader is referred to the Oxygen/Ventilation Pathway of the SLAM Universal Adult Airway Flowchart (SUAAF) for the remainder of this chapter. Respiratory arrest or respiratory distress from any cause is a common reason for emergency care of the patient. Respiratory arrest precludes the use of devices, such as a simple breathing mask or nasal cannula, and dictates the use of positive pressure ventilation through the use of an anesthesia mask, supraglottic airway device, endotracheal tube, or a cricothyrotomy. However, the emergency patient who is breathing spontaneously can often be oxygenated adequately by using supplemental oxygen and those simple measures described in the oxygenation/ventilation pathway of the SUAAF.[5,6]

Elevating the upper body may lead to both subjective and objective improvement of the patient with respiratory compromise. Gastric distension is a common problem during positive pressure mask ventilation. The gas takes the route of least resistance down the esophagus instead of the trachea. This problem is often unavoidable during mask ventilation, even when the rescuer is using a good technique, but use of an oropharyngeal or a nasopharyngeal airway coupled with lower tidal volumes delivered at lower pressure will usually decrease the extent to which it happens. When gastric distention does occur, it is best to decompress the stomach through the use of a naso- or orogastric tube because gastric distension increases the risk of vomiting and aspiration and restricts descent of the diaphragm and lung expansion, further exacerbating respiratory failure.[7]

Oxygen administration is indicated for all patients in shock and those at risk of going into shock. Patients with dyspnea or respiratory distress from any cause should also receive oxygen. A number of methods exist for administering oxygen in the spontaneously breathing patient (Table 3-3). Although caution should be exercised in administering high concentrations of oxygen to patients with chronic obstructive pulmonary disease (COPD), it should still be given in emergency situations. Careful monitoring of

Table 3-3 Sources of Oxygen[7,8]

Device or Method	Description	Flow (liters/min)	% O$_2$	FiO$_2$
Mouth-to-mouth ventilation	Oxygen is provided by the exhaled breath of the rescuer, which generally provides between 16% and 18% oxygen mixed with exhaled carbon dioxide.	NA	16% to 18%	0.16 to 0.18
Ambient air	Atmospheric air provides 21% oxygen.	NA	20.84%	0.21
Nasal cannula	Paired catheters of relatively small caliber that are placed just within the nostrils. At flow rates above 6 L/min, the nasal mucous membrane becomes very dry and can even ulcerate. However, patients generally tolerate the lower flow rates well. Nasal cannula are indicated for low-to-moderate oxygen requirements and for long-term oxygen therapy. The delivered oxygen concentration depends on how much the patient breathes through the mouth rather than the nose.	1 to 6	24% to 32%	0.24 to 0.32
Simple face mask	Indicated for patients requiring moderate oxygen concentrations, this mask tends to seal poorly. Side ports allow room air to enter the mask during inspiration, which dilutes the oxygen concentration. Flow rates over 10 L/min do not enhance oxygen concentration beyond around 50%.	6 to 10	40% to 50%	0.40
Partial rebreather mask	This is essentially a simple face mask with the addition of a reservoir bag that is fed a continuous flow of oxygen. However, the reservoir bag does not possess a one-way valve, and the patient's exhaled breath is allowed to mix with the gas in the bag. When the patient inhales, much of the inhalation volume comes from the reservoir bag. This type of mask can provide oxygen concentrations of up to 60%. It is indicated for patients requiring moderate-to-high oxygen concentrations when satisfactory clinical results are not obtained with the simple face mask.	10	50% to 60%	0.50 to 0.60
Nonrebreathing mask	This mask is similar to a partial rebreather mask, except that it has a one-way valve on the reservoir bag preventing it from filling with exhaled air, which is vented through side ports. The side ports are also guarded by one-way valves that prevent the entry of room air during inspiration.	10 to 15	75% to 80%	0.75 to 0.80

Table 3-3 Sources of Oxygen[7,8] (continued)

Device or Method	Description	Flow (liters/min)	% O_2	FiO_2
	This type of mask can provide oxygen concentrations of 75% or even higher at high oxygen flow rates. It is not indicated as long-term support for poor respiratory effort and severe hypoxia; however, it can be placed initially in an attempt to preoxygenate such patients while preparations are made for intubation, unless initial ventilatory support by positive pressure mask ventilation and 100% oxygen is indicated.			
Venturi mask	A high-flow face mask that uses a Venturi system and delivers relatively precise oxygen concentrations, regardless of the patient's rate and depth of breathing. As oxygen passes into the mask through a jet orifice in the base of the mask, it entrains room air. The device then delivers the resulting mixture to the patient. Some Venturi masks have dial selectors to control the amount of ambient air taken in; others have interchangeable caps. It is particularly useful for COPD patients, who benefit from careful control of inspired oxygen concentration. Typically, these devices deliver 24% to 28% oxygen at 4 L/min and 35% to 40% oxygen at 8 L/min, but they are designed for the controlled clinical environment rather than for emergency use in the field.	6 to 10	24% to 50%	0.24 to 0.50
Bag-valve mask	The BVM is an oval self-inflating silicone or rubber bag with two one-way valves (an air/oxygen-inlet valve and a patient valve) and a transparent plastic face mask, which is available in various sizes.	15		Maximum 0.40 with oxygen but without reservoir
	Without oxygen supplement	0	21%	0.21 (ambient air)
	With supplemental oxygen	15	40%	0.40
	Supplemental oxygen and reservoir bag/tubing	15	95%	0.95

the patient's oxygen status and breathing should then alert the rescuer to the need for an advanced method of ventilation and/or oxygenation.

Oxygen is a basic requirement of life. A properly functioning respiratory system is needed to supply it to tissues and cells. The initial assessment of the airway and breathing should be brief but thorough. After determining that no immediate threat to life exists, a more extensive examination may be conducted. The effectiveness of ventilation is clinically more subjective. To assess the adequacy of ventilation, the rescuer should assess for the presence of equal breath sounds, adequate chest rise and fall, and a regular expiratory CO_2 waveform if capnography is available and being utilized.[2]

Initial assessment is directed at identifying any life-threatening conditions resulting from compromise to airway, breathing, and circulation. Be alert for: nasal flaring (excessive widening of the nares with respiration), intercostal muscle retraction, use of the accessory respiratory muscles of respiration, cyanosis, pursed-lip breathing, and tracheal tugging (retraction of the tissues of the neck due to airway obstruction or dyspnea).[9]

Table 3-4 Signs of Possible Life-Threatening Respiratory Problems[9]

- Alterations in mental status
- Severe central cyanosis
- Absent breath sounds
- Audible stridor
- One- to two-word dyspnea (need to breathe between every word or two)
- Tachycardia $\geq$130 beats per minute
- Pallor and sweating
- Presence of intercostal and suprasternal and supraclavicular retractions
- Use of accessory muscles of respiration

Modified from reference 9.

 PEARLS Initial assessment should check for the presence of equal breath sounds, adequate chest rise and fall, and a regular expiratory carbon dioxide waveform if capnography is available.

Assessment of the patient, his or her respiratory status, and presence or absence of airway patency determine which oxygenation/ventilation method to use. Signs of possible life-threatening respiratory problems are listed in Table 3-4. If you note airway obstruction, do not waste time: get available assistance and rapidly apply basic airway management techniques to open the airway and restore oxygenation and ventilation. Bledsoe et al. have stated five clinical principles to keep in mind when assessing breathing and the airway:[9]

- Noisy breathing nearly always means partial airway obstruction.
- Obstructed breathing is not always noisy.
- The brain can survive only a few minutes in asphyxia.
- Artificial respiration is useless if the airway is blocked.
- A patent airway is useless if the patient is apneic.

Simple methods for administration of supplemental oxygen (Table 3-3) are indicated for use in spontaneously breathing patients with intact airway reflexes. Constant monitoring of the patient's respiratory status (Table 3-5), the oxygen saturation by pulse oximetry, and how much oxygen is being used assist in determining what type of oxygenation/ventilation assistance is needed. For example, if, after several hours of breathing an FiO_2 of 0.9 with a nonrebreathing mask, the patient's work of breathing is increasing, his or her oxygen saturation is dropping, respiratory rate is increasing, and respirations are more shallow and labored, then serious consideration should be given to intubating the patient as soon as possible.[8]

In the critically ill patient or a patient with multiple trauma, positive-pressure ventilation should be provided by means of a bag-valve-mask device, using 100% oxygen with or without an oropharyngeal airway (OPA) or bilateral nasopharyngeal airways (NPA), or both, in an attempt to maintain an SpO_2 of >92%.[5,6] Alternatively, a nonrebreathing mask may be used in spontaneously breathing patients who cannot be intubated, or it may be used for preoxygenation in preparation for tracheal intubation or insertion of an adjunctive supraglottic airway device.

Table 3-5 Assessment of Respiratory Status[7]

Position	Consider the patient's position. Patients with respiratory diseases tend to tolerate an upright posture better than a supine one. Indications of severe respiratory distress include a patient who is sitting upright with feet dangling over the side of the bed. In the most severe cases, the patient will assume the tripod position in which he or she leans forward and supports body weight with the arms extended.
Color	Patients with severe respiratory distress display pallor and diaphoresis. Cyanosis is a late finding and may be absent even with significant hypoxia. Peripheral cyanosis (bluish discoloration involving only the distal extremities) is not a specific finding and is also found in patients with poor circulation. Peripheral cyanosis reflects the slowing of blood flow and increased extraction of oxygen from red blood cells. Central cyanosis (involving the lips, tongue, and truncal skin) is a more ominous finding seen in hypoxia.
Mental status	Briefly assess the patient's mental status. The hypoxic patient will become restless and agitated. Confusion is seen with both hypoxia (deficiency of oxygen) and hypercarbia (excess of carbon dioxide). When respiratory failure is imminent, the patient will appear severely lethargic and somnolent. The eyelids will begin to droop, and the head will bob with each respiratory effort.
Ability to speak	Assess the patient's ability to speak in full, coherent sentences. Determine the ease with which the patient can discuss symptoms. Patients with respiratory distress will be able to speak only one to two words before they need to pause to catch their breath. Rambling, incoherent speech indicates fear, anxiety, or hypoxia.
Respiratory effort	As described, normal ventilation is an active process. However, the use of accessory muscles in the neck (scalenes and sternomastoids) and the visible retraction of the intercostal muscles indicate significant breathing effort.

 When assessing respiratory movement, expose both chest and abdomen, then look at the abdomen and chest from the position of the patient's feet. This vantage point greatly enhances the ability to see small differences in expansion of the two sides of the chest, as well as a flail segment.

 Increased resonance on percussion (bongo drum) indicates hyperinflated lungs or air in the pleural cavity. Decreased resonance suggests consolidation of lung tissue, such as in pneumonia or tumor. Fluid in the pleural cavity gives a flat, dull sound.

To provide the highest concentration of oxygen possible, a well-fitting nonrebreathing mask (Figure 3-8) with a flow of 8–15 lpm should be used, which should give an oxygen concentration of around 90%. In contrast, nasal cannulae or nasal prongs provide only a maximum oxygen concentration of approximately 32%. However, if a patient does not tolerate or refuses an oxygen mask, nasal cannulae or blow-by oxygen by insufflation may initially be the best option. It may be helpful in coherent patients who will not tolerate an oxygen mask to inform them that the additional oxygen should make their breathing easier or may actually save their lives.

Masks may cause some patients to become claustrophobic. Loosening the mask or switching to a face tent (Table 3-3) may improve the situation. In some clinical situations (e.g., closed-space rescue, lack of experience, equipment limitations, signs or history of a difficult airway), and provided that spontaneous ventilation is present, the only available option in the initial stages may be to provide supplemental insufflated oxygen (Figure 3-9).[3]

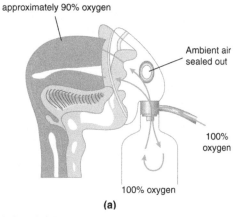

Delivered concentration
approximately 90% oxygen

Ambient air
sealed out

100%
oxygen

100% oxygen

(a)

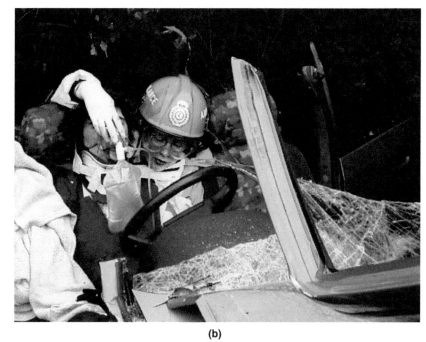

(b)

FIGURE 3-8

(a) Nonrebreathing mask.

(b) A spontaneously breathing conscious casualty, trapped in her vehicle. A paramedic is maintaining the head and neck in neutral alignment while administering oxygen via a nonrebreathing mask.

(Courtesy of Dr. Andrew M. Mason)

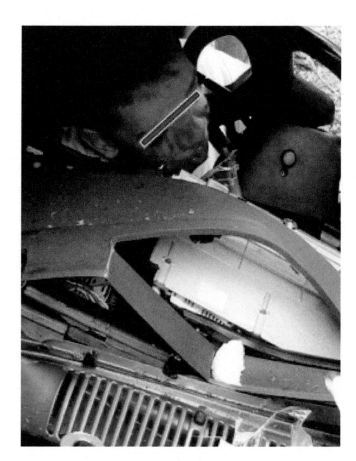

FIGURE 3-9

A critically injured victim of a motor-vehicle crash is pinned in his car and requires sedation and rescue ventilation for safe extrication. He receives preoxygenation by nonrebreathing mask prior to induction of anesthesia.

(Courtesy of Dr. Peer G. Knacke)

Basic Oxygen/Ventilation Techniques

The rescuer should always begin by considering simple measures to improve oxygenation. Opening the airway by using the jaw-thrust or head-tilt/chin-lift maneuver, together with insufflation of the highest concentration of oxygen possible, should be the minimum standard of care in patients with respiratory insufficiency. All techniques used to secure the airway should be directed toward the maintenance of airway patency and delivery of adequate oxygenation.

> **Note**
>
> The head-tilt maneuver and neck manipulation are best avoided in all patients with suspected trauma of the cervical spine, but if the only alternative is asphyxia, the provision of a patent airway by careful manipulation of the head and neck has to take precedence.

Causes of airway obstruction include the tongue, foreign bodies, local edema or hemorrhage, laryngeal spasm, and aspiration.[7] At the level of the oropharynx, the most common extrinsic causes of airway obstruction are secretions, food, or other foreign objects. The base of the tongue can also fall back in obtunded patients who are lying in a supine position (Figure 3-10). To clear an airway, secretions and foreign objects must be removed. Foreign body removal may require direct visualization and the careful use of Magill forceps. If the tongue is occluding the airway, a head-tilt/chin-lift or jaw-thrust maneuver can pull the base of the tongue away from the retropharyngeal wall (Figures 3-11 and 3-12). Simple airway devices such as the oropharyngeal airway or nasopharyngeal airway can help maintain the open airway.

Use of Continuous Positive Airway Pressure (CPAP) and Bilevel Positive Airway Pressure (BiPAP)

CPAP is used by millions of patients for the treatment of obstructive sleep apnea because it maintains the patency of pharyngeal structures throughout the entire respiratory cycle. In the acute situation, it can also be used in appropriately selected, awake, spontaneously breathing patients suffering from acute pulmonary edema (APE). It offers a therapeutic option between standard oxygen therapy and endotracheal intubation. The goal is to keep the alveoli open by using a continuous positive airway pressure (CPAP). CPAP differs from positive end expiratory pressure (PEEP), which is applied only at the end of the respiratory cycle; CPAP functions throughout the complete respiratory cycle. Additionally, PEEP is used in intubated patients, and CPAP is administered using a mask.

Standard oxygen therapy does not open collapsed alveoli; however, CPAP, by maintaining continuous positive pressure during the entire respiratory cycle, can maintain their patency. The advantages of CPAP include, but are not limited to (1) recruits collapsed alveoli, (2) restores a satisfactory level of residual capacity, and (3) improves gas exchange. It is

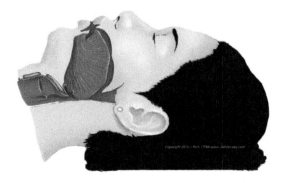

FIGURE 3-10
An unconscious patient's tongue may fall and obstruct the upper airway.

ADULT

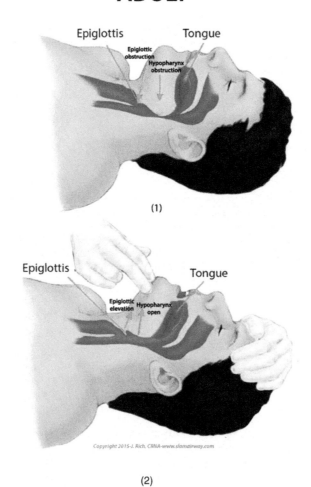

(1)

(2)

FIGURE 3-11
The head-tilt/chin-lift maneuver is used to open the airway of a patient.

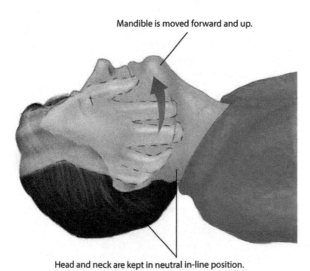

FIGURE 3-12
In a patient with suspected cervical-spine injury, the jaw-thrust maneuver is used to open the airway.

usually used for a period of one-half hour to two hours. As the patient's work of breathing decreases and he or she is showing improvement, the patient can be weaned off the CPAP by incrementally decreasing the CPAP pressure.

The advantages of CPAP include the following:

- It decreases preload and afterload in CHF.
- It improves lung compliance in CHF.
- It decreases the work of breathing.
- In the treatment of APE, CPAP reduces venous counterpressure by increasing intrathoracic pressure as well as increasing pulmonary volume.
- It increases partial oxygen (O_2) pressure in the alveoli.
- It leads to an improvement of gas exchange (elevation of functional residual capacity (FRC), and it decreases ventilation/perfusion mismatch, with reabsorption of alveolar liquid in the interstitial space of the patient with APE.
- In the event of hypoxia, it improves partial pressure of arterial oxygen (PaO_2) without the need for endotracheal intubation.
- In serious infectious conditions with hypoxemia, the complications related to intubation justify using a face mask at the beginning of ventilatory therapy, particularly in immunodeficient patients, because intubation exposes them to an increased risk of secondary pulmonary infection.

The disadvantages of CPAP include the following:

- Possible need for high flows of up to 140 L/min for standard CPAP systems.
- Need for an oxygen concentrator or generator.
- Capital equipment cost and maintenance.
- Bulkiness and weight.
- High CPAP pressure can cause barotrauma or inhibit ventricular filling, thus leading to decreased cardiac output.

Acute indications for CPAP include:

- Patients with acute pulmonary edema (APE).
- Signs of ventilatory distress and/or respiratory frequency >35 respiratory cycles/min and/or oxygen saturation with O_2<90%.
- Hypercapnic APE with no indication for endotracheal intubation in emergency condition.
- Common APE with no response to medical treatment.
- Cardiopulmonary resuscitation.

Contraindications to CPAP include:

- Gastric distension.
- Disease in one lung.
- Nondrained pneumothorax.
- Hypovolemia.
- Painful abdominal disorders.
- Intracranial hypertension.
- Major emphysema.
- Muscular fatigue.

CPAP should be discontinued in cases of excessive hypercapnia, vomiting, discomfort (e.g., patient cannot tolerate the face mask), insufficient oxygen saturation in the blood, signs that the patient is exhausted, and inability to maintain consciousness.

Boussignac CPAP System

A simple to use and disposable "open" CPAP system has recently been introduced in the United States. It was developed by a French physician, George Boussignac, and is marketed as the Boussignac CPAP System (Vitaid, Ltd., Williamsville, NY). Advantages from its use include:

- Only 15–25 LPM flow for CPAP of 5–10 cmH$_2$O.
- Requires only an oxygen source and a flowmeter.
- Disposable single-use system.
- Eliminates rebreathing.
- Accommodates patient's high peak inspiratory demand.
- Permits patient suctioning without removing the mask.
- Allows use of a nebulizer.
- CPAP is easily titratable by adjusting the oxygen flow.
- Easy to store because the entire system weighs only 6.8 ounces and measures 6″ by 5″ by 4″.

When CPAP is initiated, the usual starting point is 10 cmH$_2$O; however, starting at 5 cmH$_2$O and working up is recommended by some practitioners. Oxygen can be delivered at high enough flow rates to maintain an SpO$_2$ greater than 92%. CPAP and BiPAP can prevent the need for tracheal intubation and decrease mortality in appropriately chosen, awake patients with acute respiratory failure. BiPAP allows for individual titration of the patient's Bi-PAP pressure at both the inspiratory and expiratory level in those who do not tolerate CPAP. The levels are adjusted based on patient comfort, tidal volume achieved, and arterial blood gas reading. Noninvasive ventilation with CPAP and BiPAP can be effectively and safely used in properly selected, awake prehospital patients with acute CHF.

Use of Oropharyngeal and Nasopharyngeal Airways

An oropharyngeal airway (OPA) can keep the airway open during spontaneous respiration or bag-valve-mask ventilation by keeping the base of the tongue away from the posterior pharyngeal wall (Figure 3-13). However, unlike the endotracheal tube and some supraglot-

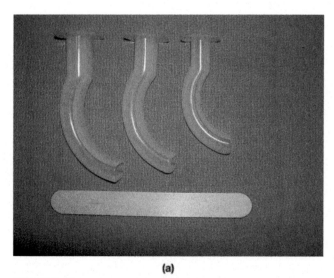

(a)

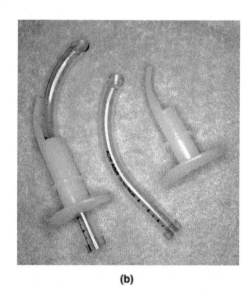

(b)

FIGURE 3-13

(a) Small, medium, and large oropharyngeal airways with tongue blade for insertion.

(b) The Chou Airway. In conjunction with the use of a regular face mask, it is to be placed orally to facilitate and maintain spontaneous or assisted breathing in emergency resuscitation situations or under general anesthesia. It is intended to overcome upper airway obstruction resulting from the presence of a large hypopharyngeal tongue, which is often associated with difficult face-mask ventilation, obstructive sleep apnea, and difficult intubation.

(Courtesy of Achi Corporation, San Jose, CA)

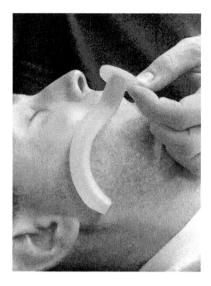

FIGURE 3-14

Proper technique for the sizing of an oropharyngeal airway. Note that the distal tip of the airway extends just beyond the angle of the jaw.

tic devices, it does not isolate the respiratory tract from the alimentary tract, so it cannot protect the patient from aspiration. It helps to prevent airway obstruction caused by collapse of the soft tissue of the oropharyngeal space, but it is of little value when airway obstruction is caused by a large floppy epiglottis overlying the laryngeal inlet. This type of obstruction is best dealt with by upward and backward pressure under the mandible, which lifts both the hyoid and epiglottis and makes ventilation easier (Figure 3-12).[2]

PEARLS If a patient can tolerate insertion of an oral airway, he or she probably meets the criteria for tracheal intubation.

The combined use of the OPA and basic airway maneuvers, such as chin lift, head tilt, and jaw thrust, are synergistic in relieving airway obstruction. However, correct sizing of the OPA is important to avoid pushing the base of the tongue back and causing further airway obstruction.[2] The OPA must rest along the tongue with its distal tip in the hypopharynx just superior to the glottic inlet. Using too large an OPA can create downfolding of the epiglottis, which can also cause airway obstruction. As a rule, the distance from the corner of the patient's mouth to the earlobe or angle of the jaw gives a good estimate of the correct size (Figure 3-14).

The OPA is usually inserted with its concavity toward the roof of the mouth. A 180-degree rotation (corkscrew motion) is then performed while simultaneously advancing the device over the base of the tongue into the oropharynx (Figure 3-15). However, to prevent trauma to the hard palate, the OPA can also be inserted in the mouth with the tip oriented toward the tongue while simultaneously sliding it on a tongue blade to decrease friction.[2]

As a general rule, an OPA should be used in all unconscious patients unless it causes gagging or retching. It is important to understand that if a patient tolerates insertion of an OPA, then he or she probably meets the criteria for tracheal intubation.[2] Following tracheal intubation, the OPA can also be used as a bite block to prevent the patient from biting the endotracheal tube.

Like the OPA, the nasopharyngeal airway (NPA) (Figure 3-16) does not afford protection against aspiration, with the exception that it can help in preventing gastric insufflation during positive pressure ventilation in a malaligned airway. In general, the NPA is less stimulating and therefore better tolerated than an OPA and can be used in patients who still possess protective airway reflexes. It is well tolerated in postictal patients or patients sedated with drugs or alcohol in the emergency situation.[2]

A number of potential problems can occur with the use of the NPA. Nasal insertion can cause bleeding, which can both obstruct the airway and decrease visualization during direct laryngoscopy and tracheal intubation. To reduce the risk of bleeding, the wider nostril

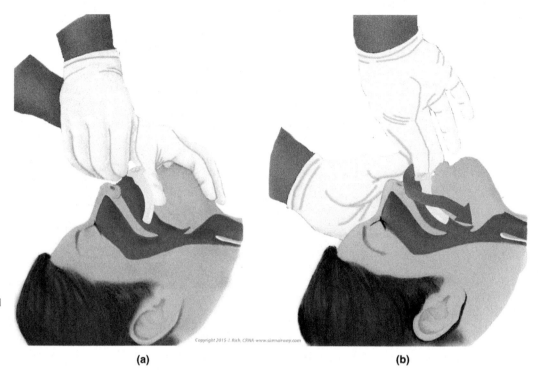

FIGURE 3-15

(a) Insert the oropharyngeal airway with the tip facing the palate. (b) Rotate the airway 180° into position.

(a)   **(b)**

should be used. The incidence of nosebleed can be reduced by spraying oxymetazline into the nostril to produce vasoconstriction of the nasal mucosa.

Additionally, the NPA should be lubricated with gel. Gels that contain a local anesthetic can increase the patient's ability to tolerate the device. It is often said that, in patients with facial trauma, insertion of tubes into the nose should be avoided to prevent entry of the tube into the brain via the fracture site. However, this probably applies more to semirigid nasogastric tubes than it does to soft nasopharyngeal airways.

Another rare complication is the migration of the entire NPA into the nasopharynx. For this reason, some NPAs have a large proximal flange, while others are supplied with a safety pin with which to transfix the device.

Traditional methods of NPA sizing relate the diameter of the device to the size of the patient's nares or little finger, but such methods are inaccurate and should not be used. Tube

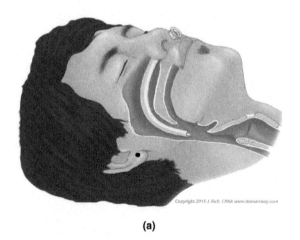

(a)

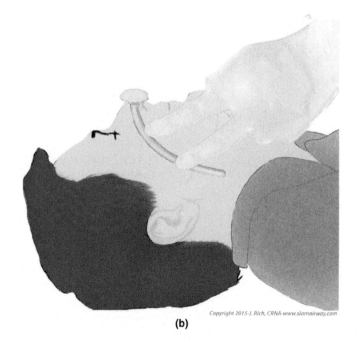

FIGURE 3-16

(a) The nasopharyngeal airway, which rests between the tongue and the posterior pharyngeal wall. (b) Proper sizing of the nasopharyngeal airway. Note that the distal tip extends beyond the angle of the jaw.

(b)

length is more important, and this is dictated by the patient's height and is independent of sex. As a guide, average-height females require a size 6 NPA, and males require a size 7. Optimal and rapid sizing of the NPA can be modified from these average sizes to account for the subject's height.[10] Alternatively, a quick method of determining the correct size is to select one with a length equal to the distance between the patient's earlobe and the tip of the nose.

Pneumothorax

A simple closed pneumothorax occurs when lung tissue is disrupted internally and a varying quantity of air leaks into the pleural space, leading to a partial or complete collapse of that lung but without interpleural tensioning. An open pneumothorax occurs when a penetrating chest wound allows outside air to enter the pleural space. A tension pneumothorax (which may be open or closed) occurs when there is an accumulation of air under pressure in the pleural space due to a one-way valve effect at the site of the leak. Signs and symptoms of a pneumothorax include shortness of breath, sudden sharp chest pain made worse by inspiration or coughing, hyperresonance of the hemithorax, and diminished breath sounds on the affected side.

Many pneumothoraces occur spontaneously due to the rupture of emphasematous bullae, but there may be evidence of penetrating or closed trauma to the chest wall, such as a stab wound or rib fractures. In the case of a tension pneumothorax, the pressure in the interpleural space increases with each breath taken until it compresses the mediastinum and begins to interfere with venous return. If left untreated, a tension pneumothorax can quickly result in cardiovascular collapse and death. Physical findings of tension pneumothorax are described in Figures 3-17 and 3-18 and include deviation of the trachea away from the affected side.

In the prehospital setting, tension pneumothorax can be treated by inserting a cannula into the interpleural space to decompress the affected side, and the most convenient site for needle entry is often in the second intercostal space, just lateral to the midclavicular line. However,

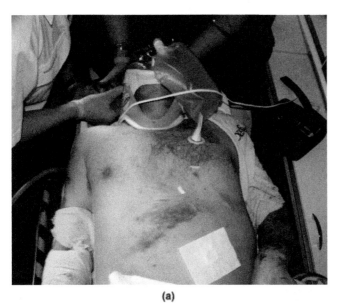
(a)

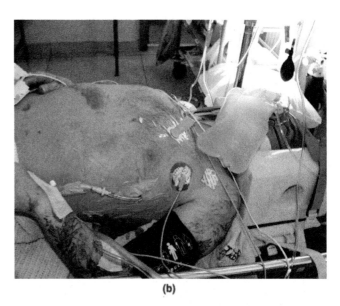
(b)

FIGURE 3-17

(a) This truck driver was crushed in his cab when he drove into the back of another truck. He sustained multiple severe injuries, including an open-book pelvic fracture, multiple rib fractures, and a ruptured liver. During transport to the hospital, he developed pulseless electrical activity due to a rapidly developing left-sided tension pneumothorax. He was treated by immediate insertion of a Cook emergency pneumothorax drain into the second left intercostal space just lateral to the mid-clavicular line. A reassuring hiss of air and immediate improvement in his clinical condition was accompanied by a return to consciousness. The catheter was stabilized within the flutter valve of an Asherman chest seal (seen already in place). Note the pattern bruising over the casualty's abdomen. (Courtesy of Dr. Andrew M. Mason)

(b) At the emergency department, the patient had a formal chest drain inserted. He underwent emergency surgery for a ruptured liver and went on to survive his injuries.

(Courtesy of Dr. Andrew M. Mason)

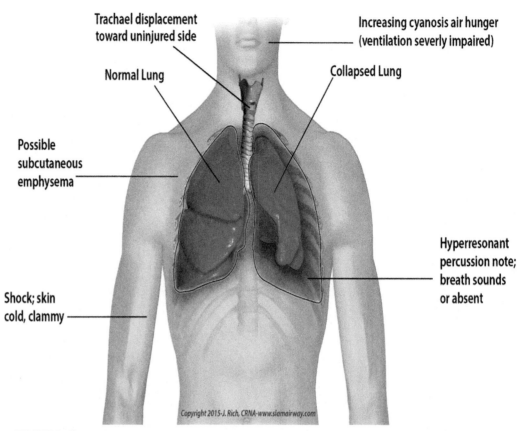

Trachael displacement toward uninjured side

Increasing cyanosis air hunger (ventilation severely impaired)

Normal Lung

Collapsed Lung

Possible subcutaneous emphysema

Hyperresonant percussion note; breath sounds or absent

Shock; skin cold, clammy

Copyright 2015-J. Rich, CRNA-www.slamairway.com

FIGURE 3-18
Physical findings of a tension pneumothorax.

ON TARGET When a proper mask fit has been obtained, care must be taken not to overventilate the patient using excessive tidal volumes or airway pressures. High airway peak pressure can overcome the decreased tone of the lower esophageal sphincter, leading to gastric insufflation. The more the stomach is inflated, the more the diaphragm is pushed upward. This can lead to a vicious cycle of further gastric insufflation, a decrease in lung compliance, and hypoventilation, which will increase the potential for regurgitation and aspiration of gastric contents.[2] The use of cricoid pressure (i.e., Sellick's maneuver) to reduce the risk of gastric insufflation and silent regurgitation should be routine during positive-pressure mask ventilation in any patient suspected of having a full stomach.

practitioners should be aware that this condition is occasionally bilateral, and in such cases, the trachea will be central, with percussion and breath sounds equal on both sides. These patients are usually in a state of collapse or are in traumatic cardiac arrest, and bilateral chest decompression should be part of the procedure for traumatic arrest where bilateral tension pneumothorax remains a possibility. On a practical point, it is vital that the needle or cannula used to decompress a tension pneumothorax is of sufficient length to penetrate the interpleural space.[11]

Positive-Pressure Mask Ventilation

Mask ventilation is probably one of the most undervalued methods of lung ventilation. Since the advent of rapid sequence intubation and supraglottic airways, it is relied on less and less in the difficult-airway situation. Nonetheless, every advanced airway practitioner should strive to be expert in providing mask ventilation. Although it can usually be performed rapidly and efficiently with minimal preparation by experienced rescuers, sufficient training in manikins and patients is needed to achieve competency. However, if positive-pressure mask ventilation fails, rescue ventilation using a Combitube or LMA should begin immediately.

Prevention of gastric aspiration during positive-pressure mask ventilation is very important. To minimize the possibility of gastric aspiration during rapid sequence intubation, Sellick's maneuver (cricoid pressure) should always be used during emergency mask ventilation, both prior to intubation attempts and between any failed attempts (Figure 3-19). (For more information on the use of cricoid pressure to prevent silent aspiration, see Chapter 7.)

Difficulties with mask ventilation can occur independent of the rescuer's skills in trauma patients with facial injuries, in older or edentulous patients, in those who are morbidly obese, in those with beards or anatomical anomalies, and in various other emergency patients.[4] Even in the operating room, experienced anesthetists are not always able to maintain adequate oxygenation using mask ventilation alone.

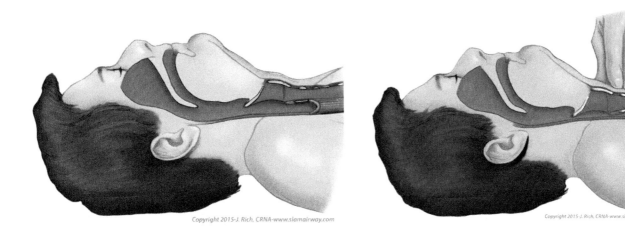

(a)   **(b)**

FIGURE 3-19

(a) The esophagus is patent before Sellick's maneuver. (b) The esophagus is occluded with Sellick's manueuver applied.

An effective way to maintain a patent airway while ventilating with a mask is by using an OPA or NPA (as described above). Use of these simple adjuncts will decrease the incidence of insufflation of air into the stomach.[2] Provision of optimal mask ventilation in conjunction with an OPA or NPA can often achieve an oxygenation saturation comparable to that obtained via an endotracheal tube.[12] Alternatively, a supraglottic airway device can be used. The less experienced the rescuer, the more important is the knowledge of additional techniques and adjuncts.[13]

Standard procedure for positive-pressure mask ventilation should be the use of supplemental oxygen and an oxygen reservoir bag (Figure 3-20). With an oxygen flow of 15 lpm, the method has the potential to provide an inspiratory oxygen fraction (FiO_2) greater than 90%. Use of a correctly sized mask to give a tight fit is imperative for achieving optimal ventilation during positive-pressure mask ventilation. Though not mandatory, use of a transparent mask will permit continuous observation of the area around the mouth for signs of regurgitation or central cyanosis.

The best position to enable the rescuer to perform effective mask ventilation and monitor the rise and fall of the chest is at the patient's head. To obtain a tight seal, the face mask is picked up between thumb and index finger (Figure 3-21). The apex of the mask is first placed over the bridge of the nose, and the mask is then lowered to cover the face and provide a seal at the point of the chin. The long finger, ring finger, and little finger grasp the patient's mandible to secure the mask, lift the chin, and tilt the head as needed. The thumb presses down on the mask in the area above the nose, and the index finger is positioned just below the nose. The mask is gripped in such a way that the thumb and index finger exert

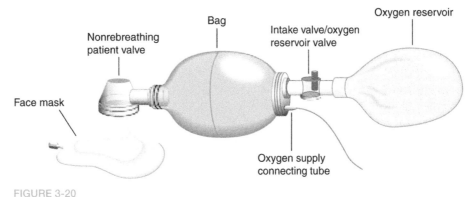

FIGURE 3-20

The bag-valve-mask device is used to provide positive-pressure ventilation.

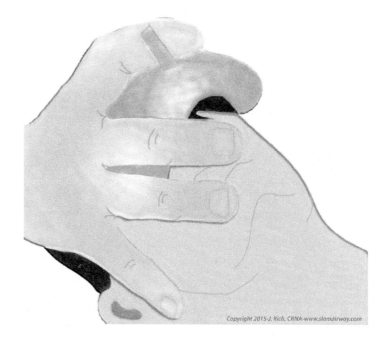

FIGURE 3-21
To obtain a tight seal, a face mask is picked up between thumb and index finger and placed over the bridge of the nose. It is then lowered to cover the face and provide a seal at the point of the chin.
(Courtesy of Dr. Harald V. Genzwuerker)

Copyright 2015-J. Rich, CRNA-www.slamairway.com

ON TARGET *Patients die from a failure to ventilate, not from a failure to intubate.*

trismus
Restriction of the mouth opening.

ankylosing spondylitis
A form of chronic inflammation of the joints of the spine and sacroiliac joints, causing pain and stiffness.

downward pressure that opposes the upward pressure of the other three fingers beneath the patient's mandible. The hand holding the mask may also be turned slightly inward and upward to improve the fit and seal the mask. The long finger, ring finger, and little finger maintain the chin lift and head tilt necessary to keep the airway open. Avoid forceful compression of the soft tissues under the chin because this can cause tissue trauma and even obstruction of the airway.

Advanced Airway Techniques

Difficult Mask Ventilation

A number of conditions and situations can make mask ventilation difficult (Table 3-6),[4] and difficulty is not always easy to predict.[13] Holding the mask in place with one hand is usually effective, but a two- or three-handed technique (requires two rescuers with one squeezing the bag) is sometimes necessary (Figure 3-22). The use of an OPA, NPA, or both

Down syndrome
Also known as trisomy 21. A congenital defect characterized by extra chromosome 21 material, leading to physical abnormalities and mild to moderate mental retardation. The Down patient may have a flat face and nose, a small mouth from which the relatively large tongue sometimes protrudes, and a short neck, all making airway management difficult.

macroglossia
Literally, large tongue.

Table 3-6 Conditions That Predispose to Difficulty with Positive-Pressure Mask Ventilation[4]	
• Full stomach	• Morbid obesity
• Cervical-spine Injury	• **Down syndrome**
• Mandibular hypoplasia	• Thick beard
• Epiglotittis	• Maxillo-facial trauma
• Layngeal edema	• Massive jaw
• Pharyngeal abscess	• Facial burns
• **Trismus**	• Neck trauma and bleeding
• Rheumatoid arthritis	• Obesity
• **Ankylosing spondylitis**	• **Macroglossia**
• Airway tumors	

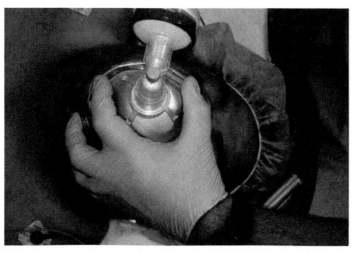

(a)

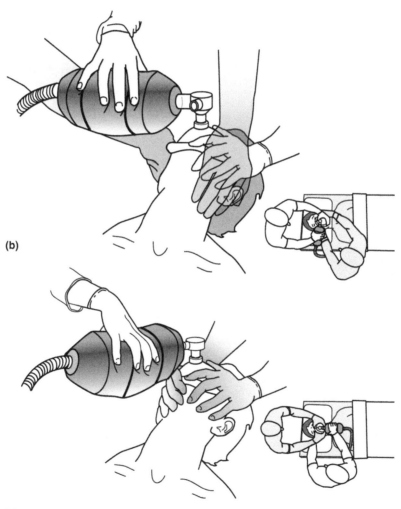

(b)

(c)

FIGURE 3-22

(a) Bag-valve-mask ventilation, proper hand position, single-rescuer technique. (b) Bag-valve-mask ventilation, three-handed, two-rescuer technique. (c) Bag-valve-mask ventilation, two-handed two-rescuer technique.

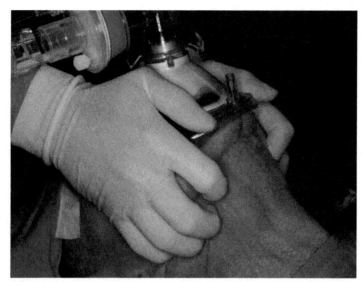

(d)

FIGURE 3-22

(continued)

(d) Deep submental insertion of fingers during two-handed BVM ventilation pulls up on the hyoid bone, which helps relieve obstruction caused by collapse of the epiglottis. (Courtesy of JM Rich, CRNA)

may be necessary to keep the airway open and provide optimal mask ventilation. If an adequate oxygen saturation cannot be achieved despite the use of optimal mask ventilation with high oxygen flow and an OPA or NPA (or both), a more invasive method of lung ventilation will be required (e.g., supraglottic airway, endotracheal tube, or cricothyrotomy).

PEARLS If it proves difficult for one rescuer to maintain a good seal and ventilate with the BVM, it may be necessary to utilize two rescuers, one to maintain the mask seal with both hands and one to squeeze the bag.

PEARLS Mask ventilation should be considered difficult when either of the following apply:[14]

- It is not possible for an unassisted rescuer to maintain the $SpO_2 \geq 92\%$ using 100% oxygen and positive-pressure mask ventilation in a patient whose SpO_2 was previously greater than 92% before intervention.
- It is not possible for the unassisted rescuer to prevent or reverse signs of inadequate ventilation during positive-pressure mask ventilation.

When either one of these conditions is met and cannot be rectified, the rescuer should switch from mask ventilation to the use of a supraglottic airway device. Alternatively, if the rescuer feels that, based on the clinical situation, he or she can quickly perform direct laryngoscopy and intubate the trachea, it is usually acceptable to make one attempt. Allowing inadequate mask ventilation and hypoxemia to continue for even a short length of time can result in disability, death, and liability for malpractice.

Large tidal volumes or a rapid ventilatory rate resulting in excessive minute ventilation should be avoided. A ventilation rate of 10 to 12 breaths per minute is generally adequate, and each ventilation should be performed over a period of approximately two seconds. This should provide a moderate rise of the chest at peak inspiration and an oxygen saturation of greater than 92%.[5,6] Use of smaller rather than larger tidal volumes will help limit the peak pressure and can reduce the risk of gastric insufflation. Ventilation of the patient without the use of oxygen is not recommended.

Alternatives to Mask Ventilation and Tracheal Intubation

Endotracheal intubation remains the gold standard for securing the airway. Placement of a cuffed endotracheal tube (ETT) with the tip lying in the mid-trachea will ensure airway patency and protect the airway from aspiration. The airway can also be suctioned through the ETT, and certain drugs can be administered down the tube during resuscitation when no intravenous access is available.[12] However, the main goal of tracheal intubation is the delivery of oxygen into the patient's lungs, so when tracheal intubation is not feasible or it is impossible, other approaches to oxygenating the patient must be adopted. It should always be remembered that patients suffer brain death and die from a failure to oxygenate and ventilate, not from a failure to intubate.[5,16-18]

The biggest challenge of tracheal intubation is obtaining a satisfactory view of the larynx by direct laryngoscopy. If the glottis cannot be visualized, insertion of the tracheal tube requires the use of advanced maneuvers; otherwise, intubation fails.[5,6,19] Following failed intubation, ventilation with a facemask is the first alternative.[20] However, to deal with any cannot-mask-ventilate/cannot-intubate situation, other alternatives must be available. As with mask ventilation and tracheal intubation, rescuers must receive adequate training in the use of alternative devices in the emergency setting.[19]

PEARLS

Use of smaller tidal volumes when ventilating helps limit peak pressures and reduces the risk of gastric insufflation. Excessive and prolonged lung expansion can interfere with blood return to the heart and reduce cardiac output.

The SLAM Universal Adult Airway Flowchart (SUAAF) preferentially recommends use of the Combitube or the LMA-Classic for provision of rescue ventilation in the face of a critical airway event. A critical airway event is indicated by:

- Any cannot-mask-ventilate/cannot-intubate (CMVCI) situation.
- Three or more failed intubation attempts or attempting intubation for more than 10 minutes (by the most experienced practitioner).
- Sustained hypoxemia that is refractory to positive-pressure ventilation with 100% oxygen.[18]

The recommendation to use the Combitube or LMA Classic is made because for a long time these were the only two supraglottic airway devices that were recommended by CPR guidelines from the American Heart Association (AHA), European Resuscitation Council (ERC), and International Liaison Committee on Resuscitation (ILCOR).[21] as acceptable and useful with good to very good supporting evidence.[22]

However, the recommendation to use the ETC and LMA Classic by the SUAAF is not intended to preclude the use of other FDA-approved supraglottic airway devices. The American Society of Anesthesiologists Task Force on Management of the Difficult Airway specifically points out that, while some devices are recommended, other new techniques or devices should not be precluded. A number of Class IIb devices (considered acceptable and useful but with only weak or fair supporting evidence) are also included in the oxygenation/ventilation pathway of the SUAAF. Growing data on devices other than the LMA and Combitube currently being researched will almost certainly increase the number of rescue ventilation devices given Class IIa status.[24]

Recommendations of the ILCOR were updated in 2005, and while the AHA upheld its recommendations (Table 3-7), the ERC added the Laryngeal. Tube as another supraglottic device that may be used as an alternative to facemask ventilation and tracheal intubation in an emergency setting.[21,23]

Alternatives to tracheal intubation and mask ventilation are playing a growing role in strategies for optimizing oxygenation in emergency airway patients. So-called supraglottic

Table 3-7 Adjunctive Supraglottic Ventilation Devices*

Device	Class IIa Device	Manufacturer
AMBU laryngeal mask	No	AMBU, Glen Burnie, MD
Cobra PLA	No	Engineered Medical Systems, Indianapolis, IN
Combitube	Yes[†]	Tyco-Healthcare-Nellcor, Pleasanton, CA
EasyTube	No	Rusch, Research Triangle Park, NC
Intubating laryngeal airway	No	Mercury Medical, Clearwater, FL
King laryngeal tube	No	King Systems, Noblesville, IN
Laryngoseal laryngeal mask	No	Tyco-Healthcare-Nellcor, Pleasanton, CA
LMA Classic (reusable)	Yes[†]	LMA North America, San Diego, CA
LMA Unique (single-use version of LMA-Classic)	No	LMA North America, San Diego, CA
LMA Fastrach (single-use and reusable versions)	No	LMA North America, San Diego, CA
LMA ProSeal (reusable)	No	LMA North America, San Diego, CA

*Based on references 1, 7, 15.

[†]AHA/ILCOR indicates American Heart Association/International Liaison Committee on Resuscitation. Devices are classified at the AHA/ILCOR conferences that occur every five years. Classification is based on review and discussion of research articles and case reports from the peer-reviewed literature. Class IIa denotes a therapeutic option for which the weight of evidence is in favor of its usefulness and efficacy.

Used by permission of reference 23.

airway alternatives—such as the esophageal-tracheal Combitube, the Easytube, the laryngeal tube, and several versions of the laryngeal mask airway—are being used in an increasing number of emergency systems to manage the difficult airway.[5,19,25-27]

The term *supraglottic* refers to the position that the device occupies within the airway, with its distal portion in the hypopharynx (i.e., below the oropharynx yet above the glottis). Supraglottic devices are specifically designed for lung ventilation, without the need of being inserted through the vocal cords. Compared to mask ventilation, these devices usually achieve better isolation of the respiratory tract from the alimentary tract and are therefore less prone to causing gastric insufflation. This yields better lung ventilation and decreases the likelihood of silent aspiration compared to bag-valve-mask ventilation. Depending on the quality of the airway seal achieved with the individual devices, the risk of gastric inflation is diminished accordingly.[18,28]

Compared to tracheal intubation, insertion of a supraglottic airway device is often faster and easier, even during critical airway events. The risk of tube misplacement is greatly reduced, and trauma to the airway is minimized. Protection from aspiration depends on the design and construction of the individual supraglottic device, but some provide protection that is almost equal to that of the tracheal tube.[18,40]

Emergency-airway training and the availability of alternative airway devices are important elements in the efficient management of emergency airway situations. Those involved must be made aware of the complexities of managing the difficult airway and taught strategies to handle these challenging situations. To address these issues, the SLAM Universal Adult Airway Flowchart[5,6] has been developed as an easy-to-follow algorithm to guide members of the rescue team. It provides important guidelines for decision making at all levels of airway management, and it acknowledges the need for maintenance of a patent airway, oxygenation of the patient at all times, and thorough preparation for each intervention.

The availability of supraglottic alternatives to tracheal intubation should be an integral part of any strategy for resolving a critical airway event. If an intubation attempt fails, reoxygenation of the patient should be attempted by face-mask ventilation in the first instance. If an SpO_2 of greater than 92% cannot be achieved, then rescue ventilation should be attempted using a supraglottic airway device. If the patient can be ventilated and adequately oxygenated by face mask following one failed intubation attempt, up to two more intubation attempts may be undertaken. The use of a modified intubation rescue technique as described in the SUAAF (Chapters 1 and 4) can greatly improve the likelihood of success during the next intubation attempt. If the patient cannot be intubated after three attempts, a supraglottic airway device should then be used to ventilate the patient. Depending on the response and the clinical situation, the rescuer must then decide whether to continue ventilating with the supraglottic device or convert it to a definitive airway using an advanced intubation technique. No more than three intubation attempts should be permitted in order to limit trauma to the airway because trauma may lead to local swelling and bleeding, endangering the ultimate goal of securing a patent airway. In addition, repeated intubation attempts mean repeated interruptions of ventilation, which jeopardizes the other important goal of keeping the patient oxygenated.

Although reverting to spontaneous ventilation is possible in some elective hospital situations, it is unlikely to be a viable alternative in the prehospital emergency setting, particularly in those patients who were not breathing or were breathing inadequately to begin with.

Supraglottic Airway Devices

Many supraglottic airway devices (SADs) have emerged in recent years, but confusion exists concerning their proper application in the emergency situation (Table 3-4) (Figure 3-23). Brain has recently classified them so that any SAD will fall into one of four categories (Figure 3-24). Having them readily available to all providers of emergency care is essential, considering the important role of these devices in overcoming critical airway situations. A common feature of

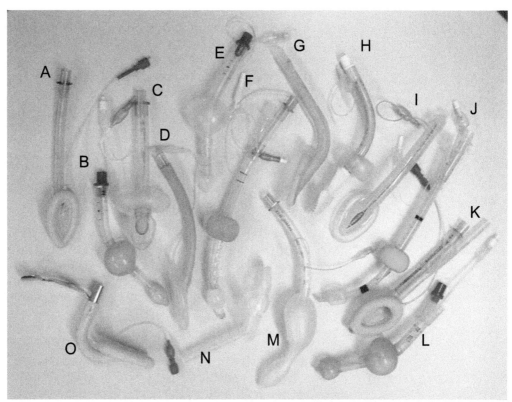

FIGURE 3-23
Various supraglottic airway devices. (a) LMA-Classic™, (b) reusable King Laryngeal Tube LT™, (c) CobraPLA™, (d) LMA-Unique™, (e) LT-D™ (Laryngeal Tube Disposable), (f) Esophageal Tracheal Combitube™ (ETC), (g) Ambu laryngeal mask™, (h) Vitalsigns PAxpress™, (i) Tyco laryngoseal™, (j) Rusch Easytube™, (k) LMA-ProSeal™, (l) King LTS™ (Laryngeal Tube Suction), (m) B+P Larryvent, (n) "SLIPA," or "Streamlined Liner of the Pharyngeal Airway", (o) Intubating-LMA™. (Courtesy of Dr. Harald V. Genzwuerker, MD)

SCHEMATIC DIAGRAM OF UPPER AIRWAY SHOWING SUPRAGLOTTIC AIRWAY SEAL STRATEGIES

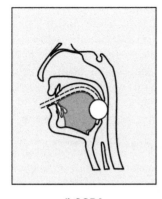
I) COPA type

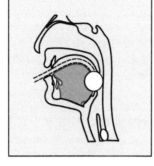
II) Combitube type

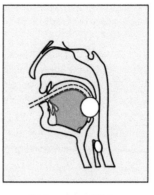
III) Laryngeal Tube type

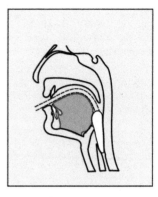
IV) Laryngeal Mask type

FIGURE 3-24

Extraglottic airway sealing strategies. (Classification by Dr. Archie I. J. Brain, redrawn by Dr. Andrew M. Mason. Used with permission.)

all supraglottic airway devices is their ability to be inserted blindly without the need for laryngoscopy. However, following insertion, it is still important to confirm correct placement and adequate ventilation. Choice of the correct size calls for specific knowledge of the device.

Training with manikins, human simulators, and cadavers as well as additional experience during elective use in the operating room, if possible, are important for successful use of any emergency airway device. Atraumatic insertion techniques reduce the risk of bleeding and swelling in the upper airway. Reinforcement of this point during training should help to ensure that the use of a supraglottic airway is effective in reducing problems and does not create new ones.

All of the supraglottic airway devices described below have both advantages and limitations. Limitations include the following:

- Insertion requires a minimum mouth opening of between 1.5 and 2.5 centimeters, depending on the device used.
- Ventilation is not possible if there is a glottic or subglottic obstruction. This situation requires a surgical airway or placement of an ETT below the level of obstruction.[29]
- Protection from aspiration is generally inferior to that of an ETT, but the level of protection does vary among devices.

A major advantage of these devices over face-mask ventilation is the better separation provided between the respiratory and alimentary tracts, reducing the risk of both gastric insufflation and regurgitation with silent aspiration. Also, the fact that they are inserted blindly does away with the need to obtain a view of the larynx. Difficult laryngoscopy and failed intubation both interrupt ventilation, and any reduction in oxygenation is often badly tolerated by those who are critically ill.

Most supraglottic airway devices are easier to insert with the patient in the sniffing position. One exception to this rule is the LMA-Fastrach, which is specifically designed to be inserted with the head and neck in a neutral position. However, with training and practice, most supraglottic devices can be inserted correctly without the need for manipulation of the head and neck, a great advantage when injury to the cervical spine is suspected.

In contrast to the careful hold that is maintained on the tracheal tube until the cuff has been inflated, the operator must learn to release the supraglottic device immediately following full insertion. This allows movement of the device into the correct position for optimal sealing of the airway during cuff inflation. Failure to observe this rule can lead to malpositioning.

As with the ETT, most supraglottic devices need to be secured using an approved method, although some devices, like the esophageal-tracheal Combitube, claim to be self-retaining.

The ideal supraglottic airway alternative should:

- Provide a good airway seal.
- Offer good protection from aspiration.
- Be easy to insert and have minimal training requirements.
- Be well tolerated by the patient.
- Be reasonably secure and not prone to dislodgment.
- Have high success rates.
- Be available in a range of sizes to fit all prospective patients.
- Be affordable.
- Be available as a single-use, disposable item.
- Give the user the option of converting the device to a definitive airway using an advanced intubation technique, should this be required.

Laryngeal Masks

The reusable laryngeal mask airway, the LMA Classic, was first introduced in 1985.[30] It was a ground-breaking device that has revolutionized both elective and emergency airway management. Its success has led to the development of several other supraglottic devices that are also effective for emergency airway management. In the United States, the LMA is not used widely in the prehospital setting, but it is used regularly in the United Kingdom, Australia, and elsewhere by basic- and intermediate-level providers with good results. It can be used in the emergency setting by providers not trained in tracheal intubation or by advanced providers faced with a difficult airway or failed intubation.[31]

Cases of difficult intubation are more frequent in emergency situations rather than in the elective setting, and the LMA can provide a fast, secure, patent airway in many patients whose airways cannot be secured by other means.[32] (Its use is fully described in Chapter 6.)

Single-use versions of the laryngeal mask are available from a growing number of manufacturers (Table 3-7). Most of these devices are copies of the reusable LMA Classic, with the LMA Unique from the same manufacturer featuring aperture bars, that are designed to prevent impaction of the epiglottis into the airway. However the necessity of the aperture bars is undergoing debate at the time of this writing.

Some manufacturers have tried to improve the product. Ambu, for example (Figure 3-23), has introduced a single-use laryngeal mask (Ambu™ Laryngeal Mask) that has a curved tube to aid insertion and a large soft cuff that slightly enhances the airway seal.[33] Insertion success and quality of airway seal are important features in emergency airway devices. As in all new devices, sufficient data or clinical performance of the device will be necessary to adequately judge the role of laryngeal masks from other manufacturers.

The LMA Fastrach™ is a variation on the LMA design that facilitates blind intubation of the trachea with a dedicated atraumatic tracheal tube. Also known as the intubating laryngeal mask airway (iLMA), the device was designed especially to overcome difficult intubation. It is described in Chapter 9

An improved airway seal can be achieved with the LMA ProSeal™ (Figure 3-23), which first appeared in 2001. The device is available in sizes suitable for small children right up to large adults. Its additional posterior cuff pushes the mask more firmly against the posterior perimeter of the larynx, creating an improved seal of 30 cm H_2O or more, whereas the LMA Classic™ is usually considered safe only up to peak airway pressures of 20 cm H_2O. Another important advantage of the ProSeal is the inclusion of a second lumen, which provides access to the alimentary tract, allowing regurgitated gastric contents to drain away and thus reducing the risk of aspiration. The gastric lumen can also be used for decompression of the stomach with a standard orogastric tube. However, the ProSeal's suitability as a rescue

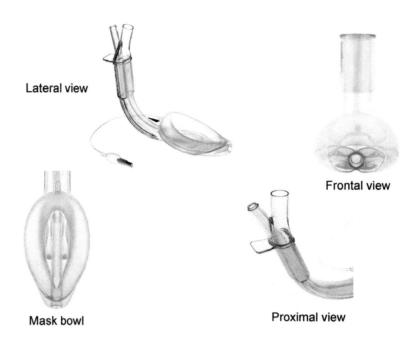

Lateral view

Frontal view

Mask bowl

Proximal view

FIGURE 3-25

The LMA Supreme™ features an integral bite block that prevents airway obstruction due to biting. The larger bicurved cuff uses higher maximum inflation volumes than previous LMA™ airways (#3:30ml; #4:45ml; #5:60ml ≤ 60 cmH₂O) and offers an improved seal. The gastric tube access port accepts 14 through 16 FG tube. The fixation tab provides quick and easy fixation and also aids in correct positioning. The fins incorporated into the mask bowl prevent airway obstruction from epiglottic impaction of the distal airway aperture (Courtesy of The Laryngeal Mask Company Limited).

ventilation device for prehospital care will require further research because initial studies have suggested that it is less easy to insert than a standard LMA, although use of the special introducer tool does address this issue somewhat.

The LMA Supreme™ (Figure 3-25) the latest addition to the range of airway devices from the Laryngeal Mask Company (LMA North America) is undergoing clinical evaluation at the time of writing. Featuring a redesigned elliptical, precurved, semirigid airway tube with an integral bite block, the LMA Supreme™ is a single-use device with a separate gastric access pathway, similar to that found on the LMA ProSeal™. The device has a totally redesigned bicurved PVC cuff providing an improved seal, and the mask bowl possesses patented fins that replace the familiar aperture bars to prevent impaction of the epiglottis into the distal airway aperture. The cuff is larger than that found on the LMA Classic™ or LMA Unique™ and requires higher inflation volumes, but the maximum recommended intracuff pressure remains the same at 60 cmH₂O. Built-in flexibility at the airway tube-mask junction is designed to accommodate variations in airway geometry among individual patients.

Unlike the LMA Proseal™, the cuff of the LMA Supreme™ does not possess an inflatable posterior element, but both devices do feature a similar gastric access pathway that opens distally at the tip of the mask. With the airway correctly inserted, and the tip of the mask lying in the upper esophageal sphincter, the presence of the gastric pathway effectively separates the patient's respiratory and gastrointestinal tracts. The gastric port allows for the easy and rapid passage of a gastric tube in order to decompress the stomach when it contains either air (e.g., after gastric insufflation following overenthusiastic BVM ventilation) or liquid (with unfasted patients). Alternatively, the port can vent air or liquid arising from the stomach during resuscitation, reducing further the already small risk of pulmonary aspiration when a standard LMA is used in emergency situations. Initially available in sizes 3, 4, and 5, and with patient sizing similar to that used with any standard LMA, the manufacturer is currently developing the device in pediatric sizes.

Laryngeal Tubes

The reusable Laryngeal Tube (LT™) (Figure 3-23) was introduced in 1999 as an airway device for general anesthesia, but it was quickly adopted for prehospital use in both Europe and Japan.[35-38] Like the LMA Classic™, the tip of this single-lumen silicone tube lies just within the esophageal inlet. The small esophageal balloon seals the esophagus, while a large pharyngeal balloon blocks the pharynx toward the mouth and nose, allowing ventilation via the openings between the cuffs. Insufflated air takes the path of least resistance and enters the glottis. Sizes of the device range from newborn to adult. A single-use device called LT-DTM (Laryngeal Tube Disposable) made from PVC was introduced in 2004.

Because of the good seal, emergency physicians recommended an additional drain tube be added to avoid excessive esophageal and gastric pressures if a patient happened to retch or gag, so the LTS™ (Laryngeal Tube Suction) was developed for emergency use.[37,38] Like the LMA Proseal™ and LMA Supreme™, it contains a second lumen allowing insertion of a gastric tube and gastric decompression. The device is comparable to the standard device as far as insertion, handling, and airway seal are concerned. Three sizes from school children (minimum weight 25 kg, less than 1.55 m) to adults are available (Table 3-8), and a PVC version was introduced in 2005.

The Laryngeal Tube is held like a pen with one hand and inserted along the hard palate, while the other hand opens the mouth. The index finger of the free hand can also be used to guide the tip of the LT™ and to lift the base of the tongue to facilitate insertion into the hypopharynx. When the tip of the tube enters the esophageal inlet, a distinct resistance can be felt. Ring marks on the tube should be aligned with the front teeth as a guide to correct insertion depth. Both cuffs are inflated simultaneously via a common inflation port using the color-coded syringe provided. The colored marks on the syringe correspond to the colors of the connectors on the different sizes of the laryngeal tube, which ensures that the correct volume of air is used to inflate the cuffs. The tube is short and S-shaped to prevent accidental tracheal insertion, which could result in complete airway obstruction. Correct position must be verified by checking for bilateral chest movements, auscultation over stomach and lungs, listening at the mouth for audible leaks, and capnography. The airway seal and the blockade of the esophagus achieved with the Laryngeal Tube are usually very good but, as with other supraglottic devices, it does not provide complete protection against aspiration.

Although the LTS™ is similar in appearance to the esophageal-tracheal Combitube, it is quite different in a number of aspects. It has a softer tip and is also latex free, and both cuffs are inflated via a single inflation line, which reduces the time until the first ventilation is performed. Only one lumen of the LTS™ is designed for ventilation, the second lumen provides access to the gastrointestinal tract, and this alone, so it cannot strictly be described as a double-lumen tube.

Table 3-8 Laryngeal Tube Sizes and Cuff Volumes

Size	Patient	Weight/Size	Connector	Cuff Volume
0	Newborn	<5 kg	Transparent	10 ml
1	Toddler	5 to 12 kg	White	20 ml
2	Child	12 to 25 kg	Green	35 ml
2.5	Child	>20 kg	Orange	45 ml
3	Large child or small adult	>25 kg <1.55 m	Yellow	60 ml
4	Adult	1.55 to 1.80 m	Red	80 ml
5	Adult	>1.80 m	Purple	90 ml

Table 3-9 *Advantages and Disadvantages of the Combitube*[7,18,40]

Advantages	Disadvantages
It provides a patent airway when conventional intubation techniques are unsuccessful or unavailable.	Suctioning of tracheal secretions is impossible when the device is placed in the esophagus (usual configuration).
Insertion is rapid and easy.	Placing of an endotracheal tube is challenging with the ETC in place.
Insertion does not require visualization of the larynx or special equipment.	Like other SADS it cannot be used in conscious patients or in those with an intact gag reflex.
The pharyngeal balloon anchors the device behind the hard palate.	Pressure from the cuffs can cause local ischemia of the mucosa of the esophagus, trachea, or hypoparynx.
The patient may be ventilated regardless of tube placement (esophageal or tracheal).	It should not be used in patients with esophageal disease or caustic ingestions.
It significantly diminishes gastric distension and regurgitation, and airway protection is similar to that achieved with an endotracheal tube.	Pediatric size not available.
It is suitable for trauma patients because the neck can remain in a neutral position during insertion and use.	Placement of the ETC is not foolproof; errors can be made if assessment skills are not adequate.
If the device is placed in the esophagus (usual configuration), gastric contents can be suctioned through the distal port to decompress the stomach.	Ventilation is impossible if wrong port is used.

Double-Lumen Tubes

In the mid-1980s, the esophageal-tracheal Combitube (ETC) was introduced to the market.[39] It was a considerable improvement over the Don Michael Esophageal Obturator Airway[18] and the advantages of the Combitube far exceed its disadvantages (Table 3-9). The ETC can be inserted blindly or with the aid of a laryngoscope. It is a single tube containing two lumens that open at separate ports at the proximal end of the device (Figure 3-23). It is capable of providing ventilation whether it is inserted into the esophagus (common) or the trachea (rare), and it provides excellent protection against aspiration.[18] (For a detailed description of the ETC, refer to Chapter 8.)

The EasyTube™ (Figure 3-23) was introduced in 2003 and is a modification of the esophageal-tracheal Combitube. It was designed to address several limitations that have been documented with the Combitube. This single-use product is latex-free and is available in two sizes, for preschool children through adults.[41] The tip of the smaller 28 Fr Easy-Tube™ is the same size as a 5.0 mm tracheal tube, and a 7.5 mm tracheal tube in the larger 41 Fr version. The narrowness of the tip makes the EasyTube™ more suitable than the ETC for insertion into the trachea. As with the Combitube, the two cuffs are inflated via separate inflation lines. While the device can be inserted blindly, use of a laryngoscope is recommended. If the vocal cords can be visualized, tracheal intubation should be attempted and ventilation performed via the first lumen; otherwise, the second lumen is used for supraglottic ventilation after insertion of the device into the esophagus.

A third double lumen device is the pharyngotracheal lumen (PtL) airway (Figure 3-26), which is similar in structure and function to the ETC. The tube is inserted blindly into the pharynx, passing either into the esophagus or the trachea, and allows ventilation in the tracheal or esophageal positions. It is disposable and is intended for single use. Advantages and disadvantages are listed in Table 3-10. Complications include pharyngeal or esophageal trauma from poor insertion technique, unrecognized displacement of the long tube from the trachea into

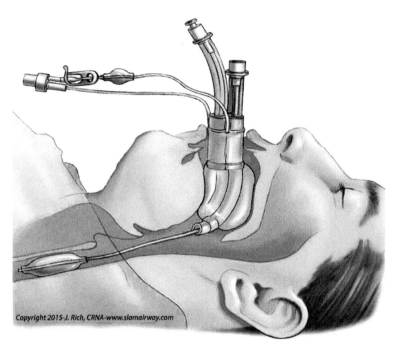

FIGURE 3-26
A pharyngotracheal lumen airway.

Table 3-10 Advantages and Disadvantages of the Pharyngotracheal Lumen Airway (PtL)[7]

Advantages	Disadvantages
It can function in either the tracheal or esophageal position.	It does not isolate and completely protect the trachea from aspiration.
It has no face mask to seal.	The oropharyngeal balloon can migrate out of the mouth anteriorly, partially dislodging the airway.
It does not require direct visualization of the larynx, so it does not require the use of a laryngoscope or additional specialized equipment.	Intubation around the PtL is extremely difficult, even with the oropharyngeal balloon deflated.
It is suitable for use in trauma patients because the neck can remain in a neutral position during insertion and use.	It cannot be used in conscious patients or those with an intact gag reflex.
It helps protect the trachea from upper airway bleeding and secretions.	It cannot be used in pediatric patients.

the esophagus, and displacement of the pharyngeal balloon. It is available in one size for adults only, and ease of use is comparable to the esophago-tracheal Combitube and EasyTube™.[31]

Other Supraglottic Airway Devices

There has been a steady evolution of supraglottic alternatives to face-mask ventilation and tracheal intubation. The devices listed above have been used successfully both in the operating room and in the prehospital setting. Other new devices will have to be evaluated for their role in emergency airway management, although initial clinical reports have suggested that the CobraPLA™ (Table 3-11) (Figure 3-23) may be a suitable alternative to the laryngeal mask airway.[42]

Table 3-11 CobraPLA™ Sizes and Cuff Volumes

Size	Patient	Weight/Size	Cuff Volume
½	Neonatal	>2.5 kg	<8 ml
1	Infant	>5 kg	<10 ml
1½	Child	>10 kg	<25 ml
2	Child	>15 kg	<40 ml
3	Child, small adult	>35 kg	<65 ml
4	Adult	>70 kg	<85 ml
5	Large adult	>100 kg	<85 ml
6	Large adult	>130 kg	<85 ml

It seems likely that some of these new supraglottic devices will eventually gain Class IIa status, but others are likely to disappear or play no role in emergency airway care.

Summary

A measured and well-prepared response to a critical airway event in or out of the hospital may well decrease morbidity and mortality for the patient as well as liability for practitioner and institution. Above all else, remember that patients suffer death and disability from lack of oxygenation and ventilation, not a lack of intubation. Do not persevere in the face of difficult mask ventilation but rather switch to a supraglottic technique to improve the oxygenation and ventilation of the patient.

REVIEW QUESTIONS

1. What are the four functions of the intercostal system?

2. Describe innervation of the intercostal muscles.

3. Describe innervation of the diaphragm.

4. What would be the result of a spinal-cord transection at the level of C7?

5. Why do patients in severe respiratory distress lean forward with their arms braced against fixed objects, such as their own knees, a wall, or table (the so-called tripod position)?

6. How does the pH of the blood alter hemoglobin's affinity for oxygen and effect the oxygen dissociation curve?

7. What are the partial pressures of oxygen and carbon dioxide in the alveoli at sea level?

8. Name four general methods used individually or in combination to ventilate the high-risk emergency patient.

9. What is the standard of care for airway management?

CHAPTER 4

Direct Laryngoscopy and Tracheal Intubation

James Michael Rich
Harald V. Genzwuerker

Chapter Objectives

After reading this chapter, you should be able to:

- Describe the indications, equipment, and techniques used for orotracheal intubation.

- Demonstrate simple methods, techniques, and equipment for rescuing a failed intubation.

- Discuss the concept of a critical airway event and how to both avoid and recover from it.

- Discuss the causes of a critical airway event.

- List common laryngoscopic pitfalls and how to both avoid and recover from them.

CASE Study _____

Medic 12 is dispatched Code 3 to a possible cardiac arrest. They arrive at the scene to find someone on the front porch waving them in. They grab their resuscitation jump bag, cardiac monitor, and stretcher and enter the house. They are directed to a bathroom where they find an elderly man lying unconscious on the floor. Family members are being instructed in CPR by the 911 dispatcher and look to be providing effective chest compressions and ventilations.

The paramedics identify themselves and ask what has happened. They are told that the 72-year-old man is known to have coronary artery disease. The wife reports that her husband said he was feeling unwell about 20 minutes earlier and went to the bathroom. After a time she heard some gurgling sounds, so she entered the bathroom and found him collapsed on the floor. She went next door to fetch her son and then called 911.

The paramedics open their airway bag and select an oral airway and bag-valve-mask (BVM) device. They attach an EKG monitor, ask the son to stop CPR briefly, and identify asystole in multiple leads. They turn up the gain on the monitor, but there is no change in the waveform, so they ask the son to resume chest compressions. They attach the BVM to oxygen and insert an oral airway. With CPR continuing, IV access is established, the appropriate ACLS medications are prepared, and the patient's airway is assessed.

There is nothing to suggest that intubation is likely to be difficult, so a laryngoscope with a #4 Miller blade, an 8.0 mm endotracheal tube (ETT), a stylet, and a 10 ml syringe are selected. The paramedics check the tube cuff and laryngoscope bulb and prepare the suction machine. Ventilations are stopped, and the oral airway is removed. The patient's mouth is opened, and the laryngoscope blade is placed on the right side of the tongue, sweeping it left. The blade is then advanced down the tongue until the epiglottis is identified. The tip of the blade is positioned to lift the epiglottis, and the laryngoscope handle is lifted up and away to avoid levering the blade against the teeth. The airway is suctioned, the glottic opening identified, and the ETT cuff is seen to pass between the vocal cords and into the trachea. The cuff is inflated and an esophageal detector bulb is compressed and then applied to the tube connector. When released, the bulb inflates rapidly.

A paramedic attaches the bag-valve device to the ETT and begins to ventilate. Breath sounds are audible in four locations, along the midaxillary lines and with no sounds over the epigastric area. The depth of insertion of the tube is recorded, and the tube is secured using a commercial tube holder with an integral bite block. The patient still shows no signs of life, so they continue with uninterrupted chest compressions while simultaneously ventilating the patient. With ACLS protocols continuing, the patient is transported to the local emergency department.

Introduction

Tracheal intubation in adults involves insertion of a cuffed tracheal tube through the glottis to seal off the airway from the alimentary tract and provide a secure means of oxygenation and ventilation. Intubation not only keeps the airway open, it protects the lower respiratory tract from aspiration of gastric contents. It also allows positive pressure lung ventilation to be applied and permits suctioning of the tracheobronchial tree.[1] A variety of methods are available for achieving tracheal intubation, but the vast majority involve the use of direct laryngoscopy, the use of a laryngoscope to expose the glottic inlet and facilitate tracheal intubation.[2] This chapter will provide an overview of direct laryngoscopy for orotracheal intubation along with simple methods to prevent and rescue failed intubation.

KEY TERMS

difficult intubation, p. 80   failed intubation, p. 80

difficult laryngoscopy, p. 79   oxymetazoline, p. 82

Overview of Tracheal Intubation

A fundamental principle that lies at the heart of good airway management is that "patients suffer brain death and die from failure to ventilate or failure to oxygenate, not from a failure to intubate."[3] Inadequate ventilation, whether due to injury, disease, sedation, neuromuscular paralysis, an obstructed or compromised airway, altered mental status, or respiratory failure can lead to brain injury or death within minutes. Always remember that providing and monitoring ventilation and oxygenation is key to the survival of the patient. This will always take priority over tracheal intubation.

Thorough preparation is essential before attempting tracheal intubation, and the first priority is to ensure an effective method for oxygenation of the patient until intubation is attempted or should intubation fail. A detailed daily check in addition to a brief inspection of all equipment and supplies before use should be carried out and documented. Additionally, the patient's position should be optimized, if possible, to improve the likelihood of successful intubation. Rapid sequence intubation (Chapter 7) should be considered for all emergency patients because the presence of a full stomach greatly increases the risk of gastric regurgitation and pulmonary aspiration. Intubation itself (i.e., the insertion of the breathing tube through the glottic inlet) is not usually a problem, and most intubation difficulties are associated with problems of direct laryngoscopy (i.e., visualization of the larynx).

Table 4-1 General Indications for Emergency Tracheal Intubation[4-6]

- Airway protection from the risk of aspiration and obstruction by:
  - Blood in the airway
  - Gastric contents
  - Secretions
  - Foreign bodies
- Apnea, soft-tissue obstruction, hypercarbia
- Impending airway obstruction: facial fractures, nasopharyngeal hematoma, and inhalation injury
- Excessive work of breathing
- Shock (SBP < 80 mm Hg)
- Persistent hypoxia (SpO$_2$ ≤92%)
- Definitive maintenance of airway patency
- Head injury and a Glasgow Coma Scale score of ≤9
- AVPU score of P or U
- Mechanical ventilation
- Respiratory failure
- Airway management during emergency surgery and requirement for general anesthesia
- Cardiopulmonary arrest secondary to illness or injury
- Application of advanced cardiac life support and drug administration
- Maintenance of oxygenation or positive end-expiratory pressure
- Hypoxemia after application of optimal attempts to ventilate the patient using 100% oxygen and positive-pressure ventilation
- Maintenance of pulmonary toilet

Indications for emergency tracheal intubation are based on the clinical situation and the need for a definitive airway in patients who are suffering from life-threatening trauma or disease (Table 4-1). Definitive airways include the nasotracheal tube, orotracheal tube, and surgical airway.

Tracheal intubation is the placement of a breathing tube through the glottis so that the distal tip lies midway within the trachea below the larynx and above the carina. It can be accomplished by inserting a tracheal tube through the mouth, nose, cricothyroid membrane, or tracheotomy incision. Direct laryngoscopy is the usual method for placement of a tracheal tube in most clinical situations and involves the direct visualization of the larynx using a rigid laryngoscope.[2] The laryngoscope is used to distract structures within the mouth and pharynx so that the glottis can be directly exposed for insertion of a tracheal tube.

Direct laryngoscopy has a significant learning curve and may require greater than 150 intubations in a concentrated period of time before a clinician becomes adept and consistently successful.[7,8] Nonetheless, diverse groups of practitioners (e.g., paramedics, nurses, anesthesia providers, and emergency medicine physicians) whose skill levels and experience vary greatly, rely on direct laryngoscopy as the primary means of tracheal intubation from the prehospital environment through all areas of patient care within the hospital. This is due to the inherent advantages of direct laryngoscopy compared with other intubation methods. These advantages include high intubation success rates, ability to provide rapid intubation, and widespread availability of equipment.[2]

difficult laryngoscopy
No portion of the glottic opening can be seen during an optimal laryngoscopic attempt.

Difficult laryngoscopy can be said to occur when no portion of the glottic opening can be visualized during an optimal laryngoscopic attempt (Cormack and Lehane Grade 3 view).[3,9] Because of the hostile nature of the prehospital emergency environment, the incidence of difficult laryngoscopy is likely to be greater there than in the controlled environment of the operating

| **Table 4-2** | Critical Airway Events* |

- Failed intubation
- Inadequate ventilation
- Cannot-mask-ventilate/cannot-intubate situation

*An untreated critical airway event can rapidly lead to long-term disability or death.[31]

 PEARLS For more extensive definitions and maxims refer to the SLAM Universal Adult Airway Flowchart at the front of the book.

room, where it is reported to occur in up to 6% of laryngoscopies.[10] However, a poor laryngeal view can often be improved by the use of simple adjuncts and maneuvers.[2,7,8,11-13]

difficult intubation
Multiple laryngoscopies, maneuvers, and/or blades are needed by an experienced practitioner to perform an intubation.

Difficult intubation occurs when multiple laryngoscopies, maneuvers, and/or blades are needed by an experienced practitioner.[14] Success with direct laryngoscopy depends on training and experience. **Failed intubation** is said to occur after three unsuccessful intubation attempts or attempting intubation for greater than 10 minutes by an experienced practitioner without intubating the trachea.[15] The reported incidence of failed intubation varies and depends on the clinical situation.[2,16-22] Wang et al. reported prehospital success rates for paramedic tracheal intubation to be 90.5% of 592 patients during a one-year period of study.[23] Another report showed that the incidence of unrecognized esophageal intubation was 5.3% of 208 out-of-hospital intubations performed by paramedics.[24] Katz reported an even larger incidence of misplaced tubes, but in a much smaller group.[25] It is, therefore, of vital importance that all tracheal intubations are confirmed using either carbon dioxide detection in patients with a perfusing cardiac rhythm or an esophageal detection device in patients with a nonperfusing cardiac rhythm.[3,26-31]

failed intubation
Intubation cannot be achieved by an experienced operator after 3 attempts, or the attempts have lasted for more than 10 minutes.

Occurrence of a critical airway event (Table 4-2) requires rapid intervention. Should failed intubation occur, it is important to provide adequate oxygenation and ventilation until an alternative or more advanced method of intubation can be applied.[3,29,30] Continuing to attempt intubation using the same failed technique can traumatize the upper airway and lead to a cannot-mask-ventilate/cannot-intubate (CMVCI) situation.

Preparation for Tracheal Intubation

Preparation prior to an emergency intubation includes checking the equipment and the patient's position, preparing drugs for patients who still have intact airway reflexes, and coordination and communication among members of the care team. It is vital that clear communication exists during the planned procedure to coordinate each phase of management. This will improve teamwork and facilitate successful airway maintenance.

Selection, Preparation, and Checking of Equipment for Direct Laryngoscopy and Tracheal Intubation

All measures must be undertaken to reduce the risk of aspiration. This includes gentle mask ventilation, if needed, to avoid gastric inflation; correct performance of Sellick's maneuver; (when indicated); and turning on the suctioning unit before starting an intubation attempt.

Equipment for Oxygenation and Ventilation
Immediate availability of equipment for oxygenation and ventilation apparatus is mandatory (Figure 4-1). High-flow oxygen must be connected to a positive-pressure bag-valve-mask manual ventilation device with an oxygen reservoir to ensure a high inspired content of oxygen.

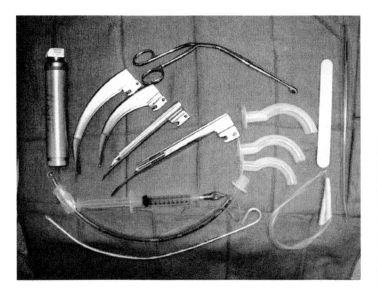

FIGURE 4-1

Basic equipment for oxygenation, ventilation, and intubation includes curved and straight laryngoscope blades, laryngoscope handle, oral airways, rigid and flexible suction catheters, Magill forceps, endotracheal tube, and malleable stylet.
(Courtesy of JM Rich, CRNA, [www.slamairway.com])

To check the ventilation device, the thumb of one hand should occlude the outflow port while the bag is squeezed with the opposite hand. Noncompressibility of the bag will ensure that adequate proximal airway pressure is present to raise the chest and ventilate the lungs. Also, listen at the outflow port to ensure that oxygen is flowing from the device and verify that reservoir tubing is attached to the distal portion of the bag. In this configuration, the bag can deliver 100% oxygen. Without reservoir tubing, the bag is unlikely to deliver more than 40% oxygen.

A properly fitting mask is necessary to provide a seal for positive-pressure lung ventilation. Ideally, the mask should be of transparent plastic and have a valve for syringe inflation or deflation of air to optimize the mask fit. A mask of medium size will usually fit most adults; however, very small adults may require a size smaller, and large adults may require a size larger. For this reason, having all three sizes available is important. A nonrebreathing mask for spontaneous ventilation should also be available.

Oxygen tanks, flow meters, and yokes should be checked to ensure that all items are properly functioning. Ideally, the oxygen tank should be full, and if it has a pressure of less than 500 psi, it should be exchanged for a full one.

The suctioning unit (Figure 4-2) should also be turned on prior to the start of airway management. Strong suction with a large-caliber hard Yankauer suctioning catheter is necessary to clear blood and viscous secretions from the airway. Both a stiff Yankauer catheter as well as a soft suction catheter (14 Fr) should be available. To ensure adequate strength of suction, attach the distal tip of the clean tubing to the skin of your forearm and immediately

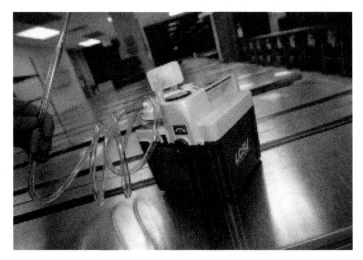

FIGURE 4-2
Portable suction unit.
(Courtesy of JM Rich, CRNA, [www.slamairway.com])

Direct Laryngoscopy and Tracheal Intubation

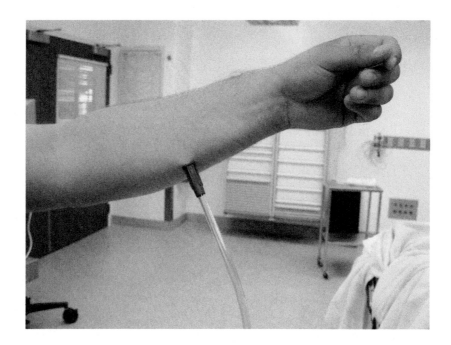

FIGURE 4-3
Checking suction. The suction should readily hold to the skin to be strong enough to move viscous secretions.
(Courtesy of JM Rich, CRNA, [www.slamairway.com])

oxymetazoline

A spray-type vasoconstrictor commonly available over-the-counter under a variety of trade names that can assist in preventing nosebleeds during instrumentation of the nares.

release it. If it holds, suction is adequate (Figure 4-3). If it will not hold fast, however, the suction strength needs to be increased. Do not hold the tubing to your skin for more than a second before letting go because negative pressure will build up in the suction line and the tubing will eventually hold fast to your skin, but this will not indicate that adequate suction is available on demand. (See Tables 4-3 and 4-4.)

Oro- and nasopharyngeal airways of various sizes should be available. In adults, oropharyngeal airways (e.g., Guedel) in sizes 70 mm, 80 mm, 90 mm, and 100 mm will provide airway patency from the smallest to the largest of adults. A tongue blade is handy for insertion of the oral airway, but it is not absolutely necessary. For patients who are postictal or simply sedated from drugs or alcohol,[2] a nasopharyngeal airway should be available in an array of sizes from 26 Fr to 34 Fr. Lidocaine jelly and **oxymetazoline** should also be available for preparation of the nasal mucosa to decrease the incidence of nosebleed.

Table 4-3 Advantages and Disadvantages of Various Types of Suction Devices

Type	Advantages	Disadvantages
Hand-powered	Lightweight, portable, inexpensive, simple to operate	Limited volume, manually powered, fluid contact components are not disposable
Oxygen-powered	Small, lightweight	Limited suction power, uses a lot of oxygen
Battery-powered	Lightweight, portable, excellent suction power, simple to operate and troubleshoot in the field	Battery memory decreases with time; mechanically more complicated than hand-powered; some fluid contact components are not disposable
Mounted	Strong suction, adjustable vacuum power, disposable fluid contact components	Not portable, cannot be serviced in the field, no substitute power source

Used with permission. From Bledsoe et al., *Paramedic Care: Principles and Practices,* Vol. 1. Upper Saddle River, NJ: Pearson Prentice Hall, 2006, p. 598.

Table 4-4	Types of Suctioning Catheters
Hard/Rigid Catheter	**Soft Catheters**
A large tube with multiple holes at the distal end	Long, flexible tube; smaller diameter than hard-tip catheters
Suctions larger volumes of fluid rapidly	Cannot remove large volumes of fluid rapidly
Standard size	Various sizes
Used in oropharyngeal airway only	Can be placed in the oropharynx, in the nasopharynx, or down the endotracheal tube
Removes larger particles	Suction tubing without catheter (facilitates suctioning of large debris)

Used with permission. From Bledsoe et al: *Paramedic Care: Principles and Practices,* Vol. 1. Upper Saddle River, NJ: Pearson Prentice Hall, 2006, p. 598.

Though mostly used during nasotracheal intubation, Magill forceps should be available at all times during provision of airway management. In the event of a foreign body being found in the airway during laryngoscopy, they can be used to remove it (Figure 4-4).

Equipment for Tracheal Intubation

Laryngoscope Handles and Blades. The conventional rigid laryngoscope has a detachable blade with a removable bulb. The blade interlocks with a handle containing a battery and activates by snapping the blade into a right angle (Figure 4-5). The illumination obtained with rigid fiberoptic laryngoscopes is generally brighter than that of conventional scopes and, in fiberoptic scopes, the light source is housed in the handle instead of the blade.

Laryngoscope blades are available in two varieties: the curved Macintosh blade and the straight Miller blade (Figure 4-6). The Macintosh blade is the most frequently used blade. During laryngoscopy, the tip of this blade is pushed into the angle formed by the base of the tongue and epiglottis (vallecula), and lifting from here indirectly lifts the tip of the epiglottis to expose the glottis beneath. The spatula of the blade has a smooth and gentle curve extending from the lock to the tip. In cross section, the construction resembles that of a reverse Z flange, facilitating greater access during intubation. A recent modification to the Macintosh English Profile blade is

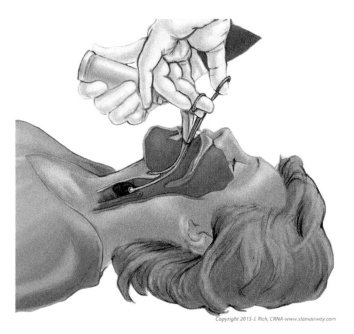

FIGURE 4-4

Removal of foreign body airway obstruction with direct visualization and Magill forceps.

Direct Laryngoscopy and Tracheal Intubation   83

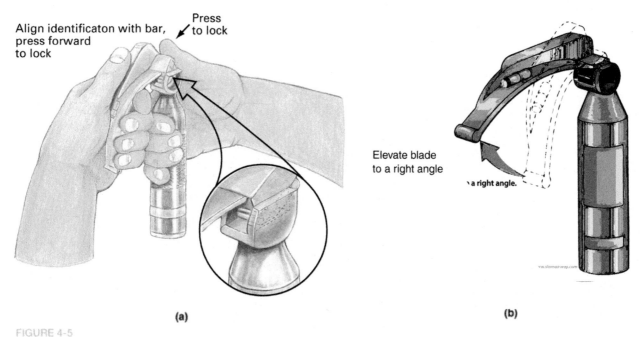

FIGURE 4-5

(a) Engaging the laryngoscope blade and handle; (b) activating the laryngoscope light source.

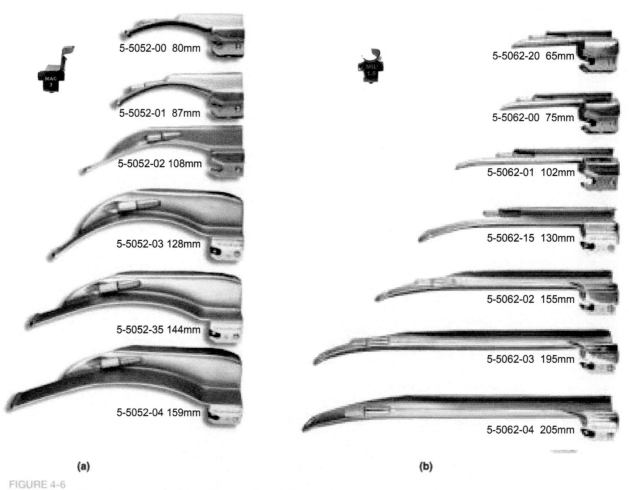

(a)

(b)

FIGURE 4-6

Laryngoscope blades: (a) curved Macintosh blade and (b) straight Miller blade.

(Courtesy of Sun Med USA, Largo, FL [www.airwaystore.com])

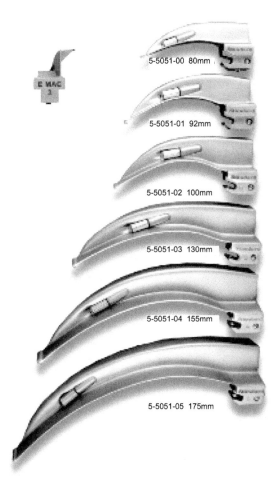

5-5051-00 80mm

5-5051-01 92mm

5-5051-02 100mm

5-5051-03 130mm

5-5051-04 155mm

5-5051-05 175mm

FIGURE 4-7

A recent modification to the Macintosh English Profile blade is the reduced flange E-Mac™.
(Courtesy of Sun Med USA, Largo, FL [www.airwaystore.com])

the reduced-flange E-Mac™ (Figure 4-7). It enables the user to exert less force on maxillary incisors while allowing more movement at the distal end to assist in visualizing the vocal cords.

The two commonly used straight blades are the Miller, which has a curved tip, and the Wisconsin (Figure 4-8) (and its modified forms), which has a straight tip.[32] The Miller, which was developed by the late Dr. Robert A. Miller of San Antonio, Texas, is the most popular straight blade. The size of the flange is reduced to minimize trauma, and the curve of the tip is extended to improve lift of the epiglottis. These improvements were incorporated to facilitate greater exposure of the larynx in difficult patients.[33] Another commonly seen straight blade is the Phillips (Figure 4-9), which integrates the preferred straight Jackson blade design[34] with the curved distal tip Miller design, providing greater visibility and an almost direct-line approach to the trachea during intubation.[33]

The smallest blade sizes are the #00 in the Miller type and the #1 in the Macintosh. The largest blade size is a #4 in both the Miller and the Macintosh. Each of the standard blades has a left-sided flange for distracting the tongue to the left and keeping it out of the line of sight, and an open side on the right for visualization of the larynx and insertion of the tracheal tube. Airway management kits should have a functioning laryngoscope with blades of various sizes. At a minimum, an adult kit should contain a #2 and #3 Miller (or another straight blade) and a #3 and #4 Macintosh blade. This will enable intubation of almost any size of adult patient. The #2 Miller blades can also be used in children, if needed. Extra batteries should also be available along with extra bulbs, and the light from the laryngoscope should be intensely bright to the point that it makes the operator squint should it be viewed directly.

Conventional handles fit only conventional blades, and fiberoptic handles fit only fiberoptic blades. Fiberoptic blades and handles usually have a green mark for rapid recognition. Regular checking of the kit should prevent mixing of the two in the same kit. If a nondisposable blade is used, it should be placed in a contamination bag (available in the kit)

Direct Laryngoscopy and Tracheal Intubation

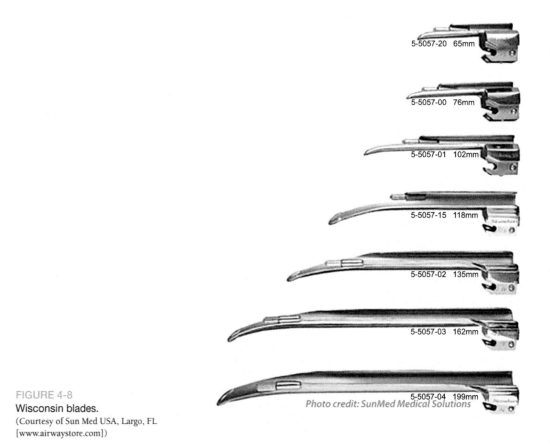

5-5057-20 65mm
5-5057-00 76mm
5-5057-01 102mm
5-5057-15 118mm
5-5057-02 135mm
5-5057-03 162mm
5-5057-04 199mm

Photo credit: SunMed Medical Solutions

FIGURE 4-8
Wisconsin blades.
(Courtesy of Sun Med USA, Largo, FL
[www.airwaystore.com])

after use and until it can be decontaminated, prior to reuse. Inexpensive disposable stainless steel[35] as well as plastic fiberoptic laryngoscope blades are now available.

Tracheal Tubes.   The tube size is measured in millimeters in the internal diameter. A tracheal tube with an internal diameter of 7 or 7.5 mm can be used in most women, and a tracheal tube with an inner diameter of 7.5 or 8 can be used in most men. In reality, a 7.5 mm tracheal tube is usually adequate for both men and women. For optimal ventilation, the largest possible diameter is desirable, but using too large a tube may cause mechanical problems during passage through the vocal cords.

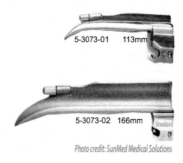

5-3073-01 113mm
5-3073-02 166mm

Photo credit: SunMed Medical Solutions

FIGURE 4-9
Phillips blades.
(Courtesy of Sun Med USA, Largo, FL [www.airwaystore.com])

Whenever a tracheal tube cannot be advanced, a smaller tube must be chosen as long as laryngospasm is not the cause of the obstruction. Subglottic stenosis, secondary to a previous tracheotomy, can narrow the trachea below the vocal cords so that the tracheal tube will pass through the cords but hold up at the stenotic lesion. Therefore, an array of different size tubes should be available in the airway kit or airway drawer. A second tube should always be available should the cuff of the first tube be damaged or defective.

The tube should be checked by opening the package at the end closest to where the 15 mm adapter lies. To prevent undue contamination, after opening the sterile wrapper, the tube should not be handled except at the adapter end during checking and intubation.[36] Pull the pilot balloon from the packaging and attach a 10 cc syringe filled with air. Grasp the cuff of the tracheal tube through the packaging and inflate the cuff with the syringe via the pilot balloon. Detach the syringe and squeeze the cuff between the thumb and forefinger of one hand while holding the pilot balloon between the thumb and forefinger of the opposite hand. When the cuff is intact, air can be felt moving back and forth between the two reservoirs. Detaching the syringe before checking the cuff will ensure that the valve in the pilot balloon is functional. Ensure that the 15 mm connector is cinched down onto the tracheal tube. These are loosely attached from the factory and, if they are not pushed in firmly, may detach during use, resulting in a breathing circuit disconnect during ventilation.

The most common tracheal tubes have high-volume/low-pressure cuffs. One of the reasons for the development of laryngeal edema is continuous undue pressure on the loosely vascular submucous tissues of the larynx and trachea.[36] The side walls of these cuffs are distributed over a large enough area to enable the cuff to seal without exerting undue pressure on the tracheal mucosa. This helps to prevent hypoxic tissue injury as a result of mucosal hypoperfusion of blood, which can occur when low-volume/high-pressure cuffs are overfilled.[36]

The tracheal tube has depth markings along the side, a system that is universal to all manufacturers and is measured from the distal tip to the marking. Depth markings run from 17 cm to 28–30 cm, depending on the internal diameter of the tube. A variety of tracheal tubes are available, and they vary with the clinical needs of the patient. The normal tracheal tube has an additional opening in the distal side wall of the tip known as a Murphy eye. The purpose of the Murphy eye is to allow gas to pass if the bevel is occluded by the wall of the trachea or by any other obstruction.[36] Its presence thus increases the chance of sufficient ventilation of the patient should the port at the distal tip of the tracheal tube face the tracheal wall, a situation that would otherwise lead to complete obstruction of the tube.

The use of a malleable stylet within the tracheal tube helps to fashion the tube into a practical shape (Figure 4-10). The recommended shape is like that of a hockey stick. This allows the tip of the tube to be directed toward the glottic inlet while keeping the shaft of the

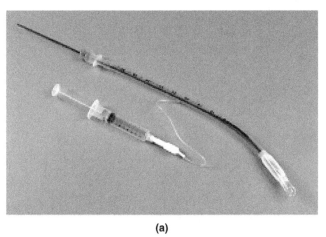

(a)

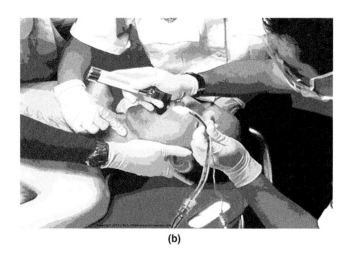

(b)

FIGURE 4-10

(a) Endotracheal tube, stylet, and syringe, assembled for intubation. (b) Oral intubation using a styleted tracheal tube. A stylet allows the operator to control the tip direction and movement of the tracheal tube.

tube lateral to the laryngoscopist's field of view during insertion. The distal tip of the stylet should be slightly recessed just short of the tip of the tube and should not protrude from the distal tip of the tube, which could cause trauma to soft tissue within the airway during insertion. Flexible stylets (e.g., gum-elastic bougie) may protrude from the tip of the tracheal tube, if necessary, and present little risk of traumatizing the mucosa or penetrating the airway with gentle insertion.

Monitoring Equipment

Monitoring equipment and disposable supplies should remain available. The minimum acceptable monitoring for airway management should include a stethoscope, pulse oximeter, sphygmomanometer, cardiac monitor, carbon dioxide detector (colorimetric or electronic), and an esophageal detector device.

 PEARLS All tracheal intubations should be confirmed using either carbon dioxide detection in patients with a perfusing cardiac rhythm or an esophageal detector device in patients who have a nonperfusing cardiac rhythm.

Drugs for Airway Management

All medications needed for tracheal intubation should be drawn up in syringes and properly labeled prior to use. Not labeling or mislabeling of drugs is one of the leading causes of medical errors. This may occur especially in the potentially chaotic prehospital environment. The intravenous line should be checked to ensure that it is not infiltrated and is flowing well into a vein. Drugs should include:

ON TARGET Before intubation, the patient should receive as much oxygen as possible. This can be achieved with a nonrebreathing mask and high oxygen flow for several minutes, or by gentle ventilation with the bag-valve-mask device. The goal is to wash out nitrogen from the lung and replace it with oxygen using the lung's functional residual capacity (FRC) as a reservoir of oxygen.

- Induction agent (e.g., etomidate, midazolam).
- Neuromuscular blocking agent (NMBA) to facilitate intubation (e.g., succinylcholine, if not contraindicated, and rocuronium).
- Appropriate NMBA to facilitate postintubation management (e.g., vecuronium).
- Adjunctive agents for sedation and analgesia during postintubation management (e.g., midazolam, fentanyl).
- Agents for control of blood pressure and heart rate (e.g., ephedrine, atropine, phenylephrine).

Agents to facilitate awake intubation should also be available. These include the sedatives and analgesics mentioned above, along with topical local anesthetics such as Cetacaine spray (Cetylite Industries, Pennsauken, NJ), 4% topical lidocaine, 2% lidocaine jelly, 5% lidocaine ointment, or 2% viscous lidocaine. Understanding the toxic dose and adverse side effects of local anesthetics is important to safe patient management. A vasoconstrictor to decrease the possibility of nosebleed, such as oxymetazoline, should also be available.

Preoxygenation

ON TARGET If the patient's oxygen saturation falls below 93%, stop the laryngoscopy and attempt to reoxygenate the patient with 100% oxygen and a bag-valve-mask device.

For every intubation, whether elective or emergency, the patient should receive maximal oxygenation before intubation is attempted. This can be achieved with a snug-fitting nonrebreathing mask and a high oxygen flow for several minutes until preparation is complete. The goal is to wash out nitrogen from the lungs and replace it with oxygen (utilizing the functional residual capacity [FRC][Chapter 3]) to avoid hypoxemia during the apneic phase when laryngoscopy and intubation are performed. In children, pregnant women, and obese patients, the FRC is reduced and oxygen saturation drops faster during the apneic period, making preoxygenation all the more important. Whenever intubation attempts fail or take excessive amounts of time, or if the patient begins to desaturate, intubation should be stopped immediately to ventilate and reoxygenate the patient.

Patient Positioning

Unless contraindicated,[37] the patient should be placed in the sniffing position. Achieving the sniffing position requires an understanding of the three axes that run through the head and neck. In the recumbent position, with the head lying on the ground, these axes are not aligned (Figure 4-11). The oral axis (OA) runs in a perpendicular line, from anterior to posterior, through the mouth to the occiput of the skull. The laryngeal axis (LA) runs from the laryngeal prominence of the thyroid to the midpoint of the crown of the head. The pharyngeal axis (PA) runs through the pharynx in a trajectory through the orbits and lower forehead. Thus, the recumbent position, with the head lying flat on the same surface as the shoulders, results in misalignment of the airway.

To better align the axes, create the sniffing position by doing the following. Raise the head approximately 10 cm with a pillow, thus creating a slight (35 degree) flexion of the neck on the chest and bringing the LA up approximately parallel with the PA. Then lift the chin to the point of extreme flexion of about 80 degrees at the atlanto-occipital joint, bringing the OA into more parallel alignment with the PA and LA. Achievement of the sniffing position in this way creates a nearly straight line between the patient's teeth (or gums) and the glottis, making direct laryngoscopy of the airway easier. However, in certain patients who are large-framed or

Head on Bed, Neutral Position

Head Elevated on Intubation Pillow, Head Extended on Neck (Sniffing Position)

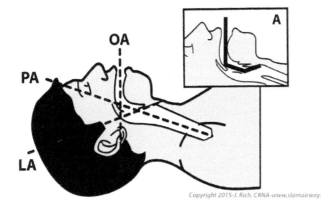
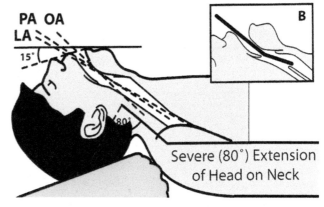

Copyright 2015-J. Rich, CRNA-www.slamairway.com

Aligning the Oral, Pharyngeal, and Laryngeal Axes to Create the Sniffing Position for Direct Laryngoscopy
The optimal position for direct laryngoscopy is the sniffing position. Aligning the oral axis (OA), laryngeal axis (LA), and pharyngeal axis (PA) normally creates a straighter line between the incisors and glottic inlet.
A—In the recumbent position, the head is in the neutral position and the airway axes are not aligned.
B—The sniffing position is created by (1) raising the head at least 10 cm on a pillow, which brings the LA and PA into better alignment; (2) providing extension of 80° of the head on the neck at the atlanto-occipital joint, which brings the OA into better alignment (Modified from Benumof JL. Conventional (Laryngoscopic) Orotracheal and nasotracheal Intubation (Single-Lumen tube), in Airway Management: Principles and Practice, ed., Benumof JL. Mosby, St. Louis, 1996, p. 263).

FIGURE 4-11
Neutral head position versus the sniffing position.
(Courtesy of JM Rich, CRNA [www.slamairway.com])

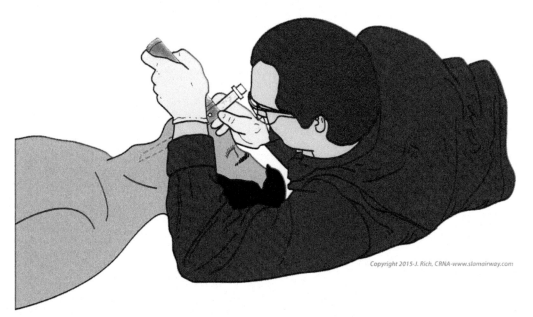

FIGURE 4-12
For patients lying supine on the ground, the trachea is easier to intubate when the intubator assumes the left lateral decubitus position rather than a kneeling position.
(Courtesy of JM Rich, CRNA [www.slamairway.com])

significantly obese, aligning the airway axes in this way is not possible because of the increased mass of tissue on the posterior neck and upper back, and special maneuvers must be employed for these patients. Such patients generally require Jackson's head-elevated laryngoscopy position (see below).[34]

In the prehospital situation, access to the patient and the head can be limited, and intubation attempts may fail because the patient's position cannot be modified. If allowable, undertaking all possible measures to optimize head and neck position is important in the emergency situation. Sometimes difficulty is created because the operator is prevented from managing the airway above the patient's head (e.g., closed-space rescue [Figure 4-12]). If the patient is suspected of having a cervical-spine injury, head extension is avoided, and the trachea is intubated while maintaining the neck in a neutral position using manual in-line axial stabilization (MIAS). With cervical-spine precautions, the incidence of difficulty with glottic visualization during conventional laryngoscopy is reported to be increased up to 42%.[37,38]

 PEARLS Unless contraindicated, the patient's head should be placed in the sniffing position to facilitate intubation.

Use of the sniffing position is contraindicated in patients with suspected or evident c-spine injury. In patients with suspected cervical-spine injury, a cervical collar may also impede the intubation attempt by limiting mouth opening. To improve the chance of success in this situation, the following procedure should be followed: (1) have a second rescuer apply manual in-line axial stabilization (MIAS [Chapter 11]), (2) loosen and/or remove the anterior portion of the cervical collar, (3) perform direct laryngoscopy and intubation while maintaining MIAS, and (4) replace the anterior portion of the cervical collar. Only then may the MIAS be released. To reiterate, MIAS must be applied constantly from before the collar is removed until the collar is replaced.

If a patient's position cannot be optimized and/or there is limited access to the patient (e.g., an entrapped car passenger), the option of maintaining spontaneous ventilation must be carefully considered over induction of anesthesia (see below and Chapter 8). Alternative airway techniques to manage the airway (e.g., rescue ventilation) in these situations must be available and may prove life-saving under these circumstances.[30,39]

Direct Laryngoscopy

Choice of Curved or Straight Blade

Until Sir Robert Macintosh invented the curved blade in the early 1940s, only straight blades were available.[40] Since that time, proponents of one blade over another have moved into either the curved-blade or straight-blade camp. The best thing is to know how to use both blades. If a straight blade is used, the tip of the blade is inserted posterior to the epiglottis so that the epiglottis can be lifted directly and trapped, exposing the glottic inlet. If a curved blade is used, the tip of the blade is inserted into the vallecula and pressed forward, where it stretches the hyoepiglottic ligament and indirectly lifts the epiglottis, thus indirectly exposing the glottic inlet. With few exceptions, the question of whether to use a curved or a straight blade for direct laryngoscopy in adults is really a matter of personal preference.

 PEARLS — Practitioners should know how to use both straight and curved laryngoscope blades.

Considerations for Curved-Blade Laryngoscopy

ON TARGET Cormack & Lehane Laryngeal Grades of the Airway. Grade 1: Entire glottic opening is visualized. Grade 2: Partial glottic view is visualized. Grade 3: Any portion of the epiglottis and/or posterior arytenoid cartilages. Grade 4: No visible laryngeal anatomy is viewed.

There is general agreement that beginners find it easier to use a curved blade, probably because it fits the shape of the tongue and has a natural stopping point in the vallecula.[2,41] The large flange of the curved blade makes it easier to control the tongue, which can improve the laryngeal view and facilitate easier passage of the tracheal tube through the oropharynx.[2,8,42,43] The large flange also makes it easier to provide instrumentation in the airway, such as when Magill forceps are used during tracheal tube exchange maneuvers.[32] Use of the curved blade is easier when novices are first learning to intubate patients with good mouth opening and no airway disproportion.[42] They are also thought to have less potential for damaging teeth and gums.[8,43] When direct laryngoscopy is performed on an awake patient, one who is lightly anesthetized, or one who is minimally sedated, the curved blade is thought to be less likely to cause laryngospasm or bronchospasm or to cause large changes in cardiac rate and rhythm[42] because it does not need to touch the sensitive posterior surface of the epiglottis, which is innervated by the superior laryngeal nerve. By contrast, the vallecula is innervated by the glossopharyngeal nerve.[8,42,43]

Reported disadvantages of curved-blade laryngoscopy include a higher incidence of Grade 3 views (only the epiglottis is visible [Cormack and Lehane Grade 3]) than with the straight blade.[10] It is also reported that the curved blade tends to impair vision during difficult laryngoscopy[41] because it compresses the base of the tongue and causes posterior displacement of the epiglottis, which can cause soft tissue to obstruct the laryngeal view.[44]

Considerations for Straight-Blade Laryngoscopy

Patients with short chins tend to have an anteriorly placed larynx. The straight blade can prove advantageous in patients like this because it lifts the epiglottis directly rather than indirectly, as with the curved blade.[32,43] For the same reason, if the patient has a long or floppy epiglottis, exposure will be improved with the straight blade because the tip of the epiglottis can be lifted directly[8,42] and the view is not obstructed by either the tongue or the curvature of the blade.[41] When mouth opening is limited, the smaller surface areas of the straight blades make them easier to insert into the mouths of patients with large maxillary teeth or limited mobility of the temporo-mandibular joint.[42] Although the straight blade may provide a better

Table 4-5 *Chevalier Jackson's Rules for Direct Laryngoscopy*

- The laryngoscope must always be held in the left hand, never in the right.
- The operator's right index finger (never the left) should be used to retract the patient's upper lip so that there is no danger of pinching the lip between the instrument and the teeth.
- The patient's head must always be exactly in the middle line, not rotated to the right or left, nor bent over sideways; and the entire head must be forward with extension at the occipito-atloid (atlanto-occipital) joint only.
- The laryngoscope is inserted to the right side of the anterior two-thirds of the tongue, the tip of the spatula being directed toward the midline when the posterior third of the tongue is reached. The epiglottis must always be identified before any attempt is made to expose the larynx.
- When first inserting the laryngoscope to find the epiglottis, great care should be taken not to insert too deeply lest the epiglottis be overridden and thus hidden.
- After identification of the epiglottis, too deep insertion of the laryngoscope must be carefully avoided lest the spatula be inserted behind the arytenoids into the hypopharynx.
- Exposure of the larynx is accomplished by pulling forward the epiglottis and the tissues attached to the hyoid bone, and not by prying these tissues forward with the upper teeth as a fulcrum.
- Care must be taken to avoid mistaking the aryepiglottic fold for the epiglottis itself, which would most likely occur as the result of rotation of the patient's head.

Modified from reference 34

view of the glottis, it provides less working area for tube insertion or instrumentation of the airway, which can make it more challenging to pass the tracheal tube.[2,41] However, practice can overcome this disadvantage.

In addition, because the straight blade has a smaller flange than the curved blade, the tongue can flop back to the right, obscuring the laryngeal view. Inserting and maintaining the blade lateral to the right side of the tongue limits the occurrence of glossal obstruction of the laryngeal view.[41] Again, practice and appropriate patient selection limits this disadvantage.

Excellent advice on performing straight-blade laryngoscopy has been available since early in the twentieth century, when it was published by the renowned laryngeal surgeon, Chevalier Jackson. His recommended two-step method (see below), as well as his "rules for direct laryngoscopy" (Table 4-5), are as applicable today as they were when he first published them.

Laryngoscopy should be done gently using only minimal force to displace the tongue and lift the epiglottis. Extensive manipulation or force must be avoided to prevent unnecessary airway trauma.[45] The easiest and most common way to open the patient's mouth for laryngoscopy is with a cross finger scissor technique using the right hand (Figure 4-13). The operator's index finger pushes the maxillary molars in a cephalad direction, and the thumb pushes the mandibular molars in the opposite direction. Using this technique, a chin lift can be easily performed by flexing the wrist during mouth opening. With practice, one can even learn to hold the tracheal tube between the first and second finger of the right hand while simultaneously opening the mouth using the cross finger scissor technique with the thumb and index finger. In this manner, the tracheal tube is immediately ready to be inserted when the glottis is exposed so that the operator's view does not have to be diverted away from the field to pick up or receive the tracheal tube. The standard technique is first to achieve a clear view of the glottic aperture, maintain this view, and then receive the tube from an assistant who correctly places it in the outstretched right hand.

Direct laryngoscopy is performed in a two-step fashion (after Jackson).[34] Step 1 exposes and identifies the epiglottis. Step 2 involves laryngoscopic elevation of the epiglottis to expose

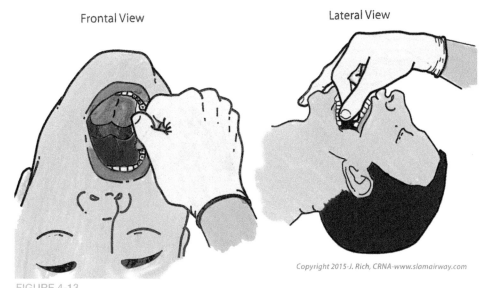

Frontal View   Lateral View

Copyright 2015-J. Rich, CRNA-www.slamairway.com

FIGURE 4-13
Opening the mouth for laryngoscopy, using the cross-finger scissor technique.

the larynx to direct view. Jackson's method involves only a slight modification when using a curved blade. Jackson states:

> *The laryngoscope is held in the left hand and the blade is inserted in the right side of the mouth along the right edge of the tongue. The blade is then advanced into the mouth continuing along the right edge of the tongue (Figure 4-14 A and B and 4-15 A). As the tip of the blade is advanced toward the base of the tongue, it is swept in a leftward direction to distract the tongue (Figure 4-14 C1 and C2 and 4-15 B). The operator continuously observes for the epiglottis to come into view. Upon seeing the epiglottis, the laryngoscope is lifted at a 45-degree angle in the direction of the patient's feet (Figure 14-4 D1, D2, D3 and 14-5 A and B). The lifting should be accomplished by elevation of the operator's left shoulder and arm and with the wrist and hand held in a straight line (without wrist flexion). Levering the laryngoscope blade on the teeth or gums by rotating and flexing the wrist will usually degrade the laryngeal view and may cause tooth damage or trauma to the lips with attendant bleeding.[42]*

As mentioned above, just prior to lifting the blade, it is swept leftward to displace the tongue and increase the space to the right for visualization of the larynx and insertion of the tracheal tube. The tip of the blade is then directed toward the epiglottis so that the epiglottis can be lifted either *indirectly* by pressing the tip of the curved blade into the vallecula, just anterior to the epiglottis (Figure 4-14 D1-D3 and Figure 2-5), or *directly* by placing the tip of the straight blade posterior to the epiglottis to lift and trap it (Figure 4-15 C inset 2 and 3 and Figure 2-6). (Curved-blade laryngoscopy is illustrated in Figure 4-14. Straight-blade laryngoscopy is illustrated in Figure 4-15.)

Pushing too deeply into the vallecula when using a curved blade may cause the epiglottis to pucker down and fold back over the glottis, thus degrading the laryngeal view (see below, under "Avoiding Laryngoscopic Pitfalls"). It is important to keep the tongue displaced to the left side during laryngoscopy so that as wide a space as possible is created for exposure of the glottis and insertion of the tracheal tube. Should the tongue flop back over to the right side of the blade, it is best to simply remove the laryngoscope and start over rather than trying to work around a poor view of the larynx that is obstructed by the tongue.

If, after lifting the epiglottis, a Cormack and Lehane (Chapter 2) Grade 1 or Grade 2 exposure of the glottis is not achieved, the right hand should be used to manipulate the larynx externally to bring the cords into view.[34] To achieve this, the thyroid cartilage is held and manipulated by the thumb, index finger, and middle finger.[2,8,11] Thyroid pressure is then

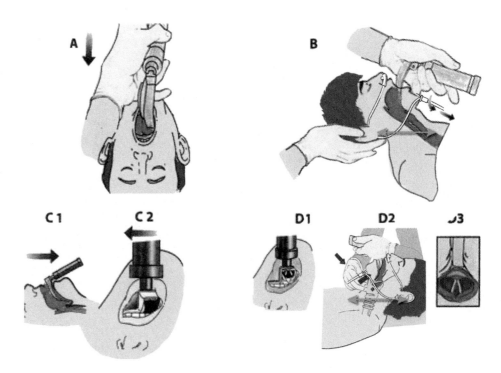

FIGURE 4-14
Curved-blade laryngoscopy.
(Courtesy of JM Rich, CRNA
[www.slamairway.com])

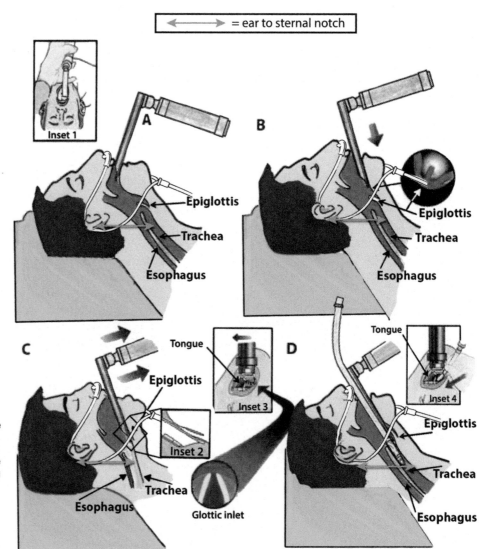

⟷ = ear to sternal notch

FIGURE 4-15
Straight-blade laryngoscopy. (a) The blade
is inserted to the right of the tongue. (b) The
tongue is swept to the left, and the epiglottis is identified. The tip of the straight blade
is then inserted behind the epiglottis. (c) The
gottic inlet is then exposed directly by lifting
the epiglottis.
(Courtesy of JM Rich, CRNA [www.slamairway.com])

Table 4-6 What Makes Intubation Easy?[7]

- Reasonably experienced laryngoscopist (150 intubations between six months and two years)
- No muscle tone
- Optimal sniffing position (may need stacking with pillows and blankets [i.e., HELP*])[12,13]
- Optimal external laryngeal manipulation (on thyroid cartilage [BURP**])
- Change blade length X 1 (e.g., Mac # 3 to Mac # 4)
- Change blade type X 1 (e.g., Mac to Miller)

*Head-Elevated Larsyngoscopy position[12,13]
**Backward-upward-rightward pressure.[47]

applied in a downward (posterior) and upward (cephalad) fashion. Known as external laryngeal manipulation,[8] this maneuver pushes the entire larynx in a posterior direction and thus can bring the vocal cords and glottis into the operator's view. Obviously, when the operator lets go, the view will be lost. Therefore, if external laryngeal manipulation improves the glottic view, the hand of an assistant should be placed at the same point prior to the operator removing his or her hand. The assistant then exerts the same direction of force on the larynx, and the operator removes his or her hand from the larynx and passes the tracheal tube through the glottic inlet under direct vision. External laryngeal manipulation is often all that is needed to optimize the laryngeal view and enable passage of the tracheal tube. It can change a Grade 4 view (only soft tissue visible) to a Grade 3 view (epiglottis only), and a Grade 3 view to a Grade 2 view (glottis visible).[46] It should be the first maneuver attempted to optimize the laryngeal view.[2,11]

The laryngoscope blade must be of an adequate length to either directly or indirectly lift the epiglottis. If the blade selected is too short to accomplish this goal, simply remove it and exchange it for a longer blade. Do not struggle with a blade that is too short. If the shape does not seem optimal, it can also be exchanged for a different shaped blade (e.g., curved to straight). A third laryngoscopy attempt should be the final and best attempt.[3,7] Benumof has developed a list to describe an optimal laryngoscopic attempt to facilitate intubation (Table 4-6). In contrast, Ovasappian has developed a list of avoidable common causes of difficult laryngoscopy (Table 4-7).

With practice and close attention to detail, the glottis can usually be optimally exposed at the first attempt. However, three attempts may occasionally be needed to obtain an adequate view for intubation (see below, under "Methods to Prevent and Rescue Failed Intubation"). The time available for laryngoscopy is limited by the patient's oxygen reserve. This emphasizes the need for preoxygenation in all patients and close monitoring of the patient's oxygen saturation using a pulse oximeter. If the patient's oxygen saturation falls below 93%, stop the laryngoscopy and attempt to reoxygenate using positive-pressure mask ventilation and 100% oxygen. If the patient's oxygen saturation cannot be raised to ≥93%, switch to rescue ventilation.

Table 4-7 Common Avoidable Causes of Difficult Laryngoscopy[42]

- Improper positioning of the head
- Inadequate opening of the mouth
- Selecting the wrong blade
- Allowing the tongue to hang over the right side of the blade
- Application of leverage rather than traction
- Obscuring the line of vision with the tracheal tube during its insertion
- Inserting the blade too deeply
- Selecting too short a blade

An intubation attempt (insertion of the blade until point of cuff inflation and removal of blade) should rarely take more than 30 seconds; otherwise, the patient should receive positive-pressure mask ventilation with oxygen, and the subsequent intubation attempt should be altered to provide better exposure of the glottis.[3,29] In addition, overly long interruption or delay of other measures such as chest compression or defibrillation during cardiopulmonary resuscitation must be avoided when attempting to secure the airway.

 Rescue Ventilation allows the difficult airway situation to be temporized until the trachea can be definitively intubated. Check out the Rescue Ventilation Pathway of the SUAAF.

Tracheal Tube Insertion

Using a stylet within the tube adds stability to the tube and provides better guidance of the tip through the vocal chords. If needed, the tube's shape can be adjusted to the individual anatomical conditions. The stylet should be slightly recessed to avoid protusion from the tip of the tracheal tube. After identification of the vocal cords, the tracheal tube should be inserted with a stylet in all emergency intubations.

Forceful blind probing with a tracheal tube during a poor laryngeal exposure can traumatize the structures of the airway and should be discouraged. Besides an increased risk of gastric inflation and aspiration when the stomach is ventilated via a misplaced tube, there is a risk of trauma to the larynx with resultant swelling and bleeding.[45] When a misplaced tube is removed, the interval without oxygenation is lengthened.

Once the glottis is exposed, the tip of a styletted tracheal tube should be passed from the right corner of the mouth through the glottis until the cuff of the tube disappears from view (Figure 4-15 D, inset 4). The tube has been passed deep enough when the cuff disappears from view beyond the vocal cords by a distance of 1 to 2 cm.

Depending on the height of the patient, this will usually be to a depth of approximately 21 cm in women and 23 cm in men (at the point of the teeth or gums). The tube is held firmly by the thumb and index finger of the right hand (with the hand lying on the cheek), and the stylet is then removed and the cuff of the tube is inflated with enough air to provide a seal during positive-pressure ventilation (usually 3 to 7 cc of air).

Securing the Tracheal Tube

After confirmation of tracheal intubation is accomplished, the tube is taped or secured firmly in place to prevent dislodgment, movement into a mainstem bronchus position, or accidental extubation. The tube can be fixed using adhesive tape, trach tape, or a commercially available fixation system. Due to body secretions, tape may not stick sufficiently to the patient's skin. The tube should be fixed at the corner of the mouth, and the position of the corresponding depth marks on the tube should be documented as a reference for comparison and to detect tube movement. After fixing the tube, the position must be rechecked due to the manipulations of the tube. The tape runs from just below and medial to the left cheek, above the upper lip, and is wrapped circumferentially around the tube at the lip. The distal edge of the tape is then affixed to just below and medial to the right cheek (Figure 4-16).

Another method involves the use of one-inch silk tape that is wrapped around the tracheal tube at the skin and then wrapped circumferentially around the head and returned to the tube from the opposite side. It is then wrapped again around the tube at the level of the lip. This is a good technique when securing a tube in a patient with a beard or for securing a nasal tracheal tube at the nose. Another method is to cinch tracheostomy tape onto the tracheal tube and then wrap it circumferentially around the head with it, tied securely.

Commercial devices to secure the tube are circumferentially wrapped around the head and firmly secured with Velcro (Thomas Tube Holder [Laerdal Medical-Wappingers Falls, NY]).

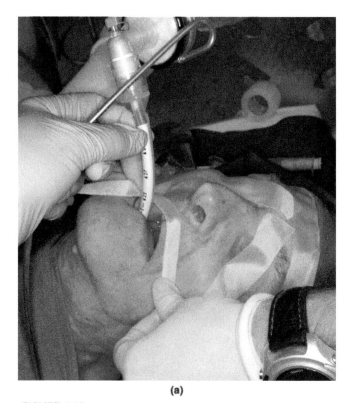
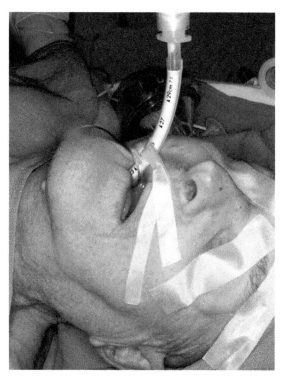

(a)   (b)

FIGURE 4-16
Securing the endotracheal tube.

They have a clamp with a setscrew that tightens the tube in the clamp. They offer the additional advantage of having a built-in bite block to protect the tube from being bitten. Care must be taken not to overly tighten the strap, which may impair blood flow to the skin and lead to pressure necrosis from the face plate.

 Use of a cervical collar after intubation can help to prevent movement of the endotracheal tube.

An additional measure to keep the tracheal tube in place is the use of a cervical collar. Immobilizing the cervical spine (even when no cervical trauma is suspected) reduces the range of motion of the head on the neck, thus preventing movement of the tracheal tube. If the head falls back during patient movement, then the distance from the corner of the mouth where the tube is fixed to the vocal cords is reduced. This may result in unintended one-lung ventilation if the tip of the tube is positioned near the carina and is moved into a mainstem bronchus. When the patient's head is flexed on the chest, then the distance from the corner of the mouth to the vocal cords increases. This may result in secondary displacement of the tracheal tube if the tip is positioned just below the vocal cords, resulting in accidental extubation.

Avoiding Laryngoscopic Pitfalls

Inserting the Blade Too Deeply

If a straight blade is inserted too deeply, it can pass behind the larynx and into the esophagus. When the laryngoscope is lifted with the blade in this position, a view of only the soft tissue can be seen. To rescue this view (i.e., paraglossal rescue technique), slowly retract the blade directly back until the larynx and epiglottis drop down onto the blade, which may well reveal an adequate view of the glottis. Insertion of a curved blade into the vallecula stretches

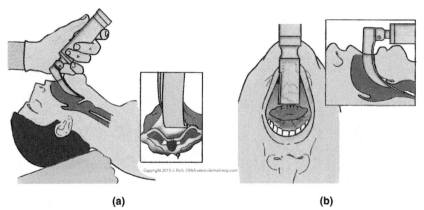

(a)   **(b)**

FIGURE 4-17

(a) Insertion of the laryngoscope blade too deeply into the vallecula may push the epiglottis down over the laryngeal inlet, diminishing exposure of the vocal cords. (b) Insertion of the laryngoscope blade too deeply into the pharynx elevates the larynx and exposes the esophagus.

(Courtesy of JM Rich, CRNA [www.slamairway.com])

the hyoepiglottic ligament so that the tip of the epiglottis normally rises and indirectly exposes the glottic inlet (Figure 2-5). However, if the operator continues to press the blade into the vallecula, the epiglottis will pucker and fold down upon the glottic inlet, thus degrading the glottic view (Figure 4-17a).[8] Deep pharyngeal insertion of the blade can cause the entire larynx to be lifted out of the line of sight, thus revealing only soft tissue or the esophageal inlet (Figure 4-17b).

Using a Blade That Is Too Short

As noted by Benumof, use of a long blade (curved or straight) is indicated in very large patients and patients with very long mandibles or long necks.[8] Should the blade not be long enough to lift the epiglottis, it is best to change the blade immediately rather than struggle with a blade that is too short, thus increasing the time of apnea during laryngoscopy as well as the risk of trauma to lips, gums, and teeth.

Not Controlling the Tongue

If the tongue flops back over the right side of the blade, the view of the larynx, will be limited (Figure 4-18).[8] Rather than struggling with an inadequate view of the larynx, it is best to remove the blade immediately and start over. Struggling to intubate with a poor laryngeal view increases the likelihood of esophageal intubation and airway trauma.

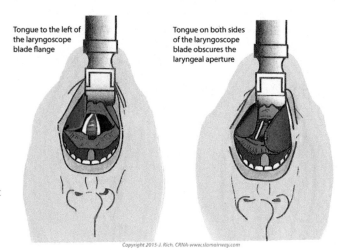

Tongue to the left of the laryngoscope blade flange

Tongue on both sides of the laryngoscope blade obscures the laryngeal aperture

FIGURE 4-18

The tongue must be kept to the left of the laryngoscope blade to provide an adequate laryngeal view

(Courtesy of JM Rich, CRNA [www.slamairway.com])

Shotgunning the Laryngoscope

The operator should keep his or her eye back from the glottis about 15 to 20 inches to maintain good depth of focus. The eye cannot focus well if it is placed directly at the proximal edge of the laryngoscope (about six inches from the glottis).[8] Shotgunning the scope also diminishes the operator's field of vision. When the operator stays back from the blade, he or she is better able to insert the tracheal tube in the right side of the mouth and better able to direct the tube tip toward the glottic inlet.

Difficult Laryngoscope Insertion in Large-Breasted or Barrel-Chested Patients

In some large-breasted or barrel-chested patients, it is difficult to insert the blade because the laryngoscope handle contacts the chest before the blade tip can be inserted into the back of the mouth.[8] To overcome this problem, the operator can insert the blade and handle at a 90 degree angle (i.e., the handle is pointing off toward the right shoulder instead of toward the feet). The handle is then swung back 90 degrees after the blade is inserted to the back of the mouth. The use of shorter laryngoscope handles can keep this problem from happening.

Assessing the Reason for Failed Laryngoscopy

If laryngoscopy fails, oxygenation of the patient is the primary goal. The laryngoscopic problem should be identified before reintubation is attempted. Ask: Is the mouth opening too small? Was the tongue displaced adequately to the left? Is external laryngeal manipulation needed? Would bougie-assisted intubation be helpful? Was the epiglottis identified? Was the epiglottis lifted adequately to allow viewing of the vocal cords? If only the epiglottis was seen, was external laryngeal manipulation applied? If the best view was a Grade 3 with external laryngeal manipulation, was bougie-assisted intubation attempted? By identifying the cause of the failure, the likelihood of correcting the problem increases. Repeating intubation attempts without reconsidering the intubation strategy rarely brings success, and possibly endangers the patient.

 Continuing to attempt intubation using the same failed technique can traumatize the upper airway and lead to a cannot-mask-ventilate/cannot-intubate situation.

Complications of Tracheal Intubation

Careful attention to detail throughout the process of tracheal intubation is necessary to minimize complications. Complications are generally divided into those observed during placement of the tube, during maintenance of the tube, and at the time of extubation (Table 4-8).

Application of Simple Methods to Rescue and Prevent Failed Intubation

Intubation-rescue techniques[11] may assist with either an unanticipated or anticipated difficult intubation. Intubation rescue is used following a failed intubation attempt, provided that no more than two to three laryngoscopic attempts have been made, laryngoscopy has been attempted for less than 10 minutes, and the patient's SpO$_2$ can be maintained at greater than 92%.[3,29,31] If laryngoscopy has been attempted for greater than 10 minutes or more than three times, or the patient's SpO$_2$ cannot be maintained at greater than 92%, intubation

Table 4-8 Various Adverse Effects Associated with Laryngoscopy and Tracheal Intubation[32,42,45,48-51]

Evident During Laryngoscopy and Tube Insertion

Aspiration
- Foreign bodies
- Gastric contents
- Teeth

Physiologic Effects
- Cardiovascular: hypertension, reflex bradycardia, tachycardia, myocardial ischemia
- Respiratory: bronchospasm, laryngospasm
- Central nervous system: increased intracranial pressure
- Ophthalmic: increased intraocular pressure or extrusion of vitreous humor

Trauma
- Evulsion/chipping/fracture: cervical spine, teeth or dental appliances
- Epistaxis
- Vocal cord injury
- Lacerations/bruising: lips, gums, tongue, pharynx,
- Ophthalmic injury: corneal abrasion
- Penetration/perforation: esophageal, laryngeal, pharyngeal with subcutaneous emphysema, tracheal pneumothorax, retropharyngeal dissection
- Dislocation: arytenoid, mandibular, cervical spine

Tube Malposition (Unrecognized)
- Bronchial intubation
- Pharyngeal intubation
- Esophageal intubation

Miscellaneous
- Bacteremia
- Hypoxemia
- Hypercarbia
- Prolonged or failed intubation

Evident During Tube Maintenance

Miscellaneous
- Aspiration
- Excoriation of nose or mouth
- Airway fire
- Sinusitis

Physiologic
- Bronchospasm
- Overventilation: hypocarbia
- Underventilation: hypercarbia, hypoxemia

Tube Obstruction
- Kinking
- Unrecognized disconnection
- Unintended extubation

Complications of Prolonged Intubation
- Infections: laryngotracheobronchitis, sinusitis, pneumonia
- Laryngeal ulceration
- Vocal cord granuloma
- Tracheomalacia
- Tracheal stenosis
- Vocal-cord paralysis

Evident at Extubation

Aspiration
- Blood
- Foreign bodies
- Gastric contents
- Secretions

Voice Changes
- Dysphonia
- Aphonia
- Hoarseness

Edema
- Glottic
- Subglottic
- Uvular

Stenosis
- Glottic
- Subglottic
- Tracheal

Paralysis
- Vocal cords
- Hypoglossal nerves
- Lingual nerves

Miscellaneous
- Difficult or impossible extubation
- Jaw dislocation
- Jaw soreness
- Laryngeal incompetence
- Laryngospasm
- Negative pressure pulmonary edema
- Sore throat
- Tracheomalacia

attempts should be stopped and rescue ventilation using a supraglottic airway device used until a definitive airway can be safely inserted using a different technique.[29,30]

Communicating and Working with a Knowledgeable Assistant

To optimize the glottic view, specific measures may be taken beyond optimizing the patient's position and the laryngoscopy technique. Good communication with an assistant while attempting intubation is of paramount importance. The assistant can make the difference between success and failure in airway management, as well as making the process difficult or easy. Think of hockey: the last player that passes the puck to the one who scores the goal gets a life-time point, the same as the player scoring the goal.[52] Having a knowledgeable assistant in the game is the key to rapid, effective, and successful airway management.

External Laryngeal Manipulation (ELM)

If proper positioning has been applied and an optimal attempt does not produce laryngeal exposure, Chevalier Jackson originally recommended nearly 100 years ago that an assistant press down on the thyroid cartilage.[34] This should be the first maneuver done to improve glottic exposure after insertion of the laryngoscope blade.[11] Backward and upward pressure on the thyroid cartilage can move the larynx and thus the vocal cords and glottis into the laryngeal view (Figure 4-19). If the initial laryngeal view is a Grade 3 view

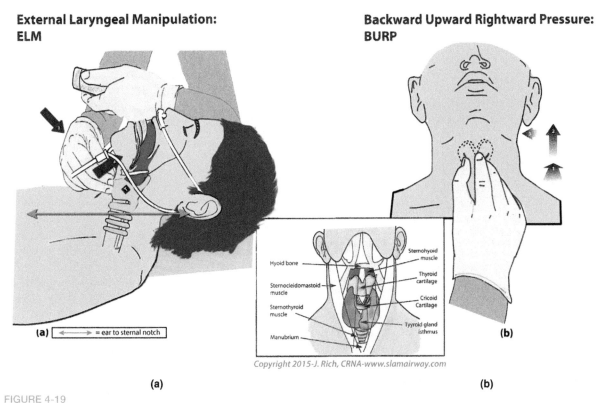

External Laryngeal Manipulation: ELM

Backward Upward Rightward Pressure: BURP

(a) ⟷ = ear to sternal notch

Hyoid bone
Sternocleidomastoid muscle
Sternothyroid muscle
Manubrium

Sternohyoid muscle
Thyroid cartilage
Cricoid Cartilage
Tyyroid gland isthmus

Copyright 2015-J. Rich, CRNA-www.slamairway.com

(a)

(b)

FIGURE 4-19

ELM versus BURP to improve the laryngeal view. (a) External laryngeal manipulation (ELM) to improve the laryngeal view is determined by the laryngoscopist by pressing on the laryngeal prominence of the thyroid cartilage simultaneously in an upward and backward direction. (b) BURP, or backward upward rightward (the patient's right) pressure on the thyroid cartilage. This essentially adds one more maneuver beyond those used for ELM. If laryngeal manipulation is successful at improving the laryngeal view, have the assistant place a hand where your hand is and proceed with intubation. Laryngeal manipulation has been documented to change Grade 4 to Grade 3 and Grade 3 to Grade 2 views.

(epiglottis only or posterior cartilages only), the use of ELM can change a Grade 3 view to a Grade 2 view (some portion of the glottic inlet is visible). This laryngeal view can usually be intubated using a hockey stick–shaped tracheal tube.[2] If the initial view is a Grade 4 view (soft tissue only), the use of external laryngeal manipulation can render a Grade 3 view.

Intubation of a Grade 3 view is difficult without employing additional maneuvers. Probing blindly behind the epiglottis or in front of the posterior cartilages can traumatize the structures near the laryngeal inlet (e.g., vocal cords) and/or could cause an arytenoid dislocation of a vocal cord.[45] When the optimal view is a Grade 3 view, the best way to insert the tracheal tube is by employing a specially designed flexible introducer or intubating stylet (eg. gum-elastic bougie) and performing a bougie-assisted intubation.

Bougie-Assisted Intubation

The gum-elastic bougie was first described by Sir Robert Macintosh in the 1940s as an aid to orotracheal intubation.[53] After invention of his curved laryngoscope blade, he found that the use of a long elastic stylet facilitated insertion of the tracheal tube during some curved-blade laryngoscopies when only a poor laryngeal view could be obtained. He found that, even though he was unable to pass the tracheal tube secondary to the poor laryngeal view, he was still able to direct and insert a flexible stylet into the trachea. He was then able to "railroad"[46] the tracheal tube over the stylet and into the trachea. Years later, Macintosh wrote a personal letter to another practitioner in which he stated, "I can honestly say that, armed with an introducer, I have never failed, providing that I have been able to see the back of an arytenoid."[46,54]

At a future point, the stylet was fashioned with a 30-degree angled coude tip and became known as the Eschmann introducer, which was manufactured by Eschmann Health Care in the United Kingdom and distributed in the United States by SIMS Portex, Inc. (Keene, NH). The common name is gum-elastic bougie, which is a misnomer because it is neither gum, elastic, nor a bougie. However, it does have the appearance of a French cathedral candle, which is called a *bougie* in French. The Eschmann introducer has been a great aid to oral intubation for over half a century but, unfortunately, remains one of the best kept secrets in airway management today.

The Eschmann introducer is 60 cm long and continues to be handmade. It is quite flexible, and the final coating is a varnishlike finish. It has to be warmed prior to shaping or bending because excessive bending or straightening of the tip at a temperature below body temperature may cause damage or deterioration. It is reusable; though it cannot be sterilized, it can receive high-level disinfection. Even so, the manufacturer states that it should not be used more than five times. It is delivered unsterile and should be disinfected prior to use. Before each use, it must be carefully inspected for external cracks or damage.[55]

Bougie-assisted intubation is an excellent method for atraumatic insertion of a tracheal tube in the presence of a Grade 3 laryngeal view (epiglottis only or tip of posterior cartilages only [Figure 4-20, inset A]). To use the device, the operator first obtains an optimal view of the larynx using direct laryngoscopy and, if required, external laryngeal manipulation. When the optimal view produced by direct laryngoscopy[7,8] is only the tip of the epiglottis, the bougie is inserted just posterior to the tip of the epiglottis so that the 30-degree angled distal tip is oriented in an anterior direction on the gently curved bougie (like a banana shape [Figure 4-20, inset B]). The distal tip is held in the midline and either inserted posterior to the tip of the epiglottis or just anterior to the posterior cartilages (depending on the view). It is then gently advanced forward.

As it enters the glottic inlet, the coude tip should bump against the c-shaped cartilaginous rings of the trachea, creating a clicking effect that is conducted up the bougie and can be felt in the fingers of the hand holding the introducer. This is the initial tactile confirmation that the glottis has been entered and is known as tracheal clicking (Figure 4-21 A).[46] If tracheal clicking is not clearly felt and there is no resistance to advancement of the bougie, continue to advance it until resistance is felt. Resistance (or holdup) should be felt initially as the bougie touches the carina (bifurcation of the trachea [Figure 4-20 B, inset 1]). The

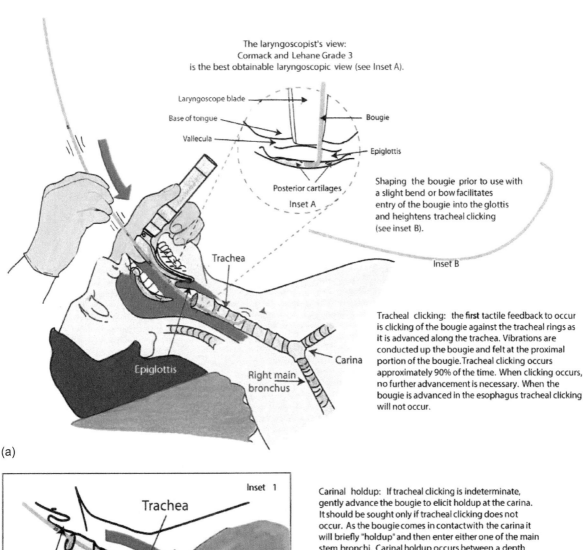

The laryngoscopist's view:
Cormack and Lehane Grade 3
is the best obtainable laryngoscopic view (see Inset A).

Laryngoscope blade

Base of tongue

Vallecula

Bougie

Epiglottis

Posterior cartilages

Inset A

Shaping the bougie prior to use with a slight bend or bow facilitates entry of the bougie into the glottis and heightens tracheal clicking (see inset B).

Inset B

Trachea

Carina

Right main bronchus

Epiglottis

Tracheal clicking: the **first** tactile feedback to occur is clicking of the bougie against the tracheal rings as it is advanced along the trachea. Vibrations are conducted up the bougie and felt at the proximal portion of the bougie. Tracheal clicking occurs approximately 90% of the time. When clicking occurs, no further advancement is necessary. When the bougie is advanced in the esophagus tracheal clicking will not occur.

(a)

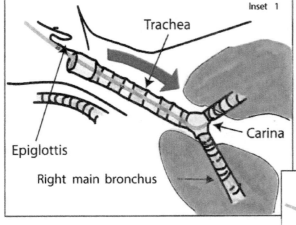

Inset 1

Trachea

Carina

Epiglottis

Right main bronchus

Carinal holdup: If tracheal clicking is indeterminate, gently advance the bougie to elicit holdup at the carina. It should be sought only if tracheal clicking does not occur. As the bougie comes in contact with the carina it will briefly "holdup" and then enter either one of the main stem bronchi. Carinal holdup occurs between a depth of 20 cm and 40 cm (mean distance 32 cm). The bougie bumps against the carina just before it is advanced into one of the main stem bronchi. When carinal hold up occurs further advancement of the bougie is not necessary or recommended.

Distal Holdup: If carinal holdup does not occur, one may cautiously proceed with very gentle advancement until distal holdup occurs. Distal holdup is sensed when the bougie encounters a small distal bronchus of a smaller diameter than the bougie. Further attempts at advancement beyond this point will damage or perforate the bronchus causing hemothorax or pneumothorax. If the bougie is in the esophagus hold up will not occur or may occur at a significantly greater depth than would occur in the tracheal-bronchial tree. Routine use of distal holdup is not recommended.

(b)

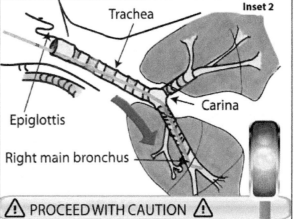

Trachea

Inset 2

Carina

Epiglottis

Right main bronchus

⚠ PROCEED WITH CAUTION ⚠

FIGURE 4-20
Bougie-assisted intubation: (a) tracheal clicking, (b) Carinal & distal holdup
(Courtesy of JM Rich, CRNA [www.slamairway.com1).

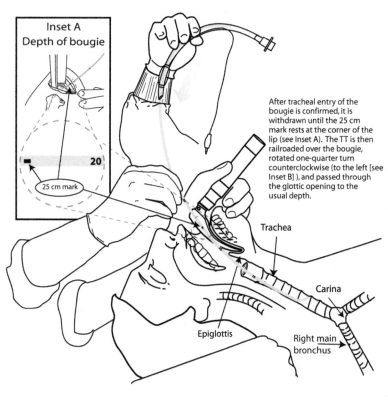

Inset A
Depth of bougie

20

25 cm mark

After tracheal entry of the bougie is confirmed, it is withdrawn until the 25 cm mark rests at the corner of the lip (see Inset A). The TT is then railroaded over the bougie, rotated one-quarter turn counterclockwise (to the left [see Inset B]), and passed through the glottic opening to the usual depth.

Trachea

Carina

Epiglottis

Right main bronchus

Two maneuvers should always be done in order to consistently slide the tracheal tube (TT) through the glottis without it catching on any supraglottic structures. First, the laryngoscope should remain in place throughout the intubation procedure. The laryngoscope distracts and tightens the slack pharyngeal tissues, which facilitates passage of the TT. Second, the TT is rotated a quarter turn counterclockwise before the tip reaches the glottic inlet (see inset B).

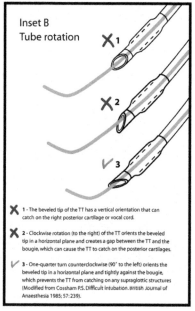

Inset B
Tube rotation

X 1

X 2

✓ 3

X 1 - The beveled tip of the TT has a vertical orientation that can catch on the right posterior cartilage or vocal cord.

X 2 - Clockwise rotation (to the right) of the TT orients the beveled tip in a horizontal plane and creates a gap between the TT and the bougie, which can cause the TT to catch on the posterior cartilages.

✓ 3 - One-quarter turn counterclockwise (90° to the left) orients the beveled tip in a horizontal plane and tightly against the bougie, which prevents the TT from catching on any supraglottic structures (Modified from Cossham P.S. Difficult intubation. British Journal of Anaesthesia 1985; 57: 239).

(c)

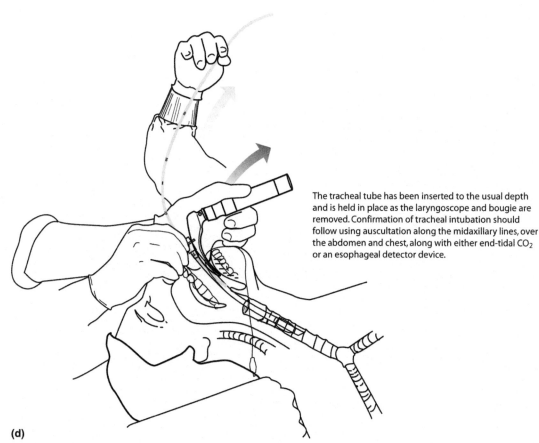

The tracheal tube has been inserted to the usual depth and is held in place as the laryngoscope and bougie are removed. Confirmation of tracheal intubation should follow using auscultation along the midaxillary lines, over the abdomen and chest, along with either end-tidal CO_2 or an esophageal detector device.

(d)

FIGURE 4-20
(*continued*)
(c) passing the tracheal tube, (d) removing blade and bougie. (Courtesy of JM Rich, CRNA [www.slamairway.com]).

brief holdup that is felt at the carina will immediately dissipate, allowing the operator to continue gently advancing the bougie until it comes into contact with a peripheral airway having a diameter less than the diameter of the bougie. At this point, the bougie will firmly hold up [Figure 4-20 B, inset 2]).[46] Advancing the bougie beyond this point could cause penetration and trauma of the airway with subsequent sequellae.[45] Holdup is the second tactile sign, confirming that the bougie has entered the trachea. Holdup should be elicited or sought only if no tracheal clicking is initially appreciated. If the bougie has entered the esophagus, no tracheal clicking or holdup should be felt.

After tactile confirmation of the trachea having been entered, the tip of the introducer should be made to rest at a depth of 25 cm from the corner of the lip and into the midtracheal region of most adult patients. On the Eschmann introducer, the 25 cm point is midway between the double and triple hash mark. (Sun Med placed a black hash line at the 25 cm mark [Figure 4-20 C]). The tracheal tube is then threaded over and railroaded down the bougie while the laryngoscope is held in place. It is best if an assistant initially threads the tracheal tube over the proximal tip of the bougie while the laryngoscopist holds the bougie and the laryngoscope in place. To make it possible for the distal tip of the tracheal tube to enter the mouth, the laryngoscopist needs to release the introducer at this point.

The operator then takes control of the tracheal tube, teasing it gently forward and into the mouth so that the proximal tip of the bougie exits the proximal tip of the tracheal tube. The assistant then grasps the proximal tip of the bougie and controls it so that it cannot be advanced during tracheal tube advancement [Figure 4-20 C]. The tracheal tube is then railroaded over the securely held bougie into the trachea to a depth that is noted at the teeth or gums of approximately 21 cm in women and 23 cm in men. With the tube held firmly in place, the bougie is then withdrawn [Figure 4-20 D], the cuff of the tracheal tube is inflated, and tracheal intubation is confirmed using capnometry or an esophageal detector device as well as a stethoscope.

The key to successful and consistent passage of the tracheal tube over a bougie introducer involves consistent application of two important steps. First, the laryngoscope should not be removed from the patient until the tracheal tube has been inserted into the trachea [Figure 4-20 C]. The laryngoscope blade keeps the pharyngeal tissue from sagging by stretching and tightening the soft tissue in the upper airway, which facilitates advancement of the tracheal tube over the bougie. The bougie is also kept taut, which facilitates passage of the tube over the bougie.[46,56] Second, after the tracheal tube is threaded over the proximal tip of the bougie, the tube should be rotated to the left a quarter turn. This changes the angle of the bevelled tip of the tracheal tube, preventing it from catching on the right posterior arytenoid cartilage. Rotating the tube causes it to slide off the posterior cartilages and eases its passage through the glottic inlet.[46] Leaving the laryngoscope in place and turning the tracheal tube nearly always ensures easy passage of the tracheal tube over the bougie and through the glottic inlet (Figure 4-20 C, inset B).

One study reported[56] that when the laryngoscope was removed and the tracheal tube was not rotated, the tube could be passed through the glottis 50% of the time. When only one or the other of the two maneuvers (scope held in place or tube rotated) was done, the tube could only be passed 75% of the time. However, when both maneuvers were performed (scope held in place and tube rotated), the tube could be advanced through the glottis 100% of the time. These are also important points to consider when encountering difficulty advancing a tracheal tube during flexible fiberoptic intubation or retrograde intubation.

Although the Eschmann introducer is extremely valuable as an airway adjunct and has an impressive clinical track record, it has several limitations. When it becomes soft from age and exposed to high ambient temperatures, it becomes difficult to direct and place the tip behind the epiglottis. Also, when it is softened due to increased heat or age, tracheal clicking is not well transmitted up the shaft. The issue of high ambient temperatures is rarely a problem during hospital use, but during prehospital use, where airway equipment and products are exposed to the environment, it is a concern. Another limitation is the length of the device. When the introducer was first produced, the length of 60 cm was adequate because most practitioners would shorten the tracheal tube by cutting it. This made it easy to grasp the proximal tip of the bougie when a short tube was passed over it. However, today most practitioners do not cut the tracheal tube prior to use. This can make it challenging to grasp and control the proximal end of the bougie when a tracheal tube is threaded over it.

An additional and important concern is infection control. The varnishlike finish on the bougie develops small cracks over time and with repeated use. It is common practice to curl the bougie and carry it in a pocket, which can also cause cracking of the surface. When this manipulation is done at room temperature, cracks may develop in the shaft of the introducer. These cracks can harbor bacteria or viruses, and possibly even prion proteins, and it is uncertain that chemical soaking will completely disinfect them.[57] A single use bougie with a coude tip has recently been introduced (Smiths Medical [Keene, NH]).

To address these limitations, the bougie was redesigned in 2003 by George Cranton, RRT (Largo, FL) and James Michael Rich, CRNA (Rowlett, TX). It was subsequently introduced on the market as the SunMed Endotracheal Tube Introducer (SunMed, Largo, FL).[35] It is as flexible as the gum-elastic bougie but not subject to the same softening by exposure to high ambient temperatures and thus retains its stiffness so that both tracheal clicking and tip placement can be easily accomplished. It is durable and can be bent and curled without cracking or degrading of the surface. With a length of 70 cm, the proximal tip of the introducer is easily accessible before the distal tip of the tracheal tube enters the mouth. The 25 cm mark on the introducer is clearly printed. It is easy to know which way the coude tip is pointing when the introducer is in the airway because the printing along the shaft is printed on the same side as the angled coude tip. Infection control is not an issue because it is delivered individually wrapped and sterile as a single-use item. It should be disposed of immediately after use to prevent cross contamination between patients. SunMed has recently introduced a pediatric version.

The Frova Intubating Introducer (Cook Critical Care, Bloomington, IN) offers the advantage of being able to facilitate jet ventilation/oxygenation through the introducer. It is supplied with and without a stiffening cannula. The pediatric version is 35 cm in length and can accommodate a tracheal tube ≥3 mm I.D. The adult version is 65 cm in length and can accommodate a tracheal tube ≥6 mm I.D. It is also a disposable device.

It is important first to practice bougie-assisted intubation in patients with normal airways, or using cadavers and airway trainers. The technique requires placing the tip of the laryngoscope blade so that a Grade 3 laryngeal view (epiglottis only or portion of the posterior cartilages only) is produced. Then insert the bougie and intubate the patient in the manner described previously. This ensures that when the bougie is needed to rescue a failed intubation, the operator will understand the sequential steps necessary to use the device expertly, and no time will be wasted.

An alternate method of bougie-assisted intubation[43] involves preplacement of the bougie in the tracheal tube prior to use so that the proximal tip of the bougie protrudes from the tracheal tube approximately 5 to 10 cm. Once an optimal laryngeal view is obtained, the bougie and tube are inserted into the mouth and airway as a single unit. The drawback of this method is that the initial presence of the tube over the bougie may decrease the conduction of the tracheal clicking; however, in the hands of a seasoned user who is skilled in bougie insertion, this is not a major disadvantage. The authors do not recommend this technique for novice users who are just learning how to perform bougie-assisted intubation. When first learning bougie-assisted intubation, it is important to learn to recognize and appreciate tracheal clicking.

A new semirigid dilating stylet (RADLyn ETG™, Lake Forest, IL) has a coude tip similar to bougie-type introducers and is designed to be used with a preloaded tracheal tube (Figure 4-21). It is placed into an endotracheal tube in the same fashion as a standard wire stylet. The two major components of the stylet, flexible tip and dilating balloon, function together, affording the laryngoscopist a single-step endotracheal tube guide (ETG), which provides direction like an Eschmann stylet yet also facilitates passage of the ETT into trachea. Difficulty passing an ETT through the glottis over an ETG, such as an Eschmann stylet, or fiberoptic bronchoscope has been well described. Problems occur after the guide is placed within the airway and the ETT is railroaded over the guide, causing the ETT to move posterior during passage and catch on the anatomy of the laryngeal inlet. Subglottic narrowing may also make passage of a standard ETT challenging. Practitioners may use excessive pressure to facilitate passage, creating potential for vocal cord injury and laryngeal-tracheal trauma.

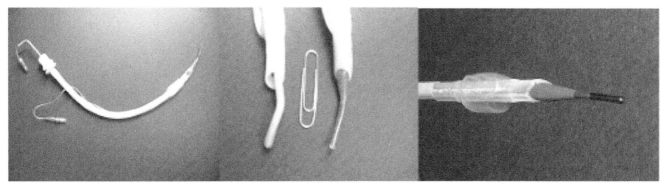

FIGURE 4-21

The RADLyn ETG™ uses a tapered balloon that is designed to open the tissue and thus allow acceptance of the ETT into the trachea and prevent the tracheal tube from catching on supraglottic structures.
(Courtesy of Lindsey A. Nelson, MD)

 It is difficult to intubate the morbidly obese patient unless the patient's shoulders are raised. Raise the shoulders by stacking blankets, pillows, or an elevation pillow to improve direct laryngoscopy of the airway.

Head-Elevated Laryngoscopy Position (HELP)

Simply creating or attempting to create the sniffing position in obese and large-framed individuals will not always facilitate laryngoscopy. Laryngoscopy in these types of patients results in an increased incidence of Cormack and Lehane Grade 3 or 4 views of the airway. What is required to improve the laryngeal view in these patients is to not only elevate the head only but also their shoulders and upper back using a ramp made of linens and pillows or a specially designed wedge elevation pillow (e.g., Troop elevation pillow, Mercury Medical, Clearwater, FL).[12] Levitan has coined the phrase that describes the position created by this procedure as the head-elevated laryngoscopy position (HELP).

The rule of thumb for how much elevation is enough is to draw an imaginary horizontal line through the patient's ear canal along the longitudinal axis of the body (Figure 4-22). The head should be elevated enough so that this imaginary line runs horizontally through the ear canal to the xiphoid process of the patient's chest. With the larger patient lying only on an intubation pillow, this line generally intersects at the midpoint of the shoulder. Performing direct laryngoscopy on such patients without using the HELP position is likely to produce a high incidence of Grade 3 views of the airway (epiglottis only). Without additional maneuvers, this can create difficulty in exposing the glottic inlet and passing a tracheal tube.

In the early 1900s, the greatest pioneer of laryngoscopy, Chevalier Jackson, recommended and used the HELP position routinely during direct laryngoscopy (Figure 4-22). He believed that a certain amount of head extension was usually desirable but that the most important thing was elevation of the upper back and shoulders.[58] He noted that the elevation of the shoulders and upper back was of even more importance than head extension. He felt that the recumbent position with shoulders flat was usually adequate for tracheal intubation; however, during difficult laryngoscopy, elevation of the shoulders provided a definite advantage.[34,58]

For decades, this knowledge lay dormat and was not taught as an option for direct laryngoscopy. However, it has been recently reintroduced by Levitan.[12] Remember that nonobese patients with a normal body mass can usually be intubated using the sniffing position and without using Jackson's raised shoulder position;[12] however, very obese, morbidly obese, superobese, and very large-framed patients almost demand this position to ensure that the glottis can be visualized during direct laryngoscopy.[13] In addition, this position facilitates spontaneous ventilation and preoxygenation in these patients.

Direct Laryngoscopy and Tracheal Intubation 107

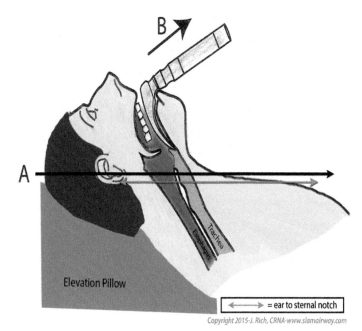

Modification of Chevalier Jackson's Head-Elevated Laryngoscopy Position: **Line-Arrow A**—an imaginary horizontal line should connect the patient's sternal notch with the external auditory meatus. For direct laryngoscopy, the back of the head should never be lower than shown here, and it is always better to have the head raised at least 10 cm above the level of the table. **Line-Arrow B**—the lifting motion is imparted to the tip of the laryngoscope as if to lift the patient by his *hyoid bone* and in the direction indicated by the arrow (Modified from Jackson C and Jackson CL. Direct Laryngoscopy: Figure 44. Schema illustrating the technic of direct laryngoscopy on the recumbent patient, in Bronchosocopy, Esophagoscopy and Gastroscopy: A Manual of Peroral Endoscopy and Laryngeal Surgery. Third Edition. W.B Saunders Company 1934, Philadelphia. Page 99).

FIGURE 4-22
Modification of Chevalier Jackson's head-elevated laryngoscopy position.
(Courtesy of JM Rich, CRNA [www.slamairway.com]).

Contingency Plans for Failed Intubation[10]

Preoxygenation provides a margin of safety should contingency plans become necessary because only a few minutes of critical oxygen deprivation are necessary to permanently injure the brain. Simple techniques such as clearing the upper airway of any possible foreign body obstruction should be done. Adjustment of head position or removal/adjustment of cricoid pressure may be all that is required to improve glottic visualization. Backward pressure over the laryngeal cartilage often improves the view at laryngoscopy, especially in conjunction with the bougie-assisted intubation. It is extremely important to appreciate that after every forceful laryngoscopic intubation attempt, the amount of airway edema and bleeding can increase, leading to a progressive decreased ability to successfully perform BVM ventilation and a change in the situation from cannot-intubate to cannot mask-ventilate. For this reason, intubation attempts should be undertaken by an experienced laryngoscopist and limited to three attempts and not to exceed more than 10 minutes.

If the patient desaturates (SpO$_2$ ≤ 92), an oral and/or nasal airway should be inserted and the patient's lungs ventilated with 100% oxygen using both jaw-thrust and chin-lift maneuvers. Extra help should be called for early. The patient's head and neck should be repositioned (if cervical-spine precautions are not in effect) to permit optimal BVM ventilation. Cervical-spine precautions must be maintained as clinically indicated. A tight seal should be obtained with the mask. Using the two-person BVM ventilation technique (Figure 3-22 B), the most experienced operator should apply the mask to the face and position the upper airway using a bilateral jaw-thrust and chin-lift maneuvers, while a second individual squeezes the bag to provide ventilation.

Cricoid pressure should be maintained continuously unless it interferes with ventilation (Figure 3-19).[59] If the SpO$_2$ cannot be maintained at greater than 92% despite use of these optimal ventilation attempts, or the trachea cannot be intubated after 10 minutes or after several optimal attempts using direct laryngoscopy (by an experienced laryngoscopist), employ rescue ventilation using a Combitube or LMA. These devices normally provide greater airway protection than that offered using a bag-valve-mask with oral or nasal airway.[37,60,61] Rescue ventilation using a Combitube or LMA should usually suffice if oxygenation is not reestablished by bag-valve-mask ventilation. A definitive airway can then be inserted using another intubation technique after the patient is reoxygenated with rescue ventilation.[3] If rescue ventilation fails, a surgical airway may be required using either transtracheal jet ventilation or cricothyrotomy. Cricothyroidotomy may then later be converted to a tracheostomy under controlled conditions.

Summary

This chapter has provided a thorough introduction to direct laryngoscopy and tracheal intubation. In intubation, all aspects are of nearly equal importance. For instance, thorough preparation and checking of equipment is just as important as proper use of the laryngoscope. As with anything, fundamentals are the key to success. Attention to detail in provision of optimal laryngoscopy, use of simple adjunctive techniques to rescue intubation, and team work improves success. Remember that providing and monitoring ventilation and oxygenation always takes priority over tracheal intubation.

REVIEW QUESTIONS

1. List five general indications for tracheal intubation.

2. Name three critical airway events.

3. Why should the patient's head be placed in the sniffing position prior to intubation, unless contraindicated?

4. At what level of oxygen saturation should the intubation attempt be stopped and the patient reoxygenated?

5. Name three laryngoscopic pitfalls.

6. How can the gum-elastic bougie assist in a difficult intubaton?

7. How is the head-elevated laryngoscopy position (HELP) employed?

CHAPTER 5

Confirmation of Tracheal Intubation and Monitoring of Lung Ventilation

James Michael Rich
Michael A. Frakes

Chapter Objectives

After reading this chapter, you should be able to:

- Describe the pitfalls to successful intubation in the prehospital environment.

- Discuss techniques for detecting misplaced ET tubes.

- Describe the advantages, disadvantages, and functions of the esophageal detector device (EDD).

- Describe the advantages, disadvantages, and functions of capnometry.

- List the requirements for adequate monitoring of ventilation during patient transport.

- Discuss oxygen saturation and how it relates to ventilation.

- Describe how to interpret a capnograph properly.

- Explain how acid-base values correlate to ventilation and how acid-base imbalances are best managed.

CASE Study _____

Medic 4 is dispatched to an unconscious person near a local bar. When they arrive, the paramedics are directed to the side of the building where a man has been found in an alley. After checking the scene for safety, they approach but get no response from the man. He is lying in a pool of vomit. The patient is deeply cyanosed, and there are no signs of breathing, so they immediately take control of the head and neck and turn the patient onto his back. While one paramedic opens the airway using a jaw-thrust maneuver, the other suctions the mouth, but large particles of food keep clogging the tip of the suction catheter.

Breathing does not return, so an oropharyngeal airway is inserted and rescue ventilation is commenced using a bag-valve-mask (BVM) device. A radial pulse is felt, so intubation equipment is prepared and direct laryngoscopy is performed with the head and neck held in neutral alignment. Despite more suctioning, secretions obscure the view of the larynx as the endotracheal tube (ETT) is inserted. A self-inflating bulb (SIB) is applied, but the refill time is delayed, so the crew decide to remove the ETT and resume mask ventilation.

After reoxygenation and further suctioning, a second attempt is made to intubate using a longer blade. This time, the vocal cords can be seen quite clearly, and the ETT is inserted without difficulty. The SIB is reapplied, and it refills rapidly. Bilateral breath sounds are heard on ventilation with no epigastric sounds.

Precautions are taken in case of spinal injury, and the patient is transferred to the ambulance. While on the way to the hospital, an end-tidal carbon dioxide (ETCO$_2$) monitor is attached, an IV cannula is inserted, and the blood glucose is found to be normal. The patient is still making no attempt to breathe and his pupils are constricted, but there is no response to IV naloxone.

After a while, the paramedic finds difficulty in bagging the patient, and a typical shark-fin waveform is noted on the capnogram. Suctioning down the tube fails to resolve the situation, and the pulse oximeter shows that the SpO$_2$ level is beginning to fall. The paramedic immediately removes the ETT and restarts BVM ventilation with good rise and fall of the chest. After reoxygenation of the patient, a new ETT is inserted, and both lung compliance and capnographic waveform are found to be normal. The original tube is examined, and its distal end is found to be partially occluded by food material. No further problems are encountered during the remainder of the journey.

Introduction

The incidence of failed intubation varies and depends on the clinical situation.[1-8] Unique pitfalls such as noise, temperature, exposure, chaotic environment, ambient light availability, entrapment, and frequent patient movements exist in the prehospital environment, making it the most challenging location for confirming tracheal intubation and monitoring lung ventilation. However, failure to detect a misplaced endotracheal tube either initially or from an unplanned extubation depends not on the clinical situation but rather on the availability and application of physical examination techniques and evidenced-based confirmation methods such as **end-tidal carbon dioxide (ETCO$_2$)** detection and esophageal detection devices (EDDs).

An early prehospital study that predates the use of portable capnography reported three undetected esophageal intubations.[9] More than two decades later, long after the availability of evidence-based detection methods, Katz et al. reported a 25% occurrence of undetected misplaced endotracheal tubes by paramedics, with 17% of all patients delivered to the hospital with an undetected esophageal intubation.[10] Wang et al. studied 783 adults undergoing prehospital intubation and reported two cases of delayed recognition of esophageal intubation, one case of unrecognized esophageal intubation, and 22 cases of tube dislodgement during patient care or transport.[11] Another important study looked at 208 field paramedic intubations (76.9% medical and 23.1% trauma patients) over a six-month period. Emergency physicians using a combination of direct visualization, EDD, ETCO$_2$, and physical examination verified endotracheal tube placement on arrival at the hospital. A total of 5.8% tracheal tubes were incorrectly placed outside the trachea: 6.3% medical patients and 4.2% trauma patients. Of the misplaced tracheal tubes, a nonphysical (evidence-based) exam verification device was used in 25% and not used in 75%.[12]

Intubation failure continues to occur to some extent across the spectrum of health care and in all practice locations.[13-15] Failure to detect misplaced tracheal tubes results from not using an evidence-based method of detection and is rarely associated with a lack of operator skill.[16]

The bottom line is that all tracheal intubations must be confirmed using a nonphysical exam technique such as ETCO$_2$ or an EDD.[17,18-26] Continuous monitoring of lung ventilation by an evidence-based method must be employed throughout the period of prehospital treatment and transport.[17]

end-tidal carbon dioxide (ETCO$_2$)

The measurement of the CO$_2$ concentration at the end of expiration.

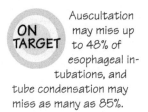

ON TARGET Auscultation may miss up to 48% of esophageal intubations, and tube condensation may miss as many as 85%.

capnography, p. 119

capnometry, p. 115

end-tidal carbon dioxide
(ETCO$_2$), p. 112

esophageal detector device
(EDD), p. 113

peak inspiratory pressure
(PIP), p. 125

Confirmation of Tracheal Intubation

Immediately after a tracheal intubation attempt, the tube position must be verified, even when the tube has been directly observed to pass through the vocal cords with a Cormack and Lehane Grade 1 view. Maintain manual control of the endotracheal tube until confirmation of midtracheal placement is confirmed and the tube is firmly secured. While one person ventilates, the responsible rescuer auscultates over the stomach. If air sounds are auscultated, cease ventilation immediately to prevent further gastric inflation and remove the tube with a suctioning catheter inserted. Oxygenation must be maintained by mask ventilation or a supraglottic alternative airway using positive-pressure ventilation along with Sellick's maneuver until intubation is reattempted. After the exclusion of sounds over the stomach, auscultation is performed bilaterally over both lungs in all four thoracic quadrants and along the midaxillary lines.

If the breath sounds differ and a pneumothorax has been excluded, then the tip of the tracheal tube is most likely positioned in one of the mainstem bronchi. After deflating the cuff, the tube is pulled back until breath sounds are equal bilaterally. Whenever tube position is unclear, laryngoscopy can be performed to determine whether the tube is lying between the vocal cords. When in doubt, remove the tube and resume oxygenation and ventilation by positive-pressure mask ventilation.

Beyond chest auscultation, clinical signs routinely used to confirm tracheal intubation include observing the rise and fall of the chest, condensation of water vapor in the tube lumen (fogging of the tube), presence or absence of abdominal distention during ventilation, and reassuring compliance of the reservoir bag used for ventilation. The use of any or all of these clinical signs alone is unreliable,[17,26-31] and their fallibility has been well described: auscultation may miss up to 48% of esophageal intubations, and tube condensation may miss as many as 85%.[31] The use of these techniques without an evidence-based nonphysical exam confirmation technique can lead to disastrous and irreversible consequences.[9,10,31,32]

During changes in location or patient position in the course of treatment, tube position must be reassessed. The tracheal tube should be held with one hand in addition to other fixation whenever the patient is moved.

esophageal detector device (EDD)

Either a syringe with an adapter that fits on an ET tube, or a bulb syringe designed to attach to the ET tube. When the plunger on the syringe is drawn back, and if the tube is properly placed, the syringe should immediately and easily fill with air. The bulb syringe is depressed and the air is forced out of it; then it is attached to the ET tube. If the tube is correctly placed, the bulb syringe should fill rapidly.

Esophageal Detector Device (EDD)

Simple, effective, and reliable, the **esophageal detector device (EDD)** works independently of, or in concert with, traditional clinical methods to determine tube location.[33-39] The EDD is effective because of the structural differences between the trachea and esophagus.[24] When an EDD is attached to an endotracheal tube that is communicating with the trachea and negative pressure is applied, it will rapidly draw in gas from the dead space of the rigidly patent trachea as well as gas within the lungs. In contrast, if the tube is communicating with the flat peristaltic esophagus, which collapses under negative pressure, the EDD is prevented from drawing in gas.[27,40] However, because the EDD will draw in gas regardless of the gas source, or not reinflate regardless of what is causing a blockage, it is considered to be only "near failsafe."[24] Nevertheless, with few exceptions, it is considered reliable for confirming tracheal intubation or detecting esophageal placement of a tracheal tube.[40-43] For this reason, it has received a Class IIa rating (recommended) from the American Heart Association Guidelines 2005 with regard to confirmation of tracheal intubation.[17]

 Failure to detect a misplaced ET tube is rarely associated with poor operator skill; rather, it occurs from failure to use an evidence-based method of tube placement verification.

 Tube position must be verified using an evidence-based system, even when the tube is observed passing through the cords. Further, the methods used to verify tube placement must be documented completely.

Wee's[38,39] original EDD consisted of a 60 cc syringe, which was attached to an endotracheal tube lying in the trachea. The syringe EDD is marketed as the Postitube (Performance Systems, Houston, TX) and the Ambu Tubecheck Syringe Type (Ambu, Ballerup, Denmark-Ballerup, Denmark). An improved variant of the EDD is the self-inflating bulb (SIB) (Figure 5-1a),[33,44] a simplification of Wee's original device[38] that offers the same evidence-based[45] effectiveness and reliability of the original device.[26,27,30,34,38,40,46] The operator squeezes the bulb, attaches it to the tracheal tube, and releases it (Figure 5-1b). A rapid refill of the bulb is indicative of tracheal intubation. No refill or a very slow refill is indicative of esophageal placement or tube obstruction. The device is inexpensive, simple, and easy to operate with one hand.

The EDD is highly reliable for confirmation of tracheal intubation and detection of esophageal intubation in healthy patients.[30,34,38,39,43,46,47] However, there are limitations and concerns with specific coexisting diseases, physiological alterations, and clinical situations.[36,37,48-53] Both false negatives (failure to confirm endotracheal intubation) and false positives (failure to detect esophageal intubation) occur. Because the EDD will not reinflate regardless of the source of an obstruction, false negative signs[37] have been reported in infants;[52] morbid obesity;[49,53,54] main stem bronchus intubation;[39] high airway resistance such as bronchospastic disease; and tube obstruction with blood, vomit, secretions, carinal tissue, or a kink.[39,50] False negatives associated with morbid obesity were less frequent when the EDD was compressed prior to being attached to the endotracheal tube (2.4% versus 4.6%). The mechanism is primarily caused by a relative reduction in airway diameter, an extreme decrease in functional residual capacity, and "collapse of large airways owing to invagination of the posterior tracheal wall when subatmospheric pressure is generated by the EDD."[53] The common denominator in all these situations is that a clinical situation exists that causes less existence of gas than normal to be available, which thus prevents rapid refill of the EDD.

The EDD must be of the correct size to accurately detect esophageal intubation. The recommended size for the EDD is 75 cc. Using a smaller diameter can elicit a false positive because the increased elastic recoil of a smaller bulb can overcome the resistance of the esophageal tissue and allow the bulb to reinflate when attached to the tracheal tube in the esophageal position.[36] Concern exists that esophageal ventilation[55] secondary to positive pressure or mouth-to-mouth ventilation prior to endotracheal intubation could distend the stomach and dilate the esophagus with gas, producing a false positive when the EDD is used. Salem et al. showed that modest insufflation of the stomach during esophageal ventilation by mask does not decrease the effectiveness of the EDD,[47] but another report found false positives when the syringe-aspiration-type EDD was used following esophageal ventilation through a tracheal tube resting in the esophagus.[56]

ON TARGET A false negative is said to exist when a test result implys a condition does not exist when in fact it does.

ON TARGET A false positive is said to exist when a test result implys a condition exists when in fact it does not.

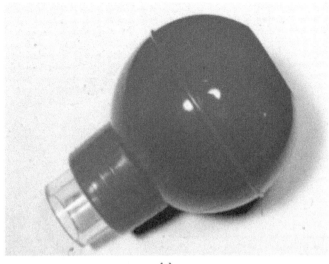

(a)

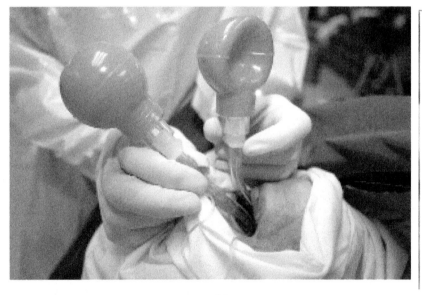

(b)

FIGURE 5-1

(a) The self-inflating bulb is used in patients with a nonperfusing cardiac rhythm and is a near-failsafe method of detecting esophageal intubation. (b) The tracheal tube with the collapsed bulb is in the esophagus, and the tracheal tube with the expanded bulb is in the trachea.

(Courtesy of JM Rich, CRNA [www.slamairway.com])

A critical clinical situation that produced a false positive with the EDD has been reported by Baraka et al.,[48] who elicited false positives in 30% of patients having cesarean sections under general endotracheal anesthesia. This was thought to be secondary to a pregnancy-induced decrease in lower esophageal sphincter (LES) tone in conjunction with lower intra-esophageal pressures and higher intragastric pressures from hormonal and mechanical factors of pregnancy. The result is retrograde gas leakage through the LES, causing the EDD to reinflate when communicating with the esophagus.[48]

Capnometry

capnometry

The measurement of expired carbon dioxide.

Capnometry measures the level of carbon dioxide (CO_2) in respiratory gases.[57] It is the gold standard for confirmation of tube placement and monitoring of lung ventilation, but its limitations must be understood.[24,43] All CO_2 detectors are classified as "near failsafe"[24] because

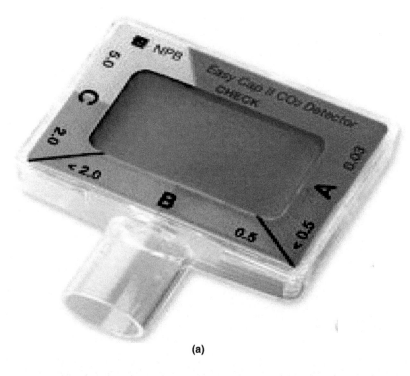

(a)

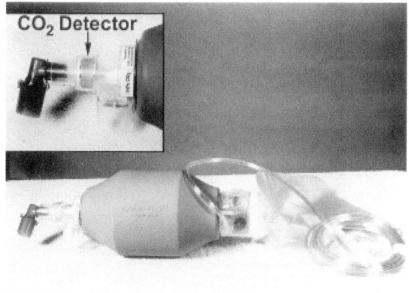

(b)

FIGURE 5-2

Examples of qualitative carbon dioxide detectors: (a) Easycap II, Nellcor Puritan Bennett. (b) Capno-Flo™ Nellcor Puritan Bennett Capnoflo™.

(Courtesy of Nellcor Puritan Bennett)

> **ON TARGET**
>
> *Capnometry is the gold standard for verification of tube placement and monitoring of ventilation.*

of the occasional occurrence of both false negatives (no detection of CO_2 in spite of the tube communicating with the trachea)[19] and false positives (detection of CO_2 with the tube communicating with the esophagus).[58] Confirming tracheal intubation and monitoring lung ventilation can be accomplished using disposable qualitative colorimetric CO_2 detectors (Figure 5-2), portable quantitative electronic CO_2 detectors (Figure 5-3), or capnographs (Figure 5-4). All three detect the presence of CO_2 in exhaled air. The colorimetric devices are qualitative only, while electronic versions are quantitative, and the capnograph displays both

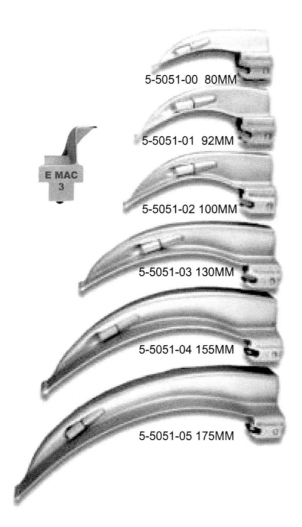

5-5051-00 80MM

5-5051-01 92MM

E MAC 3

5-5051-02 100MM

5-5051-03 130MM

5-5051-04 155MM

5-5051-05 175MM

FIGURE 4-7
A recent modification to the Macintosh English Profile blade is the reduced flange E-Mac™.
(Courtesy of Sun Med USA, Largo, FL [www.airwaystore.com])

the reduced-flange E-Mac™ (Figure 4-7). It enables the user to exert less force on maxillary incisors while allowing more movement at the distal end to assist in visualizing the vocal cords.

The two commonly used straight blades are the Miller, which has a curved tip, and the Wisconsin (Figure 4-8) (and its modified forms), which has a straight tip.[32] The Miller, which was developed by the late Dr. Robert A. Miller of San Antonio, Texas, is the most popular straight blade. The size of the flange is reduced to minimize trauma, and the curve of the tip is extended to improve lift of the epiglottis. These improvements were incorporated to facilitate greater exposure of the larynx in difficult patients.[33] Another commonly seen straight blade is the Phillips (Figure 4-9), which integrates the preferred straight Jackson blade design[34] with the curved distal tip Miller design, providing greater visibility and an almost direct-line approach to the trachea during intubation.[33]

The smallest blade sizes are the #00 in the Miller type and the #1 in the Macintosh. The largest blade size is a #4 in both the Miller and the Macintosh. Each of the standard blades has a left-sided flange for distracting the tongue to the left and keeping it out of the line of sight, and an open side on the right for visualization of the larynx and insertion of the tracheal tube. Airway management kits should have a functioning laryngoscope with blades of various sizes. At a minimum, an adult kit should contain a #2 and #3 Miller (or another straight blade) and a #3 and #4 Macintosh blade. This will enable intubation of almost any size of adult patient. The #2 Miller blades can also be used in children, if needed. Extra batteries should also be available along with extra bulbs, and the light from the laryngoscope should be intensely bright to the point that it makes the operator squint should it be viewed directly.

Conventional handles fit only conventional blades, and fiberoptic handles fit only fiberoptic blades. Fiberoptic blades and handles usually have a green mark for rapid recognition. Regular checking of the kit should prevent mixing of the two in the same kit. If a nondisposable blade is used, it should be placed in a contamination bag (available in the kit)

Direct Laryngoscopy and Tracheal Intubation

Table 5-1 Language of Capnography

- **Capnometry.** The measurement of expired CO_2. It typically provides a numeric display of the partial pressure of CO_2 (in Torr or mmHg) or the percentage of CO_2 present.
- **Capnography.** A graphic recording or display of the capnometry reading over time.
- **Capnograph.** A device that measures expired CO_2 levels.
- **Capnogram.** The visual representation of the expired CO_2 waveform.
- **End-tidal carbon dioxide ($ETCO_2$).** The measurement of the CO_2 concentration at the end of expiration.
- **$PETCO_2$.** The partial pressure of end-tidal CO_2 in a mixed gas solution.
- **$PaCO_2$.** Represents the partial pressure of CO_2 in the arterial blood.

Used with permission from Bledsoe et al., *Paramedic Care: Principles and Practice*, Volume 1, page 532.

PEARLS An end-tidal CO_2 detector may stop functioning correctly if the paper in it becomes moist. from a humidified gas mixture or vapor in the exhaled gas.

Disposable qualitative colorimetric carbon dioxide detectors (e.g,. Easycap II, Tyco Nellcor Puritan Bennett, Pleasanton, CA) (Figure 5-2a) chemically elicit a color change in the presence of carbon dioxide. The intensity of the color change is directly proportional to the level of CO_2, and three ranges of CO_2 can be measured by matching the color of the filter to the reference colors on the dome. Depending on the source of ambient light, the color changes may be lessened or increased. The detector's color chart is for use in fluorescent lighting, and a separate color chart is included for use with incandescent lighting. The detector has a shelf life of fifteen months in the unopened factory-sealed foil package. Once opened, it may function for as little as fifteen minutes if the patient is breathing a humidified gas mixture or for much longer with minimal humidity.[24,57,62]

Colorimetric detectors have also been manufactured as a device contained within the exhalation port of bag-valve devices (Capno-Flo™ Single-Patient-Use Resuscitation Bag, Tyco Nellcor Puritan Bennett, Pleasanton, CA) (Figure 5-2b). The Capno-Flo resuscitator is useful in the initial confirmation of ETT position but may be indeterminate for monitoring of lung ventilation during postintubation management because, unlike the Easycap II, color change can become difficult to recognize after initial confirmation of intubation.[63]

False negative results from capnometry occur when a tracheal tube communicates with the trachea and lungs but there is no detection of carbon dioxide. A low or absent CO_2 measurement does not, in and of itself, indicate lack of lung ventilation. Clinical situations in which CO_2 may not be detected by any type of CO_2 detector include low cardiac output states and the presence of very fast ventilatory rates.[24,57,62] Hemodynamic instability secondary to cardiac arrest, ineffective CPR, or profound hypovolemic shock decreases the amount of blood in the pulmonary circulation and thus the amount of CO_2 available for detection.[24,62] Therefore, in profound shock or CPR, a low or absent CO_2 measurement during ventilation does not necessarily indicate absence of lung ventilation. Accordingly, CO_2 detectors may be less reliable in monitoring lung ventilation in patients with nonperfusing cardiac rhythms or low cardiac output states.[18,19,24,62] In these situations, the additional information from a capnograph may be more helpful than a qualitative colorimetric or electronic device.

A false positive reading happens when CO_2 is detected from a tube that is communicating with the esophagus and stomach. The stomach may occasionally harbor residual carbon dioxide from esophageal ventilation of expired air into the stomach during mouth-to-mouth rescue breathing, during positive-pressure mask ventilation,[64] or after ingestion of carbonated beverages or antacids containing bicarbonate.[58] When CO_2 resides in the stomach or

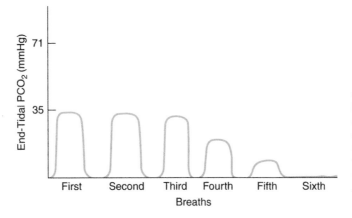

FIGURE 5-5

Cola complication. CO_2 is initially detected following esophageal intubation. A counterfeit CO_2 waveform initially appears but, after five to six ventilatory cycles, it diminishes and then disappears as carbon dioxide is cleared from the stomach.

the esophagus from any of these sources, it can be detected and briefly sustained by a carbon dioxide detection device during positive-pressure ventilation via a tube placed in the esophagus. However, a capnographic device in this situation will produce a waveform that is inconsistent with the typical shape generated by exhalation from the lung (e.g., cola complication, Figure 5-5).[58] Nonetheless, six to twelve ventilations are recommended[24,65] prior to completely relying on a colorimetric CO_2 detector[24,65-67] and no fewer than five ventilations[24,41,58] before relying on an electronic CO_2 detector. Continued CO_2 detection after these ventilations adequately confirms proper tube placement and lung ventilation.[24,37,65]

PEARLS A patient who has received rescue breathing or ingested a carbonated beverage or antacid containing bicarbonate recently prior to intubation may have carbon dioxide in the stomach, which may register a false positive in the event of an esophageal intubation. Therefore, the rescuer needs to give 6 to 12 ventilations before a reliable CO_2 level reading can be obtained.

ON TARGET A PetCO$_2$ of less than 10 mm Hg is a reliable predictor of nonsurvival of cardiac arrest.

In comparing EDD and ETCO$_2$ devices, some express concern about the performance of ETCO$_2$ measures for patients in cardiac arrest. Bozeman et al., for example, found the EDD more accurate than ETCO$_2$ monitoring in the emergency patient population because of greater accuracy in cardiac-arrest patients.[40] Others have reported that ETCO$_2$ successfully detects endotracheal tube placement in cardiac arrest[68] and have concluded that EDD and ETCO$_2$ are of equal reliability.[69,70] Overall, capnometry is 93% sensitive and 97% specific in detecting tracheal intubation.[71]

Use of an Intubating Stylet to Confirm Tracheal Intubation or Detect Esophageal Intubation

The use of an bougie introducer to distinguish between esophageal and tracheal placement of a tracheal tube has been described;[64] however, it has not been investigated for reliability and safety. One of this chapter's contributors, James Michael Rich, has used this technique with success when a self-inflating bulb (SIB) was indeterminate in a morbidly obese patient with a nonperfusing cardiac rhythm. The coude tip of the stylet normally clicks as it bumps against the tracheal rings. In the esophagus, no such clicking is appreciated. If the tracheal tube (TT) is in the trachea, holdup of the stylet should occur at a shallower depth than it would occur if the TT were in the esophagus (Figure 5-6). As the stylet is advanced, carinal holdup should be experienced at approximately 28 to 32 cm in the adult.[64] The depth markings on the stylet indicate at what depth holdup is first appreciated. This method is only of value only when

FIGURE 5-6
Use of a 70-cm coude-tipped intubating stylet (SunMed Bougie Introducer, Largo, FL, www.airway-store.com) to distinguish tracheal from esophageal tracheal tube placement. Holdup occurs much deeper in the esophageal-placed tracheal tube and occurs at a much shallower depth in the tracheally placed tracheal tube.
(Courtesy of JM Rich, CRNA [www.slamairway.com])

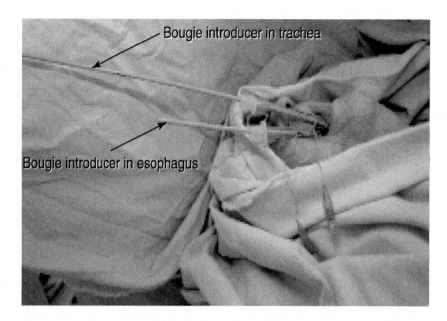

Bougie introducer in trachea

Bougie introducer in esophagus

capnography
A graphic recording or display of the capnometry reading overtime.

capnography or an EDD is indeterminate and is not otherwise recommended. If this method is employed, the stylet should be advanced gently to prevent bronchial perforation. It must always be remembered that taking a second look after intubation and visualizing laryngeal anatomy around the tube is considered failsafe in confirming tracheal intubation.[24]

Ongoing Monitoring of Lung Ventilation

Continuous monitoring of lung ventilation should commence with positive-pressure mask ventilation and continue after confirmation of tracheal intubation.[72] The potential for unplanned events and patient deterioration during transport is well documented: nearly two-thirds of patients experience adverse physiological changes during intrahospital transport, and equipment failures complicate up to 13.4% of those transports.[73-76]

Respiratory changes are particularly common during the transport of intubated patients because arterial carbon dioxide tension and pH changes occur in 70% to 100% of such patients. Although the use of a transport ventilator reduces the likelihood of such changes, it does not prevent them. Hyperventilation and hypoventilation occur, but an unintentional respiratory alkalosis is at least 2.5 times as common as an unintentional respiratory acidosis.[77-80] Hemodynamic changes may correlate with the blood gas changes: hyperventilation can result in increased intrathoracic pressures and decreased preload, while myocardial pH changes are arrhythmogenic and can adversely affect cardiac function.[78]

PEARLS Unintentional respiratory alkalosis is 2.5 times more likely to occur than an unintentional respiratory acidosis in the intubated patient.

Adequate monitoring of the intubated patient includes careful tracking of the vital signs, level of consciousness, oxygen saturation, PETCO$_2$, and mechanical ventilator parameters, if a mechanical ventilator is used.

Vital Signs

Monitoring of routine vital signs can provide an indication of respiratory system changes or respiratory distress. In the presence of acute respiratory failure, the respiratory rate usually increases but the tidal volume becomes shallower. If the respiratory failure is due to the effects of narcotics or other drugs that depress the respiratory center in the brain, the respiratory rate and tidal volume usually decreases. Heart rate generally increases in the face of progressive respiratory failure because the heart compensates to take more oxygen to the tissues. Beyond this, the patient's level of consciousness also plays a role in monitoring. Is the patient lethargic or agitated? Is he or she able to communicate appropriately, or does he or she have a decreased level of consciousness? If the patient does have a decreased level of consciousness, is it a result of hypoxia, fatigue, or something else? Without monitoring, it is difficult to get good answers to clinical questions or to assess the patient or evaluate the effect of treatment.

Oxygen Saturation

Advantages of the pulse oximeter include its portability, availability, and accuracy. However, a clear understanding of the oxyhemoglobin dissociation curve is necessary for correct interpretation of the readings obtained (Figure 5-7). Oxygen saturation reflects the percentage of hemoglobin that is bound with oxygen, and it must be clearly understood that it is not the same as the pO_2, the partial pressure of oxygen dissolved in plasma.

The low oxygen saturation alarm of most pulse oximeters is defaulted to alarm at 90% because as the saturation decreases below that level, the PaO_2 begins to rapidly decline. Therefore, if the patient's SpO_2 begins to trend downward, measures should be taken to increase the oxygen saturation. One other important point is that pulse oximetry is generally within ±2% of the true saturation of hemoglobin measured from an arterial blood sample (SaO_2). Clinically, this means that an SpO_2 of 90% could actually represent an SaO_2 from 88% to 92%.

Hypoxemia is generally considered to be present when SaO_2 is below 90%, so to ensure that the vast majority of patients have an SaO_2 higher than 90%, it is probably best to maintain their SpO_2 at greater than 92%. This is why the SLAM Universal Adult Flowchart uses a sustained SpO_2 of ≤92% as the threshold for changing a treatment option and why Mason's PU-92 concept (Chapter 1 and SUAAF flowchart) uses an SpO_2 of ≤92% as one of the indications of a crash airway.[20,23,81]

 PEARLS Hypoxemia is generally considered to be present when SaO_2 it at or below 90%.

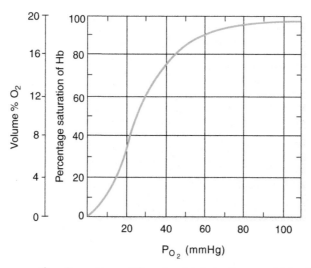

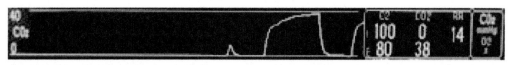

FIGURE 5-8
A capnographic waveform instantly reappears after a previously disconnected breathing circuit is reconnected and ventilation is reestablished.

(Courtesy of JM Rich, CRNA [www.slamairway.com])

End-Tidal Carbon Dioxide ($ETCO_2$)

Endotracheal tube migration or circuit integrity interruption can be as catastrophic as an undetected esophageal intubation, especially for patients with inadequate spontaneous breathing. Disconnection of the ventilator circuit generally changes the capnogram frequency and $PetCO_2$ (Figure 5-8).[59] End-tidal changes in hypoventilating patients precede pulse oximetry changes and can provide sufficient advance warning to prevent patient deterioration.[82,83]

The capnogram and $PetCO_2$ demonstrate other abnormalities as well. The normal capnogram has a characteristic square shape (Figure 5-9), and the different portions of the waveform correlate with different phases of the breathing cycle. In Figure 5-9, the normal capnogram has a horizontal baseline during inhalation (segment A-B) because it is carbon dioxide–free. The wave rises with the start of exhalation as carbon dioxide begins moving across the sensor (segment B-C). As exhalation continues (segment C-D), the CO_2 waveform is a gently rising plateau. At the end of that plateau, point D on the figure, the $PETCO_2$ is measured. When inhalation begins, there is a rapid downstroke on the capnograph as inspired air moves across the sensor and replaces exhaled carbon dioxide (segment D-E).

If the ETT is partially obstructed by secretions or a kink, the waveform changes from the characteristic square shape to one with an increasingly sloped alveolar plateau as expiratory resistance increases (Figure 5-10). These changes precede changes in the $PetCO_2$ value itself, which requires that the tube be occluded by at least half.[40,84] The slope of the expiratory plateau also correlates well with expiratory obstruction from bronchospastic disease.[85] An

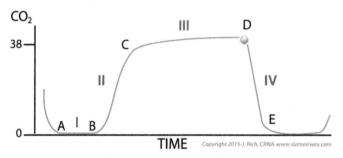

FIGURE 5-9
Normal capnogram.

AB = Phase I: late inspiration, early expiration (no CO_2).
BC = Phase II: appearance of CO_2 in exhaled gas.
CD = Phase III: plateau (constant CO_2).
D = highest point ($ETCO_2$).
DE = Phase IV: rapid descent during expiration.
EC = respiratory pause.

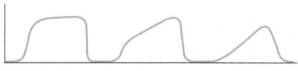

FIGURE 5-10
Capnogram with partial endotracheal tube obstruction. The alveolar plateau slopes upward in relationship to the increased expiratory resistance.

(Courtesy of Michael A. Frakes)

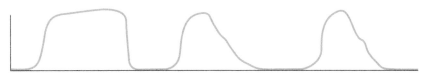

FIGURE 5-11
Downsloping capnographic waveform. Capnogram reflecting expiratory leak in endotracheal tube cuff or ventilator circuit. Rather than normal exhalation as demonstrated in the first wave, exhaled gas leaks out rapidly, and the normal plateau shape is lost.
(Courtesy of Michael A. Frakes)

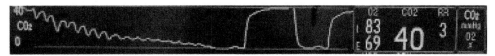

FIGURE 5-12
Cardiogenic oscillations of the diaphragm are seen during very slow ventilation rates.
(Courtesy of JM Rich, CRNA [www.slamairway.com])

expiratory leak in the circuit or the ETT cuff results in a premature return of the exhaled waveform to the baseline as well as a loss of the expected square shape (Figure 5-11).[59,86]

A waveform with an oscillating pattern on the exhalation C-D (III) portion of the capnogram is seen during low ventilation rates and is known as cardiogenic oscillations. It is a manifestation of the heartbeat causing oscillations of the diaphram (Figure 5-12). Finally, lost minute ventilation from an air leak increases $PetCO_2$ with a normal waveform, while rebreathing due to an expiratory time that is too short or an inadequate inspiratory flow rate will increase $PetCO_2$ and show a rising capnogram baseline (Figure 5-13).[59,87] Table 5-2 summarizes the correlations between capnographic changes and clinical conditions.

In addition to monitoring the airway circuit, capnometry can provide useful physiological information about ventilation and perfusion. Arterial carbon dioxide levels are affected by both metabolic and ventilatory changes, and ventilation is a primary method of managing acid-base balance.

Oxygen saturation does not equal arterial oxygen tension, and end-tidal carbon dioxide measures do not equal arterial carbon dioxide tensions. The alveolar end-tidal carbon dioxide gradient $[P(a-ET)CO_2]$ is generally 3 to 5 mm Hg. Changes in pulmonary dead space and other factors affect this difference. The anatomical space that is ventilated but not perfused (other than the pharynx, trachea, and bronchi) is the physiologic dead space. It is measured nearly perfectly by the $P(a-ET)CO_2$ gradient, which widens as dead space increases.[59] When pulmonary blood flow decreases for any reason, dead space increases. Decreased cardiac output decreases pulmonary blood flow and increases pulmonary dead space. Causes include cardiac dysfunction, positive end-expiratory pressure (PEEP) use, hypovolemia, pulmonary emboli, and patient position. Other factors, such as age, smoking, general anesthesia, and major systemic disease, can also change the gradient, increasing it to as high as 20 mm Hg in patients with severe disease. The gradient can also be negative in some cases.[59,88-92] When studied specifically in patients during out-of-hospital transport, the mean gradient was between 7.3 and 12.9 mm Hg, with relationships that worsened as underlying disease worsened.[93,94]

For the relatively short duration of most patient transports, capnometry is a useful patient monitor. Over the course of a transport, patients are generally maintained in the same position, and transport is generally short enough to preclude a substantial metabolic change.

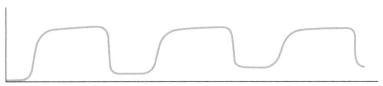

FIGURE 5-13
Rising baseline reflecting increased $PETCO_2$ from rebreathing CO_2 due to an inadequate inspiratory flow rate.
(Courtesy of Michael A. Frakes)

Confirmation of Tracheal Intubation and Monitoring of Lung Ventilation

Table 5-2 Basic Rules of Capnography

Symptom	Possible Cause
Sudden drop of $ETCO_2$ to zero	• Esophageal intubation • Ventilator disconnection or defect in ventilator • Defect in CO_2 analyzer
Sudden decrease of $ETCO_2$ (not to zero)	• Leak in ventilator system; obstruction • Partial disconnect in ventilator circuit • Partial airway obstruction (secretions)
Exponential decrease of $ETCO_2$	• Pulmonary embolism • Cardiac arrest • Hypotension (sudden) • Severe hyperventilation
Change in CO_2 baseline	• Calibration error • Crack in sampling tubing • Sampling tubing connection not well seated • Water droplet in analyzer • Mechanical failure (ventilator)
Sudden increase in $ETCO_2$	• Accessing an area of lung previously obstructed • Release of tourniquet • Sudden increase in blood pressure
Gradual lowering of $ETCO_2$	• Hypovolemia • Decreasing cardiac output • Decreasing body temperature; hypothermia; drop in metabolism
Gradual increase in $ETCO_2$	• Rising body temperature • Hypoventilation • CO_2 absorption • Partial airway obstruction (foreign body); reactive airway disease

Used by permission from Bledsoe et al., *Paramedic Care*, Volume 1, page 533.

Thus, end-tidal carbon dioxide changes during transport are most likely related to changes in pulmonary blood flow or minute ventilation. If the patient is transported with careful monitoring of blood pressure and cardiogram to exclude pulmonary blood flow changes, continuous capnometry should be a good reflection of minute ventilation. Thus, capnometry can be useful in maintaining consistent ventilation. The use of capnometry to establish ventilation parameters without a baseline blood gas or other hemodynamic information and monitors, however, is probably not appropriate.[72]

Although discussed here in the context of monitoring an intubated patient, capnometry and capnography can also be monitored in a nonintubated patient. The sample is collected through a nasal cannula attached to the capnometer, and the principles, values, limitations, and waveforms are the same as they are for an intubated patient in whom the sample is collected from the airway circuit. As capnometric changes precede changes in oxygen saturation, $PETCO_2$ monitoring in nonintubated patients may be particularly helpful in evaluating patients for impending respiratory failure from disease or from incautious sedative administration.[82,83]

Another role for capnometry is as a reflection of cardiac output. With consistent ventilation, capnometry provides a gross, breath-to-breath indicator of cardiac output. The extreme example of this is seen in the patient believed to be in cardiac arrest. More than 80% of patients believed to be in pulseless electrical activity (PEA) have synchronous cardiac wall motion and over 40% have a measurable aortic pulse pressure.[95,96] Capnometry can help to distinguish between PEA and very low cardiac output arrest states and may help to detect suboptimal chest compressions during resuscitation.[97-99]

Survival from out-of-hospital cardiac arrest is under 3%, and the annual cost of futile resuscitation efforts has been estimated at over \$1 billion.[100] Several studies have demonstrated relationships between end-tidal carbon dioxide measurements and outcomes in arrest. Sanders et al. found no survivors with a value under 10 mm Hg.[98] Another study found that a value of 15 mm Hg had the best sensitivity and specificity, with a 91% positive and negative predictive value, but included four resuscitated patients with a $PETCO_2$ under 10 mm Hg.[101] A large evaluation of 150 arrests showed that a $PetCO_2$ of 10 mmHg or less at 20 minutes into the resuscitation was 100% sensitive and specific for survival.[100]

Transport Ventilator Monitoring

Mechanically ventilated patients require constant monitoring, with evaluation of **peak inspiratory pressure (PIP)**, exhaled tidal volume, and minute ventilation, at a minimum. PIP varies with lung compliance and airway resistance, and changes can reflect patient improvement or serious problems. Increased PIP may indicate endotracheal tube occlusion, pneumothorax, increasing bronchospasm, or pulmonary edema, and high peak pressures are clearly associated with lung tissue injury. Decreased PIP can indicate resolving airway disease but can also suggest a ventilator-circuit leak, disconnection, unplanned extubation, or an insufficient gas supply.[102-104] Exhaled volume evaluates both spontaneous and mechanical ventilation. An exhaled tidal volume much lower than the set tidal volume indicates a loss of ventilator-circuit integrity, an air leak around the endotracheal tube, or an inadequate expiratory time due to obstructive lung disease or ventilator-patient asynchrony.[105] Minute ventilation has an inverse relationship with arterial PCO_2. Ongoing monitoring is needed to prevent unintended acid-base disturbances.

Summary

This chapter has demonstrated that monitoring of lung ventilation and confirmation of tracheal intubation are continuous processes that require constant vigilance and an understanding of clinical situations that can lead to false negatives or false positives. No one monitor should be relied on completely but, at a minimum, tracheal intubation should be confirmed using end-tidal carbon dioxide in patients with a perfusing cardiac rhythm or an EDD such as the SIB in patients with a nonperfusing cardiac rhythm.[17] The patient's vital signs and level of consciousness can also play a significant role in monitoring of the patient.

REVIEW QUESTIONS

1. What is the significance of an SaO_2 of 90%?

2. Which occurs first, end-tidal carbon dioxide changes in the hypoxic patient or pulse oximetry changes?

3. Discuss false positive and false negative considerations when using near-failsafe devices for confirmation of tracheal intubation.

4. Why are 6 to 12 ventilations recommended before relying on a colorimetric CO_2 detector reading?

5. Name three situations in which CO_2 detector devices may give false readings.

6. Name three conditions that can be indicated by an increase in peak inspiratory pressure (PIP).

Pharmacology of Airway Management

Tareg Bey
Charles E. Smith

Chapter Objectives

After reading this chapter, you should be able to:

- Define pharmacokinetics and pharmacodynamics.
- Review the indication for thiopental, etomidate, midazolam, and ketamine as induction agents.
- Discuss the use of fentanyl as a pharmacologic adjunct.
- Review the pharmacology of succinylcholine and rocuronium.

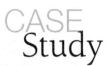
CASE
Study _____

A 38-year-old man arrives by EMS unconscious at the emergency department. He collapsed at work, holding his head, while saying, "I think my head is going to explode." During the transport, he seizes and vomits once. The paramedics administer midazolam 5 mg IV and oxygenate the patient by bag-valve-mask (BVM) with cricoid pressure. An initial attempt at tracheal intubation without the use of a muscle relaxant is unsuccessful. Because he is otherwise healthy and unresponsive, they elect to use succinylcholine to improve muscle relaxation. They first administer lidocaine 100 mg IV while they gently ventilate him by BVM with continued cricoid pressure. About 2 minutes later, succinylcholine 100 mg is administered. Sixty seconds after administration, direct laryngoscopy reveals a Cormack and Lehane Grade 2 view of the airway. A 7.5 mm tracheal tube is passed through the cords under direct vision, and the cuff is sealed. Chest auscultation and end-tidal carbon dioxide confirm tracheal intubation. The patient is subsequently administered vecuronium 5 mg for postintubation management. Vital signs remain stable, and oxygen saturation is maintained at 98%. The remainder of the transport is uneventful, and the patient is transferred to the care of the emergency department team at the local medical center.

Introduction

This chapter describes drugs used for airway management and their intended and adverse effects. Sedative hypnotics are often combined with opioids such as fentanyl, both at lower doses to minimize side effects. Most of the drugs were originally studied in healthy volunteers or patients. However, when used in critically ill patients with hypovolemia, fever, sepsis, or liver failure, these drugs may have very different pharmacologic profiles. The knowledge of pharmacokinetics and pharmacodynamics helps to understand the mechanism of action and the contraindication of these drugs.

KEY TERMS

depolarizing relaxant, p. 132   nondepolarizing relaxant, p. 133

Pharmacokinetics and Pharmacodynamics

The term *pharmacokinetics* refers to the science that describes absorption, distribution, biotransformation, and elimination of a drug in the body. In essence, pharmacokinetics describes what the body does to the drug.[1] For example, the extraction of a drug in the liver and its biotransformation falls under pharmacokinetics.

The term *pharmacodynamics* refers to the science that describes the mechanism of drug action and the relationship between the drug concentration and effect,[2] such as the action of a drug at a specific receptor site. An example is benzodiazepines at the GABA ionophore complex.

The pharmacokinetics of drugs that have a high to intermediate extraction ratio from the liver are dependent on the liver blood flow. Most of the drug is removed from the blood as it flows through the liver.[3] This is called a perfusion-limited or blood flow-limited clearance.[3,4] One classic example for a drug with a high hepatic clearance is propofol.[5] In contrast to the perfusion-limited clearance, the capacity-limited clearance is more dependent on the enzymatic activity of the liver than on hepatic blood flow.[3,4] A classic example for capacity-limited drug clearance is thiopental.[6]

In low flow states where perfusion of the liver and splanchnic system is limited, drug clearance is decreased. Conditions such as hypovolemia, cardiogenic shock or dysfunction, and endogenous or exogenous adrenergic stimulation all decrease the splanchnic and hepatic blood flow and have profound effects on the pharmacokinetics of anesthetics and sedatives with high and intermediate liver extraction ratio.[7]

Intravenous Drugs Used for Induction of Anesthesia and Endotracheal Intubation

Induction Agents

Thiopental

Thiopental is a short-acting thiobarbiturate (Table 6-1). Onset is rapid, and duration of action is short. The usual dosage is 3 to 5 mg/kg and should be reduced to between 0.5 and 2 mg/kg in the presence of hemodynamic compromise. Rapid induction occurs within 30 seconds because of maximal brain uptake.[8] The maximum effect of thiopental is seen within 60 seconds. This is followed by a rapid redistribution to other vessel-rich tissues, which accounts for the rapid offset. White points out that loss of consciousness occurs 10 to 15 seconds following induction doses of 3 to 6 mg/kg.[9] Thiopental is normally prepared as a 2.5% solution after reconstitution from a powder, which corresponds to a drug concentration of 25 mg/mL. The standard dose of thiopental for intubation purposes when used in combination with an opioid for healthy adults is normally 5 mg/kg.[10] The dose regimen has to be adjusted for age, health status, and body weight.

Table 6-1 Important Aspects of Various Airway Drugs

- Thiopental
  - Excellent drug for induction of the head-injured or seizing patient.
  - Avoid in patients with hypovolemia, hypotension, hepatic encephalopathy, and porphyria.
- Midazolam
  - Can be used as a sedative, induction agent, or anticonvulsant.
  - Relatively slower onset of action for induction and can cause cardiovascular and respiratory problems, especially in the elderly and very young patients.
  - The half-life duration of action and recovery times after midazolam are prolonged significantly when the hepatic cytochrome P450 system is inhibited by drugs like cimetidine.
- Propofol
  - Is an ultra-fast-acting anesthetic that provides good suppression of airway reflexes.
  - Should be avoided in hypotensive and hypovolemic patients.
  - Can cause bradycardia and conduction blocks.
  - Propofol solutions should be used up immediately because of the potential for bacterial contamination.
- Etomidate
  - Among all sedative hypnotics, provides the best hemodynamic stability and is the preferred induction agent for hypovolemic patients and those in shock.
  - Has been shown to suppress adrenal cortisol synthesis.
- Ketamine
  - Produces a state of dissociative anesthesia.
  - As an induction drug, can increase circulating catecholamines, arterial blood pressure, and intracranial pressure and should be avoided in patients with coronary artery disease, patients with closed and open head injuries, and in pheochromocytoma.
- Fentanyl
  - Is a synthetic opioid agonist used for pain control and as an adjunct induction drug for intubation.
  - Can cause respiratory arrest, hypotension, bradycardia, and muscular rigidity. Administration should be titrated in small doses between 25 and 50 micrograms (0.5 to 1 mL) in adults. It will take approximately 5-7 minutes to obtain a noticeable effect.
- Succinylcholine
  - Depolarizing muscle relaxant.
  - Is the fastest acting drug among all neuromuscular blockers.
  - Should be avoided in hyperkalemia and in critical ill patients and those with neuromuscular diseases.
- Rocuronium
  - Is a fast-acting nondepolarizing muscle relaxant.
  - When used for RSI, should be used at higher dose (0.9 mg/kg) to shorten the onset of action.

The classic teaching is that barbiturates have an antalgestic or hyperalgesic effect, meaning that these substances increase pain perception.[9] Currently, this topic is controversial, and several authors have not found any supporting evidence for the hyperalgesic effects of barbiturates.[11,12] During thiopental induction, coughing and reaction to laryngeal stimuli may occur. Fuchs-Buder et al. compared the intubation conditions of thiopental (5 mg/kg) versus etomidate (0.3 mg/kg). They compared two groups of 30 patients who also received alfentanil (10 mcg/kg) and rocuronium (0.6 mg/kg). The etomidate group had a more favorable profile for attenuating reactions to laryngeal stimuli than thiopental.[13]

Thiopental may cause myocardial depression and hypotension. Cardiovascular collapse may occur, especially in the hypovolemic patient.[8,9,14] Thiopental decreases cerebral metabolic oxygen consumption, cerebral blood flow, and intracranial pressure (ICP) and is an excellent drug to achieve neuroprotection in the brain-injured patient who has increased ICP.[3,6,8,9] Thiopental is an ideal choice as an induction agent for the hypertensive, normovolemic, brain-injured patient with increased cerebral metabolic demands and elevated ICP. Christensen and Andreasen suggest that the dose of thiopental be reduced by up to 40% in patients with congestive heart failure to avoid serious cardiovascular side effects.[15]

Barbiturates are commonly used to treat seizures and epilepsy.[16] Seizures may accompany severe head injuries and can complicate endotracheal intubation by creating more difficult intubation conditions.

Thiopental can produce severe tissue necrosis if inadvertently injected into an artery.[17] Angel et al. discouraged the use of urokinase to treat accidental intra-arterial thiopental injections. In animal experimental studies, they found an increase of tissue necrosis by 100%.[18]

Etomidate

Etomidate is a carboxylated imidazole derivative with short duration.[8] As a nonbarbiturate sedative-hypnotic, it has a very rapid onset of action within 30 seconds after injection.[8,9] The usual induction dose of etomidate is 0.3 mg/kg.[19] Etomidate causes minimal hemodynamic changes during the induction and injection phase; however, in the face of hemodynamic compromise, the dose should be reduced to between 0.1 to 0.2 mg/kg.

Unlike thiopental and propofol, etomidate has minimal or absent cardiac depressant effects. The lack of cardiovascular effects is most likely due to etomidate's lack of effect on the sympathetic nervous system and autonomic reflexes.[20] Etomidate decreases cerebral metabolic oxygen consumption, cerebral blood flow, and ICP. Etomidate offers an excellent safety profile in hypotensive patients and is useful in patients with shock, unstable cardiopulmonary status, and head injury,[21] although the dose should be reduced during conditions of hypovolemia and hemorrhagic shock. After laryngeal manipulation and endotracheal intubation, etomidate can cause an increase of systolic blood pressure.

In a study by Skinner et al., 36 patients receiving etomidate (0.3 mg/kg) were compared to 35 patients receiving propofol (2.5 mg/kg).[22] All patients received rocuronium (0.6 mg/kg) but no opioids. Patients in the etomidate group had no significant changes in systolic blood pressure and pulse rate before and after induction. Systolic blood pressure and heart rate were significantly elevated following intubation. In patients with significant coronary artery disease, an increase of blood pressure and heart rate should be avoided because of the risk of relative ischemia to the myocardium. Etomidate, when used in combination with an opioid like fentanyl, can provide hemodynamic stability during induction and after intubation.[23]

Problems with etomidate include irritation and phlebitis in the injected vein, myoclonic movements, and nausea and vomiting after extubation.[24] Myoclonus and injection-site pain can be minimized with lidocaine and is abolished by giving the neuromuscular relaxant during rapid sequence induction (RSI). Myoclonus is not associated with epileptiform activity, but the muscle movements can be confused with seizures.

Etomidate can inhibit the steroidogenesis by blocking the enzyme 11-beta hydroxylase in the adrenal cortex.[25] Fellows studied a small group of multiple-injury patients in the intensive care unit.[26] After a single dose, adrenal suppression lasted only six to eight hours.

Ledingham et al. found an increased mortality with a prolonged infusion in critically ill trauma patients compared to patients sedated with morphine and benzodiazepines.[27] These were both early studies from the 1980s, and etomidate was tested in the intensive care setting and in critically ill patients.[26,27] Vitamin C has been shown to restore cortisol levels after etomidate administration.[28]

Patients with adrenal dysfunction and those regularly taking steroids should be monitored for signs of adrenal insufficiency even after a single dose of etomidate.

Propofol

Propofol is a rapidly acting intravenous anesthetic. It is a lipid-soluble-substituted isopropylphenol.[8,29] Propofol is not water-soluble and comes in oil-in-water solution in soy oil.[29]

Contamination of propofol is of concern. Magee et al. found coagulase-negative staphylococci and Acinetobacter species in syringes containing propofol as early as two hours after the agent was drawn up from the ampule.[30] The authors recommend that propofol be used immediately after it is drawn up.

Propofol is rapidly distributed in the body and has a half-life of about two minutes.[31] A blood–brain equilibration half-life of 2.9 minutes has been calculated, and the liver is probably the main eliminating organ.[5] Grounds et al. found that, in unpremedicated patients, the induction dose for anesthesia was 2.5 mg/kg.[32] Doenicke points out that propofol produces a more profound drop of systolic and diastolic blood pressures than etomidate. In isolated cases, blood pressure may decrease up to 40% to 50%.[29] Propofol has more pronounced side effects, such as decline of blood pressure and respiratory arrest in hypovolemic patients. Compared to etomidate, under rapid sequence conditions, propofol produces better intubating conditions due to greater suppression of upper airway reflexes.[22] However, propofol's effects on cardiac output, blood pressure, and cerebral perfusion pressure make it a poor choice for trauma patients with hypovolemia or patients with cardiovascular compromise.

Ketamine

Ketamine belongs to the group of arycyclohexylamines and is chemically related to the illicit drug phencyclidine.[9] Ketamine is highly lipid-soluble and can achieve induction of anesthesia in less than 60 seconds.[8] The induction dose is 1 to 2 mg/kg, which should be reduced to between 0.5 and 1 mg/kg in the face of hypovolemia, hemodynamic instability, or cardiovascular compromise. It produces sympathetic nervous system stimulation with increases in heart rate, blood pressure, cardiac output, and myocardial oxygen demand. If catecholamine stores are depleted or if there is exhaustion of sympathetic system compensatory mechanisms, hypotension can theoretically occur after ketamine because of direct myocardial depression.

Ketamine is a potent cerebral vasodilator and can increase ICP. However, it is a noncompetitive NMDA (N-methyl-D-aspartate) receptor antagonist that could theoretically reduce excessive excitotoxic stimuli and brain ischemia following head injury, thereby providing neuroprotection.[33,34] Ketamine produces dissociative anesthesia and analgesia while it maintains spontaneous respiration.[35] Ketamine also increases ICP as a result of increased systemic blood pressure, cerebral artery dilation, and increase in cerebral metabolic rate ($CMRO_2$).[9,33] Ketamine is not recommended for neuroanesthesia or situations with increased ICP.

Ketamine also increases salivation and bronchial secretions.[3,35] It causes bronchodilation and can be used to facilitate tracheal intubation in spontaneously breathing asthmatics requiring mechanical ventilation.[36] Indeed, ketamine is the recommended induction agent in patients with life-threatening asthma requiring RSI because of its potent bronchodilator effects. Dreaming and hallucinations may occur, the frequency of which can be reduced by benzodiazepines. Because ketamine tends to increase blood pressure and heart rate by cardiovascular stimulation, it can be used in patients suffering from hypovolemic shock.[8,9,35]

Ketamine for anesthesia induction purposes is given at a dose of 1 to 2 mg/kg intravenously. Christ et al. point out that ketamine exhibits negative cardiovascular effects in patients with catecholamine-dependent heart failure.[37] It is not recommended as a first-line drug for long-term sedation of patients with impaired ventricular function. In an in vitro study with isolated human heart muscles, Sprung et al. found that ketamine had reduced ability to increase contractility even in the presence of increased beta-adrenergic stimulation.[38] Ketamine should therefore be used with caution in catecholamine-dependent patients (e.g., in late and severe shock), especially in those patients with impaired cardiac contractility.

Midazolam

Midazolam is a short-acting benzodiazepine with sedative, anxiolytic, amnestic, and anticonvulsant properties.[39] Midazolam has been used successfully as an induction agent for general anesthesia and endotracheal intubation. Other benzodiazepines like diazepam and lorazepam are not commonly used for induction of anesthesia due to their slower onset of action and less predictable dose relationship.[9] The dose for intravenous induction for midazolam is 0.2 to 0.4 mg/kg, and the onset of action is 30 to 90 seconds.[3] In the face of hemodynamic instability, the dose should be reduced by 50%. Elimination half-life is one to four hours.[40] When dosed below 0.2 mg/kg, midazolam provides sedation but not always good conditions for endotracheal intubation or general anesthesia. Small incremental doses, 1 to 2 mg IV, are useful for providing sedation before and after RSI. The effects of midazolam are rapidly reversed by flumazenil. In an earlier trial, Baber et al. studied midazolam as an intravenous anesthetic induction agent in 57 patients using 0.15 mg/kg and achieved satisfactory anesthesia in only 78% of patients. The remainder of the patients needed either further doses of midazolam or an alternative induction agent.[41] When compared to the barbiturates such as thiopental or methohexital, midazolam was associated with a slower onset of action and a longer recovery period.

Midazolam may cause respiratory arrest, especially in the elderly and children.[42,43] The majority of these arrests were delayed and occurred in patients receiving coadministration of opioids such as fentanyl. Close monitoring of ventilation and oxygenation, especially during the recovery period, is therefore mandatory to recognize the respiratory arrest and provide appropriate treatment. Elderly and critically ill patients require lower doses of midazolam.[9]

Midazolam is extensively metabolized in the liver by the cytochrome P450 system.[39] Drugs such as cimetidine or macrolide antibiotics, which inhibit the cytochrome P450 system, can significantly prolong the duration of action of midazolam. Fee et al. found a bioavailability increase of about 30% with cimetidine and ranitidine.[44] A careful medication history is therefore important to adjust dosing of midazolam for induction of anesthesia or to switch to another type of induction agent if faster recovery is important.

Neuromuscular Blocking Agents

Avoidance of muscle relaxants generally results in inferior intubating conditions, unless one employs large doses of induction agents such as propofol, which is not usually appropriate for prehospital administration.

Succinylcholine

depolarizing muscle relaxant

A muscle relaxer that causes muscle depolarization at the postsynaptic neuromuscular cleft. Succinylcholine is the only depolarizing agent available today.

Succinylcholine is the only available **depolarizing relaxant** for clinical use. Succinylcholine consists of two molecules of acetylcholine, which are linked together via methyl groups. The onset of action of succinylcholine is about 30 to 45 seconds, and the duration is five to ten minutes.[8] Succinylcholine is widely used for RSI. In patients with atypical forms of plasma cholinesterase, duration of action of succinylcholine may be increased to three to four hours.[45] Succinylcholine exhibits its action much like acetylcholine: by muscle depolarization at the postsynaptic neuromuscular membrane. It first causes muscle fasciculation followed by muscular paralysis by depolarization.

The intubating dose of succinylcholine is 1 mg/kg for adults. Naguib et al. found in a double-blind study with 200 patients that 98% of patients receiving succinylcholine had acceptable intubation conditions after 60 seconds.[46] The authors also tested succinylcholine doses of 0.0, 0.3, and 0.5 mg/kg. All patients received propofol 2 mg/kg and fentanyl 2 mcg/kg. The authors concluded that a succinylcholine dose of 0.56 mg/kg produced acceptable intubation results and should allow a more rapid return of spontaneous respiration.[46] It should be noted that this study was performed under operating room conditions and that in emergency situations, fast and reliable muscle paralysis is more important than rapid return of airway reflexes. In a meta-analysis, Perry et al. compared succinylcholine with rocuronium under RSI conditions.[47] They found that succinylcholine created superior intubation conditions to rocuronium when looking at excellent intubation conditions.[47]

Most of the literature on adverse side effects of succinylcholine originates from case reports or case series. One of the major side effects of succinylcholine is hyperkalemia.[8] Succinylcholine should be avoided in critically ill patients, patients with recent burns, neuromuscular diseases such as muscular dystrophy, near drowning, and conditions with high serum potassium such as renal failure.[8,48,49] Succinylcholine is contraindicated in patients with myopathies and severe crush or degloving injuries because of the risk of hyperkalemia. Hyperkalemic cardiac arrest after succinylcholine is due to up-regulation of nicotinic acetylcholine receptors (AchR) and/or rhabdomyolysis.[50] Administration of small subparalyzing doses of nondepolarizing relaxants prior to succinylcholine prevents fasciculation but does not prevent the development of life-threatening hyperkalemia. Up-regulation represents increased numbers of altered nicotinic acetylcholine receptors across the entire muscle membrane when acetylcholine is not involved in endplate interactions.[50]

Succinylcholine-induced bradycardia and asystole may occur following repeat doses of this agent in adults. Pretreatment with atropine is necessary. Masseter muscle rigidity after succinylcholine may make intubation difficult and indicate the potential for malignant hyperthermia.

PEARLS

Unless contraindicated, succinylcholine is the drug of choice for use in rapid sequence intubation.

The concept of succinylcholine-induced hyperkalemia in the emergency care setting has been recently challenged by Zink et al., who found no cardiac arrests in a prospective uncontrolled study of 100 patients receiving succinylcholine for intubation.[51] Succinylcholine also has a relative contraindication in patients with brain injuries and increased ICP. In contrast to this classic teaching, Brown et al. found in a double-blind, randomized, crossover study that, under intensive care conditions, succinylcholine did not significantly alter intracerebral pressures, mean arterial pressures, or cerebral perfusion pressures.[52] Unless contraindicated (see Chapter 7 for more information on complications, contraindications, and precautions), succinylcholine is the drug of choice for use in rapid sequence intubation.

Rocuronium

nondepolarizing muscle relaxant

A muscle relaxant that inhibits neuromuscular transmission by competitively blocking (as opposed to depolarizing) nicotinic sites on the postsynaptic cleft. Nondepolarizing relaxants do not cause hyperkalemia.

Nondepolarizing relaxants competitively inhibit neuromuscular transmission. In contrast to succinylcholine, nondepolarizers do not cause hyperkalemia, cardiac bradyarrhythmias, or malignant hyperthermia, nor do they increase intraocular, intracranial, or intragastric pressure.

Rocuronium, like vecuronium, is a nondepolarizing muscle relaxant. Rocuronium has a shorter onset of action than vecuronium. The duration of action of rocuronium is about 30 to 45 minutes, much longer than that of succinylcholine.[8] In a study of 120 children, Cheng et al. compared intubation conditions after 60 seconds for succinylcholine (1.5 mg/kg) and two different doses of rocuronium (0.6 mg/kg and 0.9 mg/kg). All children received alfentanil 10 mcg/kg and thiopental 5 mg/kg for induction of anesthesia.[53] The authors found that in children, high-dose rocuronium (0.9 mg/kg) provided similar intubation conditions when compared to succinylcholine (1.5 mg/kg), whereas rocuronium at a dose of 0.6 mg/kg was inadequate.[53] Using meta-analysis, Perry et al. analyzed 26 articles comparing rocuronium with succinylcholine.[47] They determined that overall, succinylcholine provided excellent intubation conditions more reliably than did rocuronium. In case a second-line agent was required, rocuronium created equivalent intubation conditions to succinylcholine when used in combination with propofol as an induction drug.[47]

Vecuronium

Vecuronium is a steroidal nondepolarizing muscle relaxant with an intermediate clinical duration. Onset of action is delayed compared with rocuronium or succinylcholine, although high-dose vecuronium (0.3 to 0.4 mg/kg) results in an accelerated onset of block of 80 to 90 seconds. Vecuronium is metabolized by the liver into three active metabolites and is excreted in the bile and urine. Cardiovascular effects are unlikely even when large doses are rapidly administered and there is no histamine release.[54] Because of its slower onset of action, it is more suited for postintubation management rather than for RSI.

Adjunctive Agents

Narcotic Analgesics

Opioids, such as fentanyl, are useful adjuncts to decrease pain and coughing associated with laryngoscopy and intubation. Opioids also blunt the stress response to pain and decrease sympathetic tone leading to venodilation. There is no myocardial depression, although centrally mediated bradycardia may occur with high doses of potent opioids. With increased doses, decreased pulmonary compliance, chest wall rigidity, and laryngospasm may occur. This could lead to difficulty with ventilation if the onset of action of the opioid precedes that of the neuromuscular relaxant.[55]

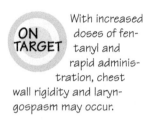

ON TARGET With increased doses of fentanyl and rapid administration, chest wall rigidity and laryngospasm may occur.

Fentanyl is a synthetic opioid used for pain management and as an adjunct for anesthesia induction. Fentanyl as an adjunct to anesthesia induction for intubation is normally used in the range of 1.5 to 3 mcg/kg.[9,46] Fentanyl has also been used as a single induction drug for endotracheal intubation before paralysis was induced. Fentanyl alone was used at a dose of 5 mcg/kg and compared to thiopental (5 mg/kg) and midazolam (0.1 mg/kg). Fentanyl provided the most neutral response during rapid sequence intubation.[56] Major side effects of fentanyl are respiratory depression and arrest, nausea and vomiting, bradycardia, hypotension, and muscular rigidity.[57]

Alfentanil has a smaller volume of distribution and shorter elimination time compared with fentanyl or sufentanil. Rapid plasma-effect site equilibration with alfentanil results in a relatively larger peak effect site concentration.[55] Sufentanil is 5 to 10 times more potent than fentanyl and has a longer distribution and elimination half-life than alfentanil.

Remifentanil is a newer opioid agent. The peak effect site concentration following remifentanil is approximately 1.5 minutes, which is very similar to that seen with alfentanil. The unique characteristic of remifentanil is its rapid clearance by plasma esterases into metabolites with nearly no activity at the μ receptor. Bolus doses of 1.0 and 1.25 mcg/kg were effective in controlling the hemodynamic response to intubation in patients receiving thiopental and succinylcholine. However, the 1.25 mcg/kg dose was associated with hypotension in 35% of patients and is therefore not recommended.[58]

Lidocaine

A number of other drugs, such as lidocaine, can be used in an effort to suppress the cardiovascular responses to tracheal intubation. Lidocaine, 1.5 mg/kg IV, two minutes before laryngoscopy and intubation did not prevent hemodynamic reactions evoked by RSI.[59]

Summary

Several types and classes of drugs are used to facilitate airway management and rapid sequence intubation. Each drug has a distinct pharmacological profile characterized by half-life, volume of distribution, onset of action, duration of action, and side effect profile (see Chapter 7 for more information on the pharmacologic profile and dosing of airway drugs for rapid sequence intubation). Although administration of these drugs for airway management is safe and effective when used under the proper conditions, failure to consider pharmacological factors may seriously jeopardize patient care and contribute to adverse outcomes. For example, the use of thiopental and propofol may cause severe hypotension in patients with shock. Similarly, the use of succinylcholine is contraindicated in patients with paralysis or muscular dystrophy, among others. The most commonly used drugs in airway management are the sedative hypnotics etomidate, midazolam, and ketamine; the opioids such as fentanyl; and neuromuscular relaxants such as succinylcholine, rocuronium, and vecuronium. All prehospital practitioners who use these drugs should be fully aware of the different effects, dosing requirements, and side effect profiles, especially under changing physiologic conditions such as hypovolemia and shock, or in different disease states. Finally, all health care personnel should know the standard dosing protocol and concentration of each drug used routinely in their own setting for airway management. Continuous medical education and regular review of existing protocols and procedures help to establish and maintain the highest standards of patient care.

REVIEW QUESTIONS

1. What conditions can cause drug clearance to be decreased?

2. What is the standard depolarizing muscle relaxant used for rapid sequence intubation?

3. What are the standard nondepolarizing muscle relaxants used in airway control?

4. Which muscle relaxants has the fastest onset time?

5. Name the most commonly used muscle relaxants and induction agents used in airway management today.

CHAPTER 7

Rapid Sequence Induction and Intubation in Adults

Charles E. Smith
Darko Vodopich

Chapter Objectives

After reading this chapter, you should be able to:

- Discuss the indications, benefits, and risks of rapid sequence induction and intubation.

- Review the equipment and techniques necessary to perform rapid sequence induction and intubation.

- Review the use of drugs for rapid sequence induction and intubation.

- Describe techniques for tracheal intubation including maximal preoxygenation and cricoid pressure.

- Review contingency plans for failed intubation.

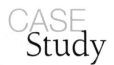

CASE Study _____

Medic 4 is dispatched to a rollover motor-vehicle incident where police officers on the scene reported a patient ejected from a vehicle. On arrival at the scene, the paramedics were directed to a ditch to find fire department personnel caring for an approximately 30-year-old male, who was being combative as they attempted to maintain c-spine precautions and place him on a long spine board. Initial assessment revealed his airway to be intact, he was breathing spontaneously, and radial pulses were strong and regular. There was no gross bleeding noted. His eyes opened spontaneously, and he was yelling inappropriate words as he was withdrawing from painful stimuli.

The paramedics elected to transport rapidly, so the patient was moved to the ambulance and taken to the level 1 trauma facility. En route, oxygen was administered via nonrebreathing mask, and vital signs revealed a blood pressure of 180/100, heart rate of 110, and respiratory rate of 20. The pulse oximeter did not give a reading.

Two large-bore intravenous lines were established. The head-to-toe exam revealed multiple abrasions to the head. There was a large hematoma to the right parietal region. There was no blood or other fluid from the nose, mouth, or ears. Pupils were equal and reactive at 4 mm. The patient's trachea was midline with no jugular venous distention. His chest excursion was equal, and breath sounds were clear bilaterally. Heart tones were normal with sinus tachycardia on the EKG monitor. His abdomen revealed a large abrasion on the right side with contracted abdominal muscles. His pelvis was stable, and he was moving all his extremities with strong equal motor responses, withdrawing from pain.

During transport the patient's mental status deteriorated. He became responsive to painful stimuli only. His respiratory rhythm was irregular, and pulse oximetry readings were 90%. Crew members began to ventilate the patient with a bag-valve device attached to 100% oxygen in preparation for a rapid sequence intubation. A rapid 6-D airway assessment was performed. The rapid sequence intubation (RSI) drugs were drawn up and labeled, and the intubation equipment was checked and readied. The desired size of the tracheal tube was opened, and a stylet was inserted. A half size larger and smaller were made available. A Combitube was set out if needed. The anterior portion of the c-spine collar was removed while manual in-line axial stabilization (MIAS) was continually applied.

After receiving lidocaine 100 mg, the patient was given midazolam 4 mg, morphine 5 mg, and succinylcholine 120 mg while Sellick's maneuver was performed. Within one minute, the pulse oxymeter was reading 97%, and the patient became easier to ventilate. Direct laryngoscopy was performed using a No. 3 Macintosh laryngoscope blade without difficulty. Tracheal tube position was confirmed as the tracheal tube cuff was inflated. There was good color change on the CO_2 detector cap after washout. The anterior portion of the c-spine collar was reattached prior to releasing MIAS. The tracheal tube was secured, and the patient was ventilated by the bag-valve device. Ventilation and oxygenation were monitored continuously using capnography and pulse oximetry. The patient started to bite on the tracheal tube, so midazolam 2 mg and vecuronium 5 mg was given. After complete muscle relaxation, the remainder of the transport was unremarkable. On arrival, report was given to the trauma team, and patient care was transferred.

Introduction

Rapid sequence induction (RSI) is one of the two intubation pathways on the SLAM Universal Adult Airway Flowchart (inside front cover).[1,2] Rapid sequence induction and intubation (RSI) is designed to provide optimal tracheal intubating conditions and minimize the risk of aspiration. Principles of RSI are that the trachea needs to be intubated, the patient is at risk of aspiration, intubation is predicted to be successful, cricoid pressure is not contraindicated, the operator is skilled at airway management, and contingency plans are available for failed intubation.

KEY TERMS

Becker dystrophy, p. 141

Duchenne dystrophy, p. 141

imidazole, p. 140

masseter muscle, p. 142

myoclonus, p. 140

nystagmus, p. 140

rhabdomyolysis, p. 142

Complications of RSI

Complications of RSI may be catastrophic and are generally due to failed oxygenation, failed ventilation, and complications of the drugs given. Major complications include unrecognized esophageal intubation, pulmonary aspiration, mainstem intubation, hypotension, hyperkalemia, pneumothorax, hypoxic brain injury, myocardial damage, cardiac arrest, and death.[3] In patients requiring emergency intubation in the field, 90% of documented aspiration occurred before administration of paralytics.[4] Compared with RSI, intubation without paralytics was associated with an increased frequency of complications such as aspiration (15%), airway trauma (28%), and death (3%) in a prospective study of RSI in the emergency setting.[5]

Preoxygenation

Maximal preoxygenation is attained when the alveolar, arterial, tissue, and venous compartments are saturated with oxygen. Preoxygenation provides the maximum amount of time a patient can be apneic without dying.[6] The traditional method of preoxygenation is providing 100% oxygen through a sealed system without air entrainment for 3 to 5 minutes of normal tidal volume ventilation. Confirmation of a sealed system includes movement of an anesthesia reservoir bag in and out with each inhalation and exhalation, presence of a normal end-tidal CO_2 waveform on a capnogram with each breath, and inspired and expired oxygen concentrations greater than 90%. Hyperventilation with eight breaths of 100% oxygen within 60 seconds through a sealed system can also be used as an alternative to the traditional 3- to 5-minute technique.[7]

In a computer apnea model, the time to critical hemoglobin desaturation (SaO_2 less than 80% and decreasing) was 8.7 minutes in a healthy 70 kg adult, assuming maximal preoxygenation.[8] Corresponding times to critical oxygen desaturation were 5.5, 3.7, and 3.1 minutes in a moderately ill 70 kg adult, a healthy 10 kg child, and an obese 127 kg adult, respectively.[8] Patients with respiratory distress, anemia, and decreased cardiac output have a reduced capacity for oxygen-loading during preoxygenation. Patients with increased oxygen extraction also desaturate more rapidly.[8]

Patients with abnormal gas exchange due to shunt or ventilation perfusion mismatch and patients with anemia or low cardiac output may not achieve the same PaO_2 with 100% oxygen and can have precipitous decreases in oxygenation during apnea.

Because maximal preoxygenation is often difficult to attain in the emergency setting, bag-mask ventilation of the patient's lungs with 100% oxygen is often done as soon as the patient stops breathing. Manual ventilation of the patient's lungs by an experienced airway provider using inflation pressures less than 20 cm H_2O and cricoid pressure is unlikely to introduce any air into the stomach[9,10] and can prevent oxygen desaturation and carbon dioxide accumulation during RSI. Some patients may be difficult to ventilate by bag-mask due to predisposing factors.[11,12] RSI in these types of patients should be undertaken with caution or, if appropriate, intubation should be undertaken using a difficult intubation technique that does not require RSI.

Aspiration Prophylaxsis

ON TARGET Cricoid pressure is not without problems. The operator should be thoroughly familiar with both the challenges and benefits of this maneuver.

Cricoid pressure occludes the esophagus during RSI to prevent passive regurgitation of stomach contents and reduce the risk of aspiration.[10] Cricoid pressure also decreases the risk of gastric insufflation during bag-mask ventilation.[10] Cricoid pressure is done by placing the thumb and middle finger on either side of the cricoid cartilage and the index finger above, thereby preventing lateral movement of the cricoid cartilage (Figure 7-1).[13] The force required to prevent regurgitation corresponds approximately to a force that is slightly painful when applied to the bridge of one's nose.

When applied prior to induction of anesthesia, cricoid pressure increases patient discomfort, activates upper airway reflexes, and may cause nausea and retching. Cricoid pressure may interfere with placement of the laryngoscope blade and cause anatomic distortion of the upper airway so that the glottic inlet is more difficult or impossible to visualize.[13] The simple maneuver of easing up, or releasing cricoid pressure during RSI under direct laryngoscope vision, may alleviate airway distortion and permit more rapid insertion of the tube through the vocal cords.[14] The benefit of rapidly inserting the tube and inflating the cuff outweighs the risk of aspiration during the brief time that the cricoid pressure is released.

Cricoid pressure interferes with laryngeal mask airway (LMA) insertion should this airway be required in the situation of failed intubation.[15]

Rare complications of cricoid pressure include esophageal rupture should active vomiting occur and disruption of the cricoid cartilage or larynx should these structures be injured.

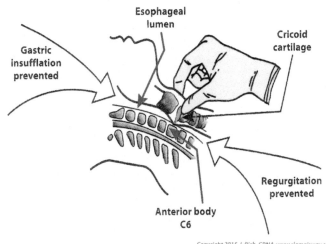

imidazole

An organic crystalline base that is an inhibitor of histamine. Many drugs contain an imidazole ring (e.g., etomidate, ketoconazole, and miconazole).

nystagmus

Involuntary movement of the eyeballs in any direction. Often occurs with drug or ETOH ingestion but may be congenital or caused by neurological conditions. There are many types of nystagmus, but all are constant and involuntary.

FIGURE 7-1
Single-handed cricoid pressure is usually done to protect the lungs from contamination with gastric contents and to prevent gastric insufflation during positive-pressure mask ventilation. The most limiting factor of cricoid pressure is anatomical distortion of the airway and interference with laryngoscope blade insertion.
(Courtesy of Dr. Charles E. Smith)

Trauma to the cricoid cartilage and larynx should be suspected in any patient with hoarseness, subcutaneous emphysema, or palpable fracture.

Drugs for RSI

As you read in Chapter 6, induction agents include etomidate, thiopental, and ketamine (Tables 7-1 and 7-2).[16,17] Propofol is usually avoided because of the risk of severe hypotension due to myocardial depression and vasodilation, especially in patients with shock.

Although rocuronium is a suitable nondepolarizing alternative for RSI, succinylcholine is the relaxant of choice for RSI (Table 7-3).[18] However, a thorough patient history coupled with understanding the absolute contraindications to the use of succinylcholine (Table 7-4)[19] as well as the reported complications (Table 7-5)[20] is paramount.

myoclonus

Twitching of muscles.

Table 7-1	Pharmacokinetics of Selected IV Induction Drugs for RSI			
Agent	Standard Dose (mg/kg)	Dose If Hemo-Dynamic Instability Is Present	Half-Life (Hours)	Comments
Thiopental	3–5	0.5–2	11.6	Rapid onset barbiturate. May cause myocardial depression and hypotension. Preferred agent for head-injured patient with hypertension.
Etomidate	0.2–0.3	0.1–0.2	2–5	Rapid onset **imidazole** agent. Hemodynamic effects unlikely. Associated with **myoclonus** and adrenal suppression. Preferred agent for hypotensive patient with head injury or coronary artery disease.
Ketamine	1–2	0.5–1	1–2	Phencyclidine agent with potent analgesic properties. May cause sympathetic stimulation, bronchodilation, dreams, **nystagmus,** and salivation. Preferred agent for hypotensive patient with asthma or cardiac tamponade.

Modified from Kingsley CP, Perioperative use of etomidate for trauma patients. In Smith CE, Grande CM, eds., *The Use of Etomidate in the Trauma Patient.* International Trauma Anesthesia and Critical Care Society Special Monograph. ITACCS, Baltimore 1997; pp. 1–7, 16.

Table 7-2 Cardiovascular and Central Nervous System Effects of Induction Drugs for RSI

Agent	Blood Pressure	Heart Rate	Cardiac Function	Cerebral Blood Flow	CMRO$_2$[†]	Intracranial Pressure
Thiopental	Decrease	Increase	Decrease	Decrease	Decrease	Decrease
Etomidate	No change	No change	No change	Decrease	Decrease	Decrease
Ketamine	Increase	Increase	Increase*	Increase	Increase	Increase

*Centrally mediated sympathetic response usually overrides direct depressant effects.
[†]CMRO$_2$ = cerebral metabolic oxygen requirements.
Modified from Kingsley CP, Perioperative management of thoracic trauma. *Anesth Clinics North America* 1999; 17(1):183–195.

Table 7-3 Selected Neuromuscular Blocking Agents for RSI

Agent	Intubating Dose (mg/kg)	Intubating Time (minutes)*	Clinical Duration (minutes)[†]	Comments
Succinylcholine	0.6–1.1	1	4–6	Associated with several side effects that may contraindicate its use.
Rocuronium	0.6–1.2	0.7–1.1	31–67	Nondepolarizer of choice for RSI.
Vecuronium	0.08–0.10	2.5–3	25–40	Onset time delayed unless high doses (0.3–0.4 mg/kg) used. Hemodynamic effects unlikely.

*Average time to good–excellent intubating conditions (>80% block).
[†]Average time to 25% first twitch recovery.
Modified from Smith CE, Grande CM, Wayne MA, ITACCS Consensus Panel, and International Review Committee. Rapid Sequence Intubation in Trauma. International Trauma Anesthesia and Critical Care Society. ITACCS, Baltimore 1998.18.

Duchenne dystrophy
A progressive disease with childhood onset that is transmitted as a sex-linked recessive trait and that causes weakness in muscles, particularly the pelvic and shoulder muscles. Most patients die before age 20.

Becker dystrophy
A disease similar to Duchenne dystrophy but less serious. It affects mainly the pelvic girdle.

Table 7-4 Conditions Associated with Exaggerated Hyperkalemia After Succinylcholine

- **Duchenne dystrophy**
- **Becker dystrophy**
- Thermal trauma
- Muscle trauma
- Upper or lower motor neuron denervation
  - Stroke
  - Spinal-cord injury
  - Guillain-Barre syndrome
- Motor nerve section
- Ventral horn disorder
- Intensive care unit milieu
  - Disuse atrophy
  - Infection
  - Pharmacologic denervation
  - Steroid use and necrotizing myopathy
- Miscellaneous receptor upregulation
  - Rhabdomyosarcoma
  - Neuroleptic malignant syndrome

From Gronert GA: Cardiac arrest after succinylcholine: Mortality greater with rhabdomyolysis than receptor upregulation. *Anesthesiology* 2001; 94:523.

Breakdown of muscle fibers leading to release of particles of muscle fiber into the circulatory system. It may be the result of crushing injury, burns, stress of muscle fibers, and other causes and can lead to kidney failure.

The muscle involved in chewing and clenching the jaw.

Table 7-5   Complications of Succinylcholine

- Hyperkalemia and cardiac arrest in susceptible patients
- Cardiac arrhythmias
- Muscle fasciculations
- Myalgias
- **Rhabdomyolysis**
- Increased intracranial pressure
- Increased intragastric pressure
- Increased intraocular pressure
- Malignant hyperthermia
- **Masseter muscle** spasm or jaw rigidity
- Prolonged apnea (1–4 hours), if atypical plasma cholinesterase

From Bevan DR, Complications of muscle relaxants. *Semin Anesthesia* 14:63, 1995, p. 20.

Avoidance of neuromuscular relaxants for RSI (Table 7-3) generally results in inferior intubating conditions unless large doses of induction agents, opioids, and lidocaine are employed. Performing RSI without the use of neuromuscular relaxants has a higher incidence of gastric aspiration.

Benzodiazepines and narcotics can also be used therapeutically in RSI (Table 7-6).[21]

A summary of the various steps involved in RSI is shown in Table 7-7.[18] Suggested drugs for RSI according to clinical setting and cardiovascular stability are shown in Table 7-8.[22,23] Management of specific complications such as hypotension or difficulty with ventilation is shown in Table 7-9.[3,22]

Table 7-6   Selected Adjunct Drugs for RSI

Agent	Standard Dose	Dose If Hemo-Dynamic Instability Is Present	Comments
Fentanyl	2–5 µg/kg	1–2 µg/kg	Minimal hemodynamic or cerebrovascular effects. Useful for blunting noxious stimuli.
Sufentanil	0.5–1.0 µg/kg	0.1–0.5 µg/kg	Similar to fentanyl but more potent.
Alfentanil	20–80 µg/kg	5–20 µg/kg	Similar to fentanyl but faster onset and offset.
Midazolam	2–4 mg	0.5–2.0 mg	Minimal cardiovascular effects when used in small doses. Useful for sedation and amnesia. Increases seizure threshold. Can be reversed with flumazenil.
Lidocaine	1.5 mg/kg	1.0 mg/kg	Useful for blunting airway reflexes. Also blunts blood pressure and intracranial pressure response to intubation, myoclonus after etomidate, and injection-site pain from etomidate.

Modified from Grande CM, Smith CE, Stene JK: Trauma Anesthesia. In Longnecker DE, Tinker JH, Morgan GE (eds), *Principles and Practice of Anesthesiology,* 2nd edition. Mosby, St Louis, 1998, pp. 2138–2164.[21]

Table 7-7 Summary of Technique for RSI

1. Evaluate the patient. Ensure that the trachea needs to be intubated, the patient is at risk of aspiration, intubation is predicted to be successful, cricoid pressure is not contraindicated, and contingency plans are available for failed intubation.
2. Assemble necessary equipment such as laryngoscope, tracheal tubes, suction, and gum-elastic bougie, and ensure that a neurological assessment including Glasgow Coma Scale score has been done.
3. Preoxygenate with 100% oxygen and attach monitors: pulse oximeter, ECG, BP cuff.
4. If cervical-spine injury is suspected, apply manual in-line axial stabilization and remove anterior portion of the rigid cervical-spine collar. Otherwise, use sniff position.
5. Give drugs as indicated by the clinical setting and hemodynamic status. Flush IV line with 10 mL of crystalloid solution after each drug to ensure drug delivery to the central circulation and to prevent precipitation within the IV line.
   - Induction agents: etomidate, thiopental, or ketamine
   - Neuromuscular blocking agents: succinylcholine or rocuronium
   - Adjunct agents: fentanyl, lidocaine, midazolam
6. Apply cricoid pressure.
7. Ventilate the lungs with 100% oxygen using inflation pressures < 20 cm H_2O to prevent or treat hypoxemia prior to intubation.
8. Intubate the trachea one minute after the neuromuscular blocking drug has been flushed in.
9. Confirm tracheal tube placement with end-tidal CO_2 detector.
10. Auscultate the lungs to confirm correct tube placement.
11. Secure the tube at a proper depth (e.g., 20 to 22 cm for women; 22 to 24 cm for men).
12. Be prepared to manage complications of RSI.

Modified from Smith CE, Grande CM, Wayne MA, ITACCS Consensus Panel, and International Review Committee. Rapid Sequence Intubation in Trauma. International Trauma Anesthesia and Critical Care Society. ITACCS, Baltimore 1998.[18]

Table 7-8 Suggested Drugs for RSI According to Clinical Setting and Hemodynamic Status

Clinical Setting	Induction Drug	Neuromuscular Blocking Agent	Adjunct Drugs
Cardiac arrest	None	None	None
Shock, SBP < 80 mm Hg	None	Succinylcholine or rocuronium	Midazolam 1–2 mg Fentanyl 0.5–1.0 μg/kg
Hypotension, SBP 80–100 mm Hg, Head trauma	Etomidate 0.1–0.2 mg/kg	Succinylcholine or rocuronium	Lidocaine 1–1.5 mg/kg Fentanyl 1 μg/kg
Hypotension, SBP 80–100 mm Hg, cardiac tamponade	Ketamine 1 mg/kg	Succinylcholine or rocuronium	None
Hypotension, SBP 80–100 mm Hg, coronary artery disease	Etomidate 0.1–0.2 mg/kg	Succinylcholine or rocuronium	Fentanyl 1 μg/kg Esmolol 10 mg (titrated)
Normotension, head trauma	Etomidate 0.3 mg/kg or thiopental 2–3 mg/kg	Succinylcholine or rocuronium	Fentanyl 2–3 μg/kg Lidocaine 1–1.5 mg/kg
Normotension, coronary artery disease	Etomidate 0.3 mg/kg	Succinylcholine or rocuronium	Fentanyl 2–4 μg/kg Esmolol 10–20 mg titrated

(continued)

Table 7-8 Suggested Drugs for RSI According to Clinical Setting and Hemodynamic Status (continued)

Clinical Setting	Induction Drug	Neuromuscular Blocking Agent	Adjunct Drugs
Hypertensive, head injury	Etomidate 0.3 mg/kg or thiopental 3–4 mg/kg	Succinylcholine or rocuronium	Fentanyl 2–4 μg/kg Lidocaine 1–1.5 mg/kg
Hypertension, coronary artery disease	Etomidate 0.3 mg/kg	Succinylcholine or rocuronium	Fentanyl 3–5 μg/kg Esmolol 10–20 mg titrated or labetalol 7.5–10 mg titrated
Asthma	Ketamine, 1–2 mg/kg	Succinylcholine or rocuronium	Fentanyl 1–4 μg/kg Lidocaine 1–1.5 mg/kg

Succinylcholine dose = 1.0–1.5 mg/kg; rocuronium dose = 1.0 mg/kg. When using rocuronium and thiopental in the same IV line, ensure that thiopental is flushed in before giving rocuronium to avoid precipitation and loss of the IV. Lidocaine 50–100 mg may be used to blunt myoclonus and injection-site pain from etomidate.

Modified from:

Smith CE: Rapid sequence intubation in adults; indications and concerns. *Clin Pulm Med* 2001; 8:147–165.[22]

Tryfus SJ, Abrams KJ, Grande CM: Airway management in neurological injuries. In: *Trauma Anesthesia and Critical Care of Neurological Injury*. Edited by Abrams KJ, Grande CM. Futura Publishing, Armonk, NY, 1997, pp. 121–151.[23]

Table 7-9 Complications During and After RSI: Diagnosis and Treatment

Complication	Diagnosis	Treatment
Manual ventilation device malfunction	Difficult to ventilate manually	Replace device.
Endobronchial intubation	Difficult to ventilate manually, decreased or absent breath sounds unilaterally	Withdraw tube to midtrachea.
Tracheal tube blockage/kink	Difficult to ventilate manually	Pass 14 or 18 F suction catheter; if still blocked, replace tube.
Tension pneumothorax	Difficult to ventilate manually, decreased or absent breath sounds unilaterally with hyperresonance, hypotension	Needle thoracostomy/chest drain.
Increased pulmonary resistance (chronic obstructive pulmonary disease, asthma, bronchospasm)	Difficult to ventilate manually, wheezing, "auto-peep," hypotension	Smaller tidal volume, respiratory rate 8–10 breaths per minute; increase expiratory time, bronchodilators.
Enlarged abdominal cavity (morbid obesity, term pregnancy)	Difficult to ventilate manually	Reverse Trendelenberg position.
Decreased venous return	Hypotension	Fluid bolus, treat other causes of hypotension (e.g., "auto-peep," spinal shock, anaphylaxis, cardiac failure).
Myocardial depression, cardiac tamponade	Hypotension	Fluid bolus, inotropes, pericardiocentesis
Cardiac arrhythmias (e.g., succinylcholine)	Bradycardia, asystole, massive hyperkalemia	Advanced cardiac life support: atropine, 1–2 mg IV for bradycardia or asystole; calcium for hyperkalemia*

*Treatment of hyperkalemia includes hyperventilation; calcium chloride, 10–20 mg/kg IV; glucose; insulin; and sodium bicarbonate.

Modified from:

Smith CE, Rapid sequence intubation in adults; indications and concerns. *Clin Pulm Med* 2001; 8:147–165.[22]

Smith CE, Walls RM, Lockey D, Kuhnigk H, Advanced airway management and use of anesthetic drugs. In *The International Textbook on Prehospital Trauma Care*. Grande CM, Soreide E (eds.), New York: Harcel Dekker, Inc., 2001.[3]

Summary

RSI is designed to provide optimal tracheal intubating conditions and to reduce the risk of aspiration. In experienced centers, RSI using muscle relaxants has a higher success rate, fewer complications, and better outcomes compared to RSI without neuromuscular relaxants and blind nasal intubation. Maximal preoxygenation can be attained by providing 100% oxygen through a sealed system for three to five minutes of normal tidal volume ventilation or by hyperventilation with eight deep breaths of 100% oxygen within 60 seconds. Cricoid pressure prevents passive regurgitation of stomach contents and reduces the risk of gastric insufflation during bag-mask ventilation.

Tracheal intubation aids, such as the gum-elastic bougie, are useful whenever difficult glottic visualization occurs. The bougie is relatively easy to insert through the vocal cords when no part of the glottis is visible and only the epiglottis or tip of the arytenoids (Grade III view) can be visualized. The tracheal tube is then threaded over the bougie, and tracheal placement is confirmed using capnography. The combined use of the BURP maneuver (Backwards, Upwards, Rightwards Pressure) over the thyroid cartilage to bring the larynx into view during laryngoscopy (Figure 4-19), in conjunction with the gum-elastic bougie can greatly increase intubation success.

Special laryngoscopes, such as the McCoy, Wuscope, and Bullard, and lighted stylets are also valuable for facilitating difficult intubation. Failure to intubate and subsequent inability to ventilate can lead quickly to death or cerebral hypoxia and brain injury. Contingency plans for failed intubation include optimal two-rescuer bag-mask ventilation, laryngeal mask airway, Combitube, and cricothyrotomy. Use of an airway algorithm such as the SUAAF (inside front cover) or others are of paramount importance.

REVIEW QUESTIONS

1. List the six principles for RSI.

2. Describe the drugs used in RSI.

3. Describe the equipment necessary for RSI.

4. Describe the special equipment available for facilitating difficult intubation.

CHAPTER 8

Rescue Ventilation

Andrew M. Mason
James Michael Rich
Michael Frass

Chapter Objectives

After reading this chapter, you should be able to:

- Identify and define the role of alternative nonsurgical airway devices for the rescue of failed tracheal intubation.

- Discuss the methods for correcting inadequate mask ventilation.

- Describe the management of the cannot-mask-ventilate/cannot-intubate (CMVCI) situation.

- Describe the indications, contraindications, and techniques for deploying an esophageal tracheal Combitube (ETC).

- Describe the indications, contraindications, precautions, and techniques for deploying a laryngeal mask airway (LMA).

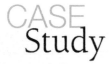
CASE
Study

Medic 7 is dispatched to a medical emergency reported as a possible stroke. The crew arrive at the scene to find an elderly man sitting in a chair. Family members state that, after eating lunch, he started calling them by the wrong names and then attempted to walk into the coat closet. On initial assessment the paramedics note that the patient is responsive only to painful stimuli and has snoring respirations. They open his airway by repositioning the head and note that the breathing pattern is irregular, with episodes of rapid respiration followed by apnoeic periods lasting around five seconds. All peripheral pulses are strong but the rhythm is irregular.

Oxygen is administered via a nonrebreathing mask, an IV line is established and the blood glucose level checked. The patient is secured to the stretcher and is loaded into the ambulance for transport to the local stroke center. Initial monitoring reveals that the cardiac rhythm is atrial fibrillation with a rate of 100 beats per minute, the blood pressure is 190/110 mmHg and the oxygen saturation (SpO_2) is 92%. Pupil size and reaction is normal and physical examination is otherwise unremarkable.

During transport, the patient becomes unresponsive and his SpO_2 falls to 85%. The paramedics insert an oral airway and begin to ventilate the patient with 100% oxygen using a bag-valve-mask device. This raises the SpO_2 to 95%. Intubation equipment is prepared, but laryngoscopy is unsuccessful and the attempt is suspended when the SpO_2 reading once again fails to 85%. A second attempt at laryngoscopy also fails to reveal adequate anatomical features to permit intubation. The paramedics therefore elect to use a Combitube (ETC) which is inserted using the laryngoscope. Inflation of the two cuffs causes the ETC to rise and seal successfully. The bag-valve device is attached to the pharyngeal port (#1) and there is good rise and fall of the chest with normal breath sounds heard equally on both sides of the chest. A colorimetric end-tidal CO_2 detector reveals satisfactory color changes and the SpO_2 reading rises quickly to 100%. Rescue ventilation is continued for the remainder of the journey and the patient is delivered to the emergency department without further incident.

Introduction

Because they are currently the only alternative airway devices with an American Heart Association (AHA) Class IIa designation, only the LMA Classic and esophageal-tracheal Combitube are covered in this chapter. The authors are aware that several other alternative airway devices are currently available (e.g., the King LTA, LMA Pro-Seal, LMA Fastrach, Cobra PLA, EasyTube, etc.), and it is intended that future revisions of this chapter will incorporate all those devices that attain Class IIa status. The chapter concludes with a comparison of the relative merits of the Combitube and LMA Classic. Surgical airway management is not discussed here, but it is covered in Chapter 12.

Cardiac arrest and other respiratory emergencies require immediate action to secure the airway and achieve adequate ventilation and oxygenation. The placement of a cuffed tracheal tube is the preferred method of providing both lung ventilation and airway protection, and this remains the gold standard of airway management. However, tracheal intubation is not always possible, particularly in the prehospital setting where neuromuscular blocking agents (NMBAs) and drugs for induction of anesthesia are not always available to rescue personnel.

The use of NMBAs has been shown to reduce the incidence of complications during emergency airway management.[1] Because the incidence of difficult intubation in routine general anesthesia under ideal conditions can be as high as 6%, it is hardly surprising that those who undertake emergency airway management in the hostile prehospital environment frequently encounter difficulties, even when such drugs are available.

Difficulty with intubation cannot always be predicted[2] and, when it does occur, it is usually the result of a complex interaction among patient factors, the clinical setting, and the skills of the practitioner.[3] The degree of difficulty varies from case to case, and problems can surface without warning during either mask ventilation or tracheal intubation. Paradoxically, some patients who are difficult to ventilate with a mask may be easy to intubate, and vice versa.[4] Regardless of whether intubation failure is secondary to a skill deficit, a patient factor, or equipment issues, the critical airway event can usually be resolved through the use of rescue ventilation.[5]

The cannot-mask-ventilate/cannot-intubate (CMVCI) situation occurs when inadequate mask ventilation and failed intubation occur simultaneously. Although relatively uncommon, a CMVCI event is one of the most challenging situations that any airway practitioner can face. Under such circumstances, repeated attempts at conventional laryngoscopic intubation may result in airway trauma with subsequent edema, which only worsens the problem. The situation requires an immediate switch to rescue ventilation to prevent hypoxemic brain damage and the death of the patient.[5]

With any critical airway event, rescue personnel should beware of the danger of falling victim to the so-called Law of Insanity, when an individual repeats the same failed strategy over and over again, each time expecting a different outcome. It is vital that those who undertake emergency airway management can switch to an effective plan B in the event of failed orotracheal intubation or inadequate mask ventilation. This will entail proficiency in the use of alternative airway devices. Such equipment must be available immediately, and emergency personnel should be able to make rapid and appropriate decisions regarding its use.

ON TARGET The cannot-mask-ventilate/cannot-intubate (CMVCI) situation occurs when inadequate mask ventilation and failed intubation occur simultaneously. This is one of the most challenging situations that any airway practitioner can face and requires an immediate switch to rescue ventilation. Because few ambulances are equipped with transtracheal jet ventilation equipment, all advanced airway practitioners should be able to perform a surgical airway intervention.

inadequate ventilation An inability to prevent or reverse hypoxemia using one- or two-person positive-pressure bag-valve-mask (BVM) ventilation in conjunction with an oropharyngeal and/or two nasopharyngeal airways and 100% oxygen.

 PEARLS The Law of Insanity is when an individual repeats the same failed strategy over and over again, each time expecting a different outcome, but getting the same failed result.

Noninvasive Alternative Airway Devices

failed intubation

Intubation that cannot be achieved by an experienced operator after three attempts, or the attempts have lasted for more than 10 minutes.

Alternative airway devices include (but are not limited to) the laryngeal mask airway (LMA) and the esophageal-tracheal Combitube (ETC). In the event of **failed intubation**, one or other (or both) of these devices should be considered before techniques such as transtracheal jet ventilation (TTJV) or surgical cricothyrotomy are tried. Other alternative airway devices have appeared over recent years but, currently, the ETC and LMA are the only two alternative airway adjuncts with an American Heart Association (AHA) Class IIa designation.[6]

AHA Class IIa status is reserved for therapeutic options for which the weight of evidence is in favor of their usefulness and efficacy.[6-8] Consequently, rescue ventilation should initially involve the use of such a device in combination with 100% oxygen and positive pressure ventilation in the face of a critical airway event. An exception to this rule is an obstruction to the airway at or below the level of the glottis because the LMA and ETC are both supraglottic devices. With obstruction at the glottic or infraglottic level, and where endotracheal intubation is not possible, rescue personnel are advised to proceed directly to TTJV or a surgical airway.[5,9]

Laryngeal Mask Airway (LMA)

ON TARGET

A critical airway event[5] can be defined as any one of the following:

1. Any cannot-ventilate/cannot-intubate (CVCI) situation.
2. ≥3 unsuccessful attempts at tracheal intubation or attempting intubation ≥10 minutes.
3. Sustained hypoxemia ($SpO_2 ≤ 92\%$) that is refractory to positive-pressure mask ventilation with 100% oxygen.

The LMA (LMA North America, San Diego, CA) was invented and first described by the British anesthesiologist Dr. Archie Brain in 1983.[10] The first commercially available LMA (LMA Classic™) appeared in 1987. This reusable model was made from silicone and was guaranteed for 40 uses or two years, and a single-use PVC version (LMA Unique™) followed in 1998.

The LMA Classic and LMA Unique (hereinafter collectively called the standard LMA) both possess a transparent semiflexible wide-bore airway tube with a universal standard 15 mm connector at the proximal end. At the distal end of the device is an elliptical mask that has an inflatable cuff around its margin. The cuff is inflated by means of an inflation line fitted with a self-sealing valve and pilot balloon (Figure 8-1).

The standard LMA is inserted via the mouth so that the mask lies in the hypopharynx with its airway opening facing the posterior aspect of the larynx. The device is self-seating and, on inflation of the cuff, the mask seals around the posterior perimeter of the larynx with its tip lying in the upper esophageal sphincter (Figure 8-2).

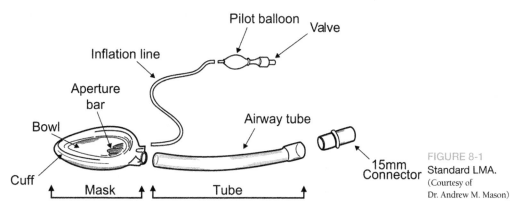

FIGURE 8-1
Standard LMA.
(Courtesy of Dr. Andrew M. Mason)

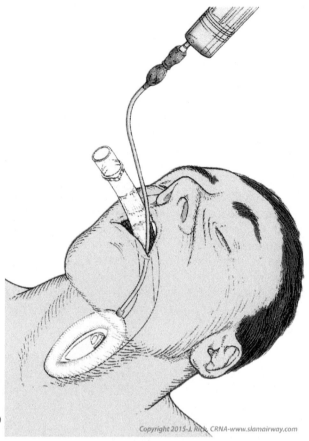

FIGURE 8-2
Standard LMA in situ.
(Courtesy of Intavent LTD, Coalville, UK)

Copyright 2015-J. Rich, CRNA-www.slamairway.com

 Patients who will accept an oropharyngeal airway without gagging will often tolerate an LMA. Agents such as etomidate, midazolam, or propofol can facilitate insertion of the LMA.

The seal remains airtight at moderate airway pressures, and the mean (range) pressure required to produce gastric insufflation has been shown to be 28 (19–33) cm H_2O, with a mean (range) pressure for oropharyngeal leakage of 31 (19–41) cm H_2O.[11] Therefore, if peak ventilatory pressures are kept below 20 cm H_2O, leakage of air is unlikely to occur when the correct size of LMA is selected.

Patient Selection

The LMA should be used only in patients who are profoundly unconscious and unresponsive, are without glossopharyngeal reflexes, and have an identified need for an artificial airway. In the emergency situation, it is useful to be aware that patients who will accept an oropharyngeal airway without gagging will often tolerate the careful insertion of an LMA. Indeed, patients emerging from routine general anesthesia are usually capable of responding to verbal commands before they begin to reject their LMA, and insertion of the device is certainly tolerated at higher levels of consciousness than the tracheal tube. To facilitate LMA insertion into those who are still responsive, sedation with an agent such as etomidate, midazolam, or propofol is required. On the other hand, muscle relaxants are not required for LMA insertion.

LMA insertion can be performed readily by a variety of practitioners[12-15] and skill retention following instruction is high, making it a suitable device for those who have limited opportunities to perform tracheal intubation. It is equally suitable for use by experienced personnel in situations where tracheal intubation proves impossible for technical or other reasons.

Indications

As a broad generalization, the LMA is indicated where use of a face mask would be appropriate, but not when a tracheal tube is advisable.[16] However, in situations where tracheal intubation is not possible (e.g., lack of equipment or training), use of an LMA can offer significant advantages over bag-valve-mask ventilation (BVMV). Indications for use of the LMA might include:

- Cardiac arrest
- Near-drowning
- Inhalation of smoke or toxic fumes
- Drug overdose with respiratory depression
- Severe blood loss
- Trauma (e.g., in patients with serious head or facial trauma who are unable to maintain an airway or oxygenation)
- Failed tracheal intubation, including CVCI situations (i.e., as a rescue ventilation device)
- Oropharyngeal/supraglottic bleeding, which obscures the glottis and prevents tracheal intubation by direct laryngoscopy or with a flexible fiberoptic bronchoscope

Contraindications

Elective use of the LMA is contraindicated where there is a significant risk of aspiration (e.g., full stomach, morbid obesity, etc.) and where high inflation pressures are necessary (e.g., low compliance of lungs/chest wall or high airway resistance).

Aspiration and the LMA

Although concern is sometimes expressed about the relative lack of protection that the LMA affords against aspiration, the risk is almost certainly overstated. In one meta-analysis study of aspiration with the LMA, the overall incidence of pulmonary aspiration was approximately two cases per 10,000,[17] with no death or permanent disability resulting. This rate is not statistically different from the incidence of pulmonary aspiration with the tracheal tube in routine anesthesia (approximately 1.7 cases per 10,000).

In the event that fluid appears in the airway tube, the LMA should neither be deflated nor removed; the rescuer should simply apply suction down the airway tube and also in the pharynx.

Naturally, the risk of aspiration when treating unfasted patients in the emergency setting is higher than that during planned procedures. Even so, in one multicenter hospital-based CPR study,[18] the incidence of aspiration with the LMA was less than 1%, much less than has been shown to occur with the unprotected airway when other ventilatory techniques are used during resuscitation.[19] In trauma, and particularly in those with maxillofacial injuries, the risk of aspiration of gastric contents is, in any case, less than the risk of aspiration of blood,[20] and the cuff of the LMA has been shown to afford effective protection against the aspiration of blood arising from the oropharynx.[21] The contraindication to use of the LMA in unfasted patients in the emergency setting is therefore relative, and the risk of aspiration has to be balanced against the advantages of the ease with which an airway can be established and the speed with which oxygenation of the patient can be commenced using the device.

It is known that regurgitation is more likely to occur if the stomach has already been inflated by mouth-to-mouth, mouth-to-mask, bag-valve-mask, or automatic resuscitator-mask ventilation applied prior to insertion of the LMA. Use of an LMA from the outset of resuscitation could therefore be advantageous. In the event of fluid appearing in the airway tube, the LMA should neither be deflated nor removed. The rescuer should simply apply suction down the airway tube and also in the pharynx.

Size Selection and Cuff Volume

The standard LMA is available in a range of sizes to suit almost any individual (Table 8-1). When it appears that two adjacent sizes of LMA might suit a particular patient, the rescuer is always advised to select the larger size initially. Cuff volume should be adjusted to the minimum required to achieve an adequate seal and should never exceed the recommended maximum cuff volume. Overinflation of the cuff simply distorts periglottic tissues and aggravates leakage of air around the mask during positive-pressure ventilation. When sizing has been performed correctly, the cuff volume producing the best seal is often half the recommended maximum cuff volume.[23] Consequently, if a leak is detected, it is often worth removing some air from the cuff, especially when it has been inflated initially to the maximum recommended volume. The manufacturer recommends that the cuff should be inflated with just enough air to obtain an intracuff pressure of 60 cm H_2O.

Cuff Preparation

Full deflation of the cuff is the key to successful insertion. When correctly deflated, the mask has a shallow concave profile with a thin leading edge. Deflation is achieved using a 50 ml syringe so that the mask forms a flat oval disc with the rim arching away from the aperture. Try to ensure that there are no wrinkles near the tip of the deflated cuff. Correct deflation can be achieved by applying a strong vacuum with the syringe while the fingers of the other hand press the mask, aperture side down, against any clean flat surface (Figure 8-3). Alternatively, available from the distributor is a special cuff deflation tool that consistently produces the ideal cuff shape for insertion. A positive flip test indicates that correct deflation has been achieved (Figure 8-4).

Table 8-1   LMA Size Selection and Cuff Volume

Size	Patient	Maximum Cuff Volume
1	Up to 5 kg	4 ml
1½	5 to 10 kg	7 ml
2	10 to 20 kg	10 ml
2½	20 to 30 kg	14 ml
3	Large child or small adult (30 to 50 kg)*	20 ml
4	Normal adult (50 to 70 kg)*	30 ml
5	Large adult (70 to 100 kg)*	40 ml
6	Extremely large adult (>100 kg)*	50 ml

*The weight of adults provides only an approximate guide to LMA size because pharyngeal geometry is only loosely associated with body weight. Although body weight is frequently employed to estimate LMA size, there is evidence that gender may be a useful guide in adults[22] as follows: size 4 for females, size 5 for males.

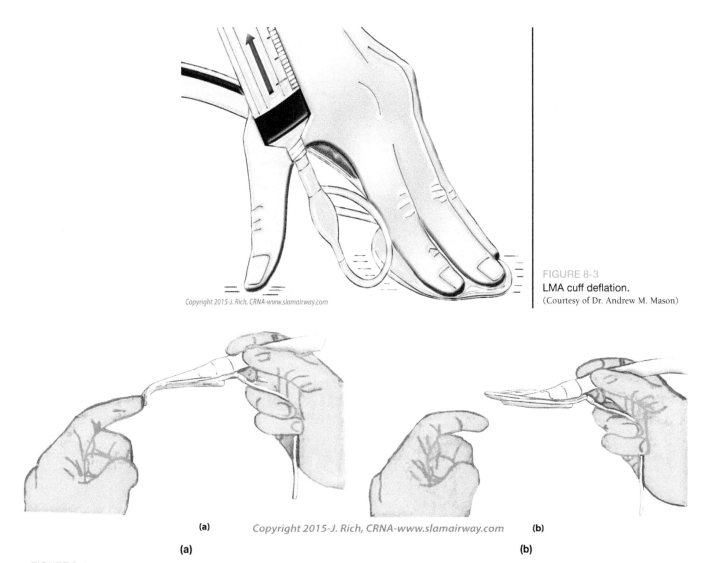

Copyright 2015-J. Rich, CRNA-www.slamairway.com

FIGURE 8-3
LMA cuff deflation.
(Courtesy of Dr. Andrew M. Mason)

(a)   Copyright 2015-J. Rich, CRNA-www.slamairway.com   **(b)**

(a)   **(b)**

FIGURE 8-4
(a) For a flip test, pull down the tip of the deflated mask with the index finger and then release. (b) The tip of the mask should flip back immediately into extension.
(Courtesy of Dr. Andrew M. Mason)

Patient Positioning for Insertion

Although neck flexion with atlanto-occipital joint extension (i.e., the traditional sniffing position) provides the best conditions for placement of the LMA, insertion is also possible with the head maintained in neutral alignment by manual in-line stabilization.[24] This may provide an advantage over the tracheal tube in the initial resuscitation of trauma patients with suspected neck injuries.

Supporting Equipment

Ensure that all support items are on hand before attempting LMA insertion. Suggested items include:

- Surgical gloves.
- 50 ml syringe.
- Water-soluble lubricating gel.
- Suction equipment.

- Bag-valve-mask manual ventilation device.
- Bite block.
- Catheter mount.
- Oxygen source.

In emergency situations where a bag-valve device is not available, mouth-to-tube ventilation can be applied in conjunction with a biological filter.

Standard Insertion Technique

Gloves should be worn while performing this technique.

1. First, apply a bead of water-soluble gel to the back of the mask close to its tip. Try to avoid getting gel on the fingers of the inserting hand because it can make it difficult to grip the LMA during insertion.
2. In the absence of suspected neck injury, position the head and neck in the sniffing position by supporting the occiput with the nondominant hand.
3. Holding the LMA like a pen, with the tip of the index finger placed anteriorly at the junction of the cuff and tube, insert the mask into the mouth, ensuring that the longitudinal black line on the airway tube is facing the patient's nose.
4. Press the tip of the mask against the hard palate and move it back and forth a few times to distribute the lubricating gel.
5. After ensuring that the mask is lying flat against the palate and the tip is not folded over, begin to advance the finger into the oropharynx, keeping the mask in firm contact with the palate.
6. With the wrist of the inserting hand well flexed, push the tip of the index finger in a cranial direction toward the palm of the supporting hand, allowing the palatopharyngeal curve to guide the mask into the hypopharynx (Figure 8-5).
7. As insertion progresses, the inserting finger should be hyperextended with its entire flexor surface in contact with the airway tube, keeping it in firm contact with the palate and tissues of the posterior pharyngeal wall. By the time any resistance is felt, the finger should be almost fully inserted into the mouth.
8. At this point, remove the supporting hand and use it to stabilize the tube before withdrawing the inserting finger from the mouth.

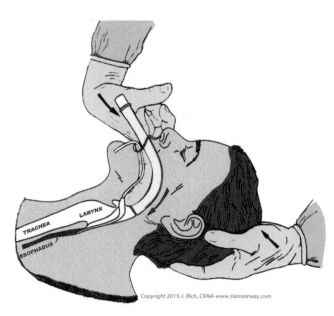

FIGURE 8-5
Standard insertion technique.
(Courtesy of Dr. Andrew M. Mason)

9. Push the LMA further into the hypopharynx until definite resistance is felt, but do not use excessive force.

10. Let go of the tube completely before inflating the cuff with the appropriate volume of air, and watch for the characteristic 1 cm rise of the airway tube with filling out of the tissues on either side of the neck.

11. Check for correct placement by observing the rise and fall of the chest during gentle hand ventilation, and perform auscultation of both lungs and the side of the neck to confirm air entry into the lungs and the absence of a leak at mask level.

12. In patients with a perfusing cardiac rhythm, it is also good practice to ensure the presence of end-tidal carbon dioxide.[5]

It is worth trying a slight lateral approach in cases where initial resistance is encountered during insertion, reverting to the midline as soon as resistance is overcome. Rotating the standard LMA through 180 degrees during insertion (as with an Guedel oropharyngeal airway) is a useful fallback technique when all else fails.

Alternative Insertion Techniques

When access to the patient's head from above is difficult or impossible, or where the presence of a cervical collar impedes insertion, the standard LMA can be inserted from below using the thumb (Figure 8-6). The principle of insertion is otherwise the same as in the standard insertion technique. It is also possible to employ a nondigital insertion technique in cases where the rescuer wishes to avoid placing a digit into the patient's mouth, and full details of both of these alternative techniques can be found in literature available from the distributor. In one randomized crossover study, insertion of the LMA Unique into paralyzed adults by inexperienced personnel (registered nurses with no hands-on clinical experience of airway management after manikin-only training) was found to be equally successful with or without digital intraoral manipulation. The overall success rate for insertion was 94% with digital intraoral manipulation, and 93% using a nondigital insertion technique.[25]

Fixation

Use of a bite block is recommended to prevent compression of the airway tube, and a roll of gauze swabs approximately 2.5 cm thick can be fashioned for this purpose. To stabilize the LMA and

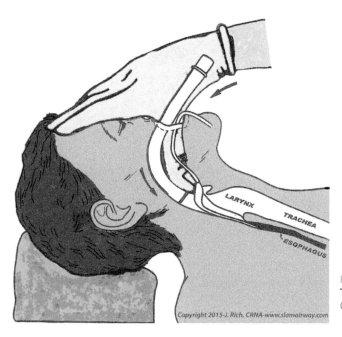

FIGURE 8-6
Thumb insertion technique.
(Courtesy of Dr. Andrew M. Mason)

Rescue Ventilation 155

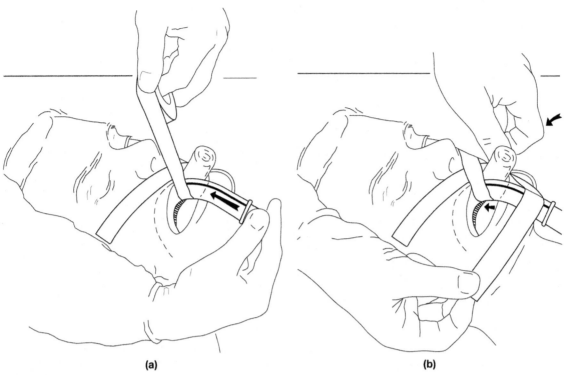

(a)   **(b)**

FIGURE 8-7

(a) Taping around the tube and bite block.
(Courtesy of Dr. Andrew M. Mason)

(b) Taping to the mandible.
(Courtesy of Dr. Andrew M. Mason)

prevent accidental dislodgement, a length of adhesive tape can be applied along one zygomatic arch, looping over and around the tube and bite block and thus binding them together, and then across to the opposite zygomatic arch. During the taping process, the natural caudal curve of the airway tube should be pushed upward into the palatopharyngeal arch. Finally, the proximal end of the airway tube is taped separately to the mandible so that the airway tube maintains good contact with the palate and the 15 mm connector points in a caudal direction (Figure 8-7). A stabilization device with an integral bite block based on the Thomas endotracheal tube holder (Laerdal Medical Corporation, Wappingers Falls, NY), suitable for use with any standard LMA, has recently become commercially available (Figure 8-8).[26] A Guedel oropharyngeal airway is not recommended for use as a bite block with the LMA because both devices are designed to sit in the midline. And the tip of the oropharyngeal airway may compromise the cuff of the LMA.

Removal

The LMA should be removed only if tracheal intubation is about to be performed or the patient has recovered with active protective reflexes. Apply suction to the pharynx before removing the LMA and keep suction on hand during the removal process. Always remove the LMA with its cuff fully inflated to help extract accumulated secretions and debris, thus preventing them from falling back onto the unprotected larynx.

 The LMA should not be removed unless tracheal intubation is about to be undertaken or the patient has regained airway reflexes. The device should be removed with the cuff fully inflated and with suction on hand.

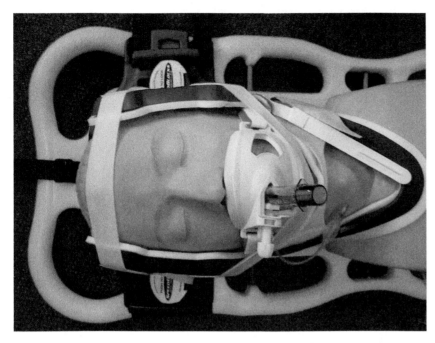

FIGURE 8-8
LMA secured with Thomas tube holder.
(Courtesy of Dr. Andrew M. Mason)

Problems Associated with Insertion

In expert hands, the failure rate for LMA insertion is less than 0.5%,[27] but this can rise to 5% or more with inexperienced personnel or when incorrect insertion techniques are used. It is occasionally advocated that the LMA should be inserted with the cuff partially inflated, and there is some evidence that this method may assist inexperienced users.[27] However, careful attention to detail in terms of size selection, cuff deflation, and insertion technique offers the best chance of success for occasional users.

The most common malposition of the LMA is associated with epiglottic downfolding, which can increase the work of breathing and, if sufficiently severe, can obstruct the airway completely. Impaction of the device with the laryngeal inlet can also lead to laryngospasm or stridor. Epiglottic downfolding is more likely to occur if the device is inserted with the cuff partially or fully inflated, or when the LMA is not pressed firmly into the posterior pharyngeal wall during insertion. The avoidance of holding the LMA tube during inflation of the cuff may be an important factor in allowing a downfolded epiglottis to revert to its normal position. In the event that epiglottic downfolding is suspected, the LMA should be removed, its cuff prepared again, and the device reinserted with careful attention to correct technique.

The most common technical errors during placement are:

- Premature release of the index finger before the mask has reached the hypopharynx.
- Failure to observe the mask inside the mouth, ensuring that it lies flat against the palate and that the tip is not folded over.
- Poor positioning of the head and neck.
- Failure to adopt a slight lateral approach if resistance is encountered.

Family of LMA Devices

The current range of LMA devices (Figure 8-9) consists of:

- LMA Classic™, a reusable model of silicone construction guaranteed for 40 uses or two years (1987).

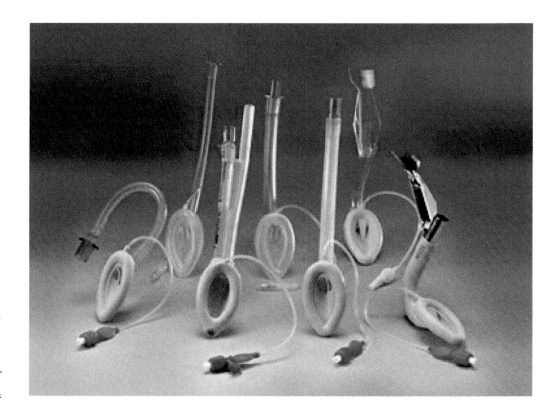

FIGURE 8-9
Family of LMA devices.
(a) Reusable LMA Flexible.
(b) Single-use LMA Flexible.
(c) Reusable LMA Proseal.
(d) Single-use LMA Unique.
(e) Reusable LMA Classic.
(f) Single-use LMA Fastrach.
(g) Reusable LMA Fastrach.
(Courtesy of The Laryngeal Mask Co., LTD., St Helier, Jersey)

- LMA Flexible^{TM}, a reusable silicone model with flexible airway tube allowing unrestricted surgical access to mouth and pharynx (1991).
- LMA Fastrach^{TM}, a reusable device with an anatomically curved metal airway tube coated with silicone, facilitating seamless progression to blind (or fiberscopically guided) tracheal intubation with a dedicated tracheal tube (1996).
- LMA Unique^{TM}, a single-use PVC version of the LMA-Classic (1998).
- LMA Proseal^{TM}, a reusable device with a modified cuff providing an enhanced airway seal (30 cm H_2O or greater) and incorporating a separate drain tube opening at the tip of the cuff in the upper esophageal sphincter that facilitates drainage of gastric secretions and passage of a gastric tube (2000).
- Single-use LMA Flexible^{TM}, a PVC version of the silicone LMA Flexible (2004).
- Single-use LMA Fastrach^{TM}, a plastic construction with a PVC cuff (2004).

The LMA Classic is ideal for extrication of patients in a closed-space rescue who require ventilation that cannot be provided by mask or tracheal tube (Figure 8-10). The LMA Proseal and LMA Fastrach both have features that suggest they may be of value in emergency situations. However, at the time of writing, the LMA Classic is the only device in the LMA range with official AHA Class IIa status.

Esophageal Tracheal Combitube (ETC)

The esophageal tracheal Combitube® (ETC; Tyco-Healthcare-Nellcor, Pleasanton, CA) is another valuable alternative airway adjunct for use in emergencies. The ETC serves as an effective rescue airway, especially when used in combination with the self-inflating bulb (SIB) and/or carbon dioxide detector.[5,28]

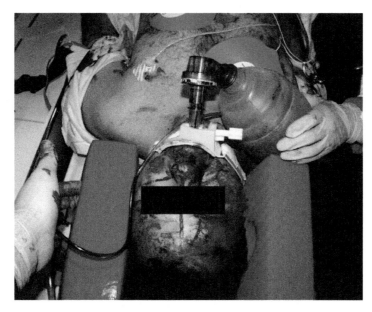

FIGURE 8-10
Prehospital use of the LMA
for rescue ventilation.
Young victim extricated from
motor vehicle with LMA
secured with Thomas tube
holder.
(Courtesy of Dr. Andrew M. Mason)

The ETC (www.combitube.org) is provided as an ETC 37F SA (small adult) to be used in patients four to six feet tall (about 120 to 180 cm), while the ETC 41F is for use in patients taller than six feet (about 180 cm), according to the investigations of Urtubia, Gaitini, Walz, Panning, and Krafft.[29-33] The kit is distributed either as a hard tray, a rollup kit, or single item. The kit includes a large syringe, preloaded to 85 ml (41F: 100 ml), and a small syringe, preloaded to 12 ml (41F: 15 ml). The blue-coded large syringe is used for inflation of the oropharyngeal balloon via the valve with the blue pilot balloon. A 10F (41F: 12F) suction catheter and a deflection elbow, to avoid soiling of the rescuer by gastric contents, are also included.

Recent studies show that the ETC may be safely reused, providing special precautions are observed. Sterilization allows more economic use of the ETC in patients undergoing elective procedures. However, in emergency situations, unused Combitubes are preferred.

Design

Frass et al. invented the ETC[34] as an improvement on the esophageal obturator airway (EOA).[28] In the 1980s, recommendations were made to replace the EOA with BVM ventilation or tracheal intubation by paramedical personnel in the United States.[35] Coincidentally, the ETC was introduced in 1987 to bridge the gap between the prehospital phase and arrival in the emergency department, as well as when ideal conditions or trained staff for tracheal intubation were not immediately available.[36]

The ETC is available in two sizes. The original 41F ETC (Combitube) is for use in patients greater than six feet tall (183 cm),[37] while the size 37F ETC SA (Combitube small adult), which was introduced in 1995 and originally approved only for patients less than five feet tall, has now been used successfully in patients between 3.9 feet and 6.5 feet (120 cm and 198 cm)[33] and is recommended for use in patients four to six feet tall[30] who are older than 12 years of age.[38] However, based on the successful use in taller patients, the 37F ETC SA is also recommended for use without any upper height limitations.[33]

ETC design (Figure 8-11) incorporates the benefit of the tracheal tube (TT) combined with the positive features of the EOA.[28,39] It is marked with double rings just distal to where the two proximal tubes combine to form a single tube with a double lumen. The ETC facilitates lung ventilation when placed in either the esophagus or trachea. Upon insertion, the patient's teeth or alveolar ridges should lie between these rings.

The large proximal oropharyngeal cuff (inflated with 85 ml of air with the ETC 37F SA and 100 ml with the ETC 41F, respectively) serves to seal the upper airway. The smaller

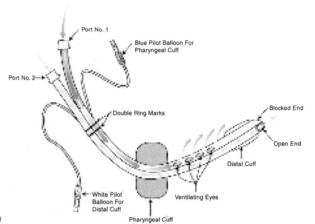

FIGURE 8-11

Cross section of the esophageal-tracheal Combitube (ETC) showing the pharyngeal (No. 1) as well as the tracheo-esophageal lumen (No. 2) and the tubes for connection to the ventilation device. The printed ring-marks indicate depth of insertion and should lie above and below the level of the upper teeth or alveolar ridges after ETC placement.

(Courtesy of JM Rich, CRNA [www. slamairway.com])

distal cuff is inflated with 5 ml to 12 ml for the ETC 37F SA, and 5 ml to 15 ml for the ETC 41F, respectively (Figure 8-12). Inflation of the proximal oropharyngeal cuff automatically adjusts the ETC to the correct position and seals the airway in the oropharynx just posterior to the hard palate. This anchors the device securely for oxygenation and ventilation during transportation, thus obviating the need for further fixation.[39-43] The proximal oropharyngeal cuff may occasionally require an additional volume of 25 ml to 50 ml of air to provide sealing in some patients;[33] however, the maximum recommended volume of the distal cuff must never be exceeded to avoid damage to the structures of the esophagus or trachea.[44,45] Small distal cuff inflation volumes of 10 ± 1 ml are usually adequate for sealing with either size of ETC.[39]

Insertion

As with the LMA, the ETC should be used only in patients who are profoundly unconscious and unresponsive, are without glossopharyngeal reflexes, and have an identified need for an artificial airway.[5,28] Depending on the location of the tip of the ETC after placement, the device seals either the esophagus or trachea, respectively, and provides airway protection, oxygenation, and ventilation comparable to that provided by routine tracheal intubation.[5,28,32,38,40,46,47]

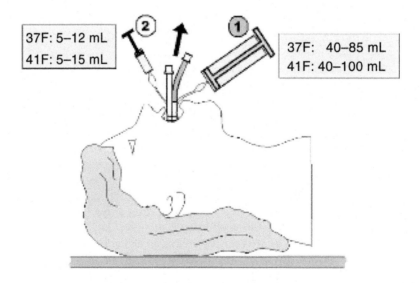

FIGURE 8-12

Inflation of the balloons: in the Combitube (ETC) 37F SA (small adult) 85 ml of air is inflated into the large oropharyngeal balloon, and 10 ml in the distal cuff (in the ETC 41F, 100 ml and 10 ml are inflated, respectively).

(Courtesy of JM Rich, CRNA [www. slamairway.com])

With special attention to detail, the ETC is normally easy to insert and, although the ETC was designed for blind insertion, use of a laryngoscope can facilitate esophageal placement[32,46-48] by holding the tongue out of the way, like the thumb is used during blind insertion.[38] Excessive force during insertion or overinflation of the distal cuff after insertion may cause injury and should be avoided.[49-51]

It is not recommended to place the patient's head in the sniffing position as is used routinely with direct laryngoscopy, but rather in a neutral, semiflexed position. A neutral head position is advantageous, especially in patients with suspected or evident cervical-spine injury. As with any airway maneuver in patients with suspected or evident cervical-spine injury, strict adherence to manual in-line axial stabilization (MIAS) is necessary to prevent injury.[5]

The position of the operator may be at either side of the patient. The back of the patient's tongue and lower jaw are grasped between thumb and forefinger of the nondominant hand, and a jaw-lift maneuver is performed. Then, the Combitube is introduced blindly by performing a gentle downward curved movement along the tongue until the two printed ring marks lie between teeth (or alveolar ridges in edentulous patients) (Figure 8-13). Unlike the LMA, the ETC is inserted along the tongue of the patient. Insertion of the Combitube using direct laryngoscopy aids in keeping the soft tissues distracted and makes it easier to insert the ETC into the esophagus.

Using the large syringe, the upper balloon is inflated with 85 ml (41F: 100 ml) of air through port No. 1 with its blue pilot balloon. Due to the self-adjusting property of the oropharyngeal balloon, the ETC rises out of the patient's mouth until the large oropharyngeal balloon seats just under the hard palate. Resistance is commonly encountered during inflation of the upper balloon and may require additional force or a two-handed inflation technique.

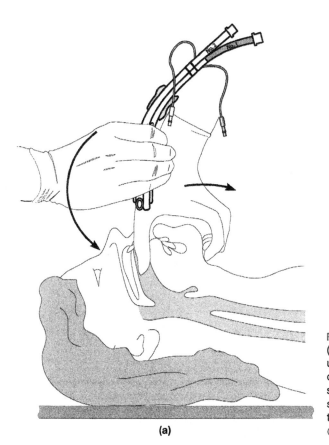

(a)

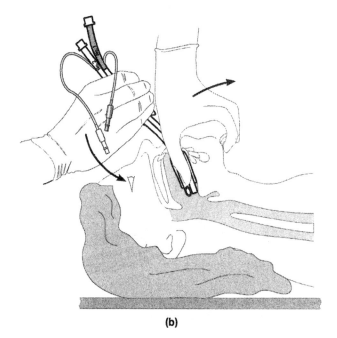

(b)

FIGURE 8-13

(a) Jaw-thrust and blind insertion of the Combitube. Perform a jaw-thrust using deep thumb insertion and advance the Combitube in a curved downward motion along the midline of the tongue. Little to no resistance should be felt. Advancement of the ETC against resistance may result in soft-tissue injury. (b) Insertion of the Combitube along the midline of the tongue facilitates placement into either the esophagus or trachea.

(Courtesy of JM Rich, CRNA [www. slamairway.com])

Recommended inflation volumes should be adhered to for emergency use. Oropharyngeal balloon inflation is 85 ml in the Combitube SA 37F, and 100 ml in the Combitube 41F. After inflation of the upper balloon, the distal cuff is inflated with 10 ± 1 ml of air through the valve with the white pilot balloon using the small syringe. This distal cuff serves to seal either the esophagus or the trachea.

Lung Ventilation

With blind insertion, there is a high probability (up to 98%) of esophageal placement (Figure 8-14a).[28,38,48,52] Initial ventilation should therefore be attempted first via the longer blue tube (No. 1) leading to the pharyngeal lumen. Since the distal end is blocked, air is forced through the ventilating eyes into the pharynx. Because the nose and mouth are blocked by the oropharyngeal balloon and the esophagus is occluded by the distal cuff, air takes the path of least resistance through the glottis into the trachea. Auscultation should be performed to confirm adequate bilateral breath sounds over the lungs and the absence of gastric insufflation. Capnography and/or use of an esophageal detection device are recommended to confirm correct placement.[5] Ventilation via a manual bag-valve device or a mechanical ventilator is then continued via this lumen. The second unused lumen allows immediate decompression of the esophagus and stomach, thereby decreasing the possibility of aspiration.

If no signs of lung inflation are present during ventilation through the long blue tube No. 1, the ETC has probably been inserted into the trachea (Figure 8-14b). In this case, ventilation is performed via the shorter transparent tube No. 2, leading to the distally patent tracheo-esophageal lumen. Lung ventilation should then be confirmed again (as noted above). When ventilation is performed through the transparent tube No. 2, the Combitube is functioning as a conventional tracheal tube.[5]

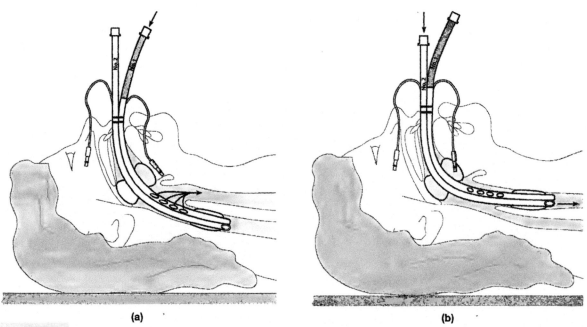

(a)   **(b)**

FIGURE 8-14
FIGURE 8-14

(a) Position of the Combitube in the esophagus. Ventilation is performed via the longer blue tube No. 1, causing air to pass into the pharyngeal lumen. Air cannot escape at the distal blocked end of the pharyngeal lumen and takes the path of least resistance via the ventilating eyes (side ports) into the hypopharynx and then enters the trachea. (b) Position of the Combitube in the trachea. Ventilation proceeds via the shorter transparent tube No. 2 into the tracheo-esophageal lumen, which communicates directly into the trachea (like an endotracheal tube).

(Courtesy of JM Rich, CRNA [www. slamairway.com])

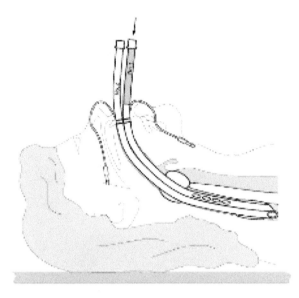

FIGURE 8-15

Malposition of the Combitube in the esophageal position. Excessive insertion depth of the Combitube causes obstruction of the glottic opening, which makes ventilation impossible. Note that the ventilating eyes are resting within the esophagus, which blocks ventilation between the cuffs (note arrows exiting ventilating eyes). After pulling the Combitube back 2 to 3 cm (note position of 2 black rings), the ventilating eyes are correctly positioned to facilitate ventilation through port No. 1.

(Courtesy of JM Rich, CRNA [www. slamairway.com])

Malposition of the ETC

Occasionally, it is impossible to ventilate through either the longer or shorter tube.[53,54] This situation occurs only with esophageal placement and is probably caused by deep insertion of the ETC into the esophagus (even though the teeth or gums are between the black rings) (Figure 8-15). In this orientation, the oropharyngeal balloon can occlude the laryngeal aperture, and the ventilating eyes become buried in the esophagus. To remedy this problem, both balloons are deflated completely, and the ETC is withdrawn approximately 2 to 3 cm, after which both balloons are sequentially reinflated. This may need to be repeated once or twice to attain correct positioning of the ETC. If after slightly withdrawing the ETC several times, it is still impossible to ventilate the lungs, the device should be withdrawn completely and reinserted, or ventilation attempted using another device.[5]

Manikin Training with the ETC

Manikin training is important to facilitate and develop proficiency with the ETC.[28,39,55-59] To facilitate insertion, the ETC and the mouth of the manikin should be sprayed with silicone or a similar substance to avoid friction.[60] Bending the ETC at the pharyngeal portion between the cuffs for a few seconds just prior to use (the so-called *Lipp maneuver*) [Figure 8-16a][5,61] enhances the preformed curvature and eases insertion. This maneuver has been modified by Urtubia et al. (Figure 8-16b).[62] To improve the blind insertion technique of the ETC in terms of efficacy and safety, Urtubia recommends keeping the ETC bent as long as possible until it enters the oropharyngeal cavity. This is done by holding the ETC between the first three fingers of the dominant hand. Maintaining the ETC bent, together with a rapid curved downward movement of insertion into the oropharyngeal cavity, enables the tip to reach the esophagus before the ETC recovers to its original, less curved shape, making insertion fast and safe.

For blind insertion, open the mouth of the manikin with the thumb and index finger of one hand and then deeply insert the thumb of the other hand into the mouth, pressing the tongue in an anterior direction. Lift the jaw so that the tongue is trapped under the thumb while the jaw is pulled forward. Pass the ETC gently into the mouth along the tongue and pull the proximal end of the ETC in a cephalad direction while advancing the tube. This positions the lower curved portion of the ETC in a parallel orientation with the manikin's chest and keeps the tip from contacting the posterior pharynx. The ETC should be inserted until the teeth of the manikin lie between the two black ring-marks.

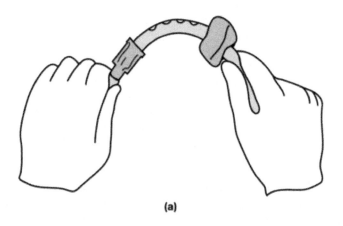

(a)

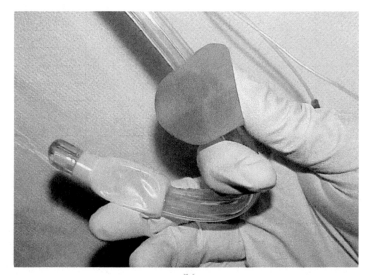

Verifying Correct Placement of the ETC

Confirmation of tube placement should include auscultation over the epigastrium and bilaterally over the midaxillary lines (axillae). In addition, a near-failsafe device (CO_2 detection device and/or esophageal detector device [EDD]) should be used. However, it should be appreciated that CO_2 detectors may fail in patients with low cardiac output. Because of insufficient evidence, neither the EDD nor CO_2 detector is recommended for confirmation of correct placement of the ETC in AHA Guidelines 2005.[63] However, the authors have found that the use of clinical signs and the use of a CO_2 detector in conjunction with the LMA and clinical signs and the use of a CO_2 detector/EDD with the ETC are adequate to confirm placement and monitor ventilation. None of these methods are failsafe, however, and may produce false negatives or false positives, facts that must be fully understood by the operator (Chapters 1 and 5).[64-66]

Advantages of ETC

The esophageal-tracheal Combitube (ETC) has many positive features and can be used by almost any provider, independent of level of training or expertise (Table 8-2) (Figure 8-17). It is useful in many emergency and difficult airway management situations, especially from the closed space prehospital situation[41] (Figure 8-18) through rescue of failed intubation in the operating room.[5]

Several studies have shown that the Combitube works well in the hands of emergency medical technicians.[57,59,73-75] EMTs assessed the ETC as the best airway with respect to

Table 8-2 Advantages of the Combitube (ETC)[5,9,28,32,34,38,40,41,46,47,59,67-72]

- Useful with patients in whom manipulation of the cervical spine is hazardous or impossible (trauma, suspected cervical-spine injury, rheumatoid arthritis).
- Controlled mechanical ventilation is possible at high ventilation pressures.
- Functions equally well with either tracheal (rare) or esophageal (usual) placement.
- Insertion using either a blind technique or a laryngoscope is possible.
- No preparation of ETC is necessary because the tube and syringes are ready to use.
- Noninvasive as compared to cricothyrotomy.
- No need for neck flexion—neutral head position is best.
- Device is secure on inflation of oropharyngeal cuff and fixation is unnecessary.
- Slim design allows insertion in patients with a small interincisor gap.
- Provides airway control when access to the patient's head is difficult (e.g., confined space rescue situation).
- Provides airway control and rescue of a failed intubation with the unexpected difficult airway.
- Provides airway control by persons previously trained in tracheal intubation who have infrequent opportunity to maintain their skills.
- Provides airway control after failed intubation due to lack of skill, equipment limitations, or anatomical abnormality.
- Provides airway control when used by persons untrained in tracheal intubation who are responsible for ventilating the patient prior to the arrival of trained individuals (i.e., first responders).
- Provides aspiration protection comparable to the tracheal tube and allows high ventilatory pressures (useful in patients with decreased lung compliance).
- Provides rapid ventilation for paralyzed patients who cannot be intubated or mask ventilated (CVCI).
- Provides superior sealing of the airway in comparison to other supraglottic airway devices.
- Quick and easy-to-use emergency airway device.
- Ventilation with the ETC in the esophageal position produces higher arterial oxygen tensions than in patients ventilated with a tracheal tube.
- Well suited for obese patients.

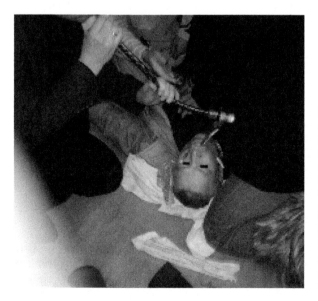

FIGURE 8-17
A patient suffered cardiopulmonary arrest in the lobby of a hospital. He was defibrillated using an AED and received rescue ventilation with a Combitube. The rescuer is ventilating the patient by blowing into a tube that contains a microbial barrier to protect the rescuer from the exhaled air of the victim.
(Courtesy of Dr. Michael Frass, M.D.)

overall performance and adequacy of airway patency and ventilation in comparison to the PTLA, LMA, and oral airway/mask. The ETC was associated with fewer problems with ventilation and was the most preferred by a majority of EMTs.[75] In the retrospective study of Tanigawa and Shigematsu, who reported on 12,020 cases of nontraumatic cardiac arrest, the ETC was found to have a better first attempt insertion rate (82.4%) than either the esophageal gastric tube airway (EGTA) or the LMA.[57] One of the studies involved 500 emergency medical technicians trained in defibrillation (EMT-D) with only manikin intubation skills. The overall successful ETC insertion rate was 79% in spite of a small run-volume of only 195 cardiac-arrest patients over an 18-month period.[59] Lefrançois and Dufour investigated 831 blind ETC insertions by prehospital EMT-Ds and found a successful placement rate of 95.4% with a successful ventilation rate of 91.4%.[74] With the ETC, ten times more case reports than with the classic LMA are reported in trauma patients (53 versus 5).[76]

The ETC is effective for use in trauma patients. With the ETC, ten times more case reports than with the classic LMA are reported in trauma patients (i.e., 53 versus 5).[76] The success rate for Combitube placement assessed in five studies was 90.9%.[77] No complications were found.

A further prospective study showed that flight nurses receiving only didactic and videotape instruction along with manikin training successfully inserted the ETC after two or more failed attempts at rapid sequence intubation (RSI) in patients suffering from different types of trauma, including mandibular fractures, facial trauma, and/or traumatic brain injury.[58] All ETC insertions were successful, and no patient died as a result of failure to control the airway.

In a recent study,[78] paramedics used the Combitube when rapid sequence intubation failed. Tracheal intubation was successful in 84.5% of 240 patients. The success rate with the Combitube in the failed intubation group was 95.1%. The authors recommend the Combitube as a salvage device in this situation. Also, nurses not trained in endotracheal intubation performed insertion and ventilation with the ETC faster than did physicians with endotracheal tubes using direct laryngoscopy.[56]

Although the LMA can substantially reduce the risk of aspiration, the ETC minimizes the risk of pulmonary aspiration similar to that of the tracheal tube.[9] In several studies, it has been shown that the two-tube, two-cuff design protects the airway from gastric contents, blood, and debris.[32,75,78,79]

Effective sealing of the ETC has been demonstrated in several studies during general anesthesia.[29,31,32,47,67] An airtight seal could be achieved at airway pressures of up to 30 cm H_2O during peritoneal carbon dioxide inflation and steep Trendelenberg position[67] and in another study, it could be achieved up to 40 cm H_2O.[80] Frass et al. also reported airtight sealing of the device in a review of 500 cases.[72] To achieve an airtight seal consistently, it is necessary to use the recommended cuff-inflation volumes for both the Combitube (100 ml) and Combitube SA (85 ml) for the proximal oropharyngeal cuff in emergency situations. In this way, maximal sealing capacity is achieved, and risk of pulmonary aspiration is minimized.

Exchanging the ETC for a Definitive Airway

When the patient's situation has stabilized, the ETC can remain in place for up to 8 hours and should then be replaced with a definitive airway.[81] Options include cricothyroidotomy, tracheotomy,[82-84] nasotracheal fiberoptic intubation,[85] or orotracheal intubation.[28,86,87] While replacing the ETC, the distal cuff of the ETC remains inflated until tracheal intubation is confirmed to avoid any danger of aspiration. The technique of exchanging an alternative airway with a definitive airway without interruption of ventilation is of special value in patients with severe pulmonary dysfunction.[85]

When the patient regains sufficient spontaneous ventilation, ventilatory assistance can be gradually reduced until the patient is breathing without any ventilatory support. Next, the oropharyngeal cuff is completely deflated, but the ETC is left in place. Supplemental oxygen can be continued as needed. Once the patient meets the criteria for extubation, the ETC is removed during continuous suctioning via the open-ended lumen No. 2.

If extubation is impossible and an extended period ≥ 8 hours of ventilatory support is expected, the ETC must be exchanged. After several hours of ETC ventilation, venous stasis and swelling of the tongue may be seen. This complication is usually harmless and resolves soon after ETC removal in most patients.[88] To minimize swelling, the oropharyngeal balloon should be inflated only to the minimal volume necessary to maintain an airtight seal.

The ETC can be exchanged for a conventional ETT using direct laryngoscopy, fiberoptic-assisted intubation (Figure 8-19), or a surgical airway. Prior to direct laryngoscopy, the proximal ETC balloon must be deflated completely, and the ETC pushed to the left corner of the mouth to make laryngoscopic visualization possible. If the intubation attempt fails, the balloon can be rapidly reinflated, and ventilation reinstituted.

Krafft et al.[87] successfully performed tracheal intubation using the fiberscope and wire in a modified ETC. In another controlled operating-room study in fasting patients, Gaitini et al.[85] studied ETC insertion utilizing a flexible fiberoptic bronchoscope to exchange the ETC for an endotracheal tube in 20 spontaneously breathing and 20 mechanically ventilated patients. After anesthesia induction and ETC insertion, Gaitini et al.[85] performed nasotracheal intubation utilizing a flexible fiberoptic bronchoscope with the oropharyngeal balloon partially deflated to improve visibility of the laryngeal structures. The exchange procedure was successful in 18 of 20 spontaneously breathing patients (mean duration 9 ± 3 min), and in 15 of 20 mechanically ventilated patients (mean duration 13 ± 4 min). Ventilatory support was maintained easily during the entire procedure (Figure 8-18).

The third possibility for definitive airway management is a surgical airway performed under anesthesia and continued positive-pressure ventilation using the ETC.[84] The advantage is that there is no airway positioned in the trachea during cricothyrotomy or tracheostomy.

Percutaneous dilational tracheostomy can also be performed, but only under bronchoscopic visualization during the entire procedure. Attempts to perform blind percutaneous needle tracheostomy can cause injury and potentially life-threatening situations. Letheren et al. reported a serious complication of this procedure that was caused by the fact that accidental transtracheal needle aspiration of free air from the distal balloon of the ETC in the esophagus was misinterpreted as proper tracheal needle positioning.[83]

Limitations and Contraindications of the ETC

The ETC has specific limitations[9,28,39] and contraindications[28,38,89] (Table 8-3) that should be understood before using it. Particular contraindications include use of the ETC SA 37F in patients less than four feet in height, elective use of ETC in patients with known esophageal pathology or who have ingested caustic substances, and use of the ETC with an intact gag reflex or a clenched jaw. Patients with an intact gag reflex or a clenched jaw cannot be intubated with the ETC unless they are first sedated or paralyzed. However, its slim design allows insertion in patients with a small interincisor gap. The ETC is not beneficial in cases of glottic or subglottic obstruction and is effective only in alleviating supraglottic airway obstructions. Resolution of a glottic or subglottic obstruction requires placement of an airway device below the level of the obstruction with an ETT, transtracheal jet ventilation (TTJV), or a surgical airway.

Complications of ETC Use

Like most other airway devices, complications have been reported when using the ETC, including the occasional inability to perform lung ventilation via either of the two proximal tubes. Complications may also involve injury to the pharyngeal and esophageal mucosa. Vézina et al. described two esophageal lacerations in the review of prehospital use of the ETC caused by overinflation of the distal cuff with 20 ml to 40 ml of air.[50,51] To reduce possible trauma, the use of the smaller ETC 37F SA is preferred over the ETC 41F.[81]

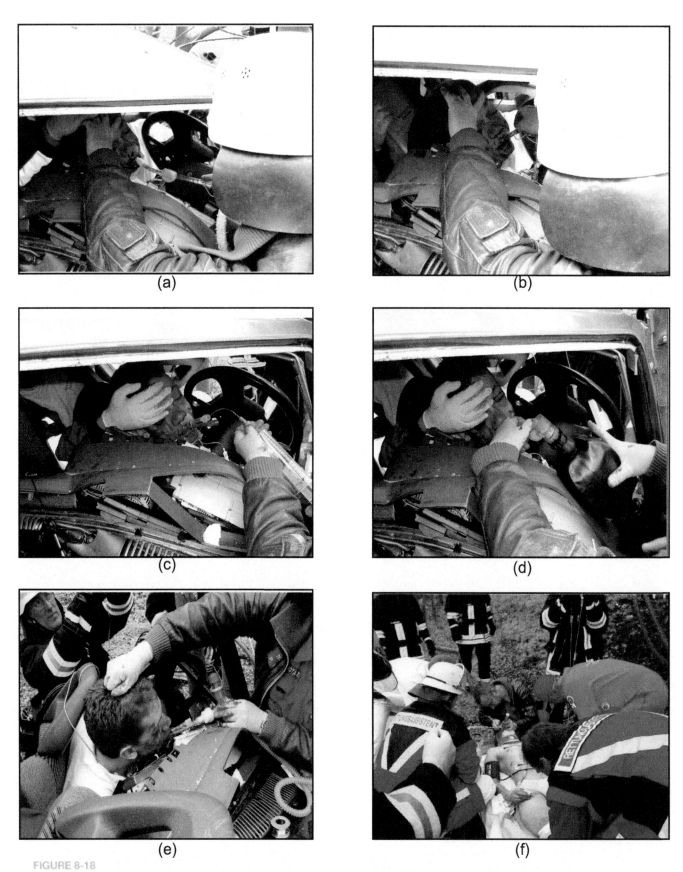

Use of the ETC for airway management during a closed space rescue. (a) and (b) After preoxygenation and induction of general anesthesia, a Combitube is inserted. (c) The ETC cuffs are inflated. (d) Rescue ventilation with a BVM. (e) After the roof of the vehicle is cut away, the patient is extricated with a secure airway and ventilation is controlled using a transport ventilator. (f) The ETC is removed and exchanged for an endotracheal tube using direct laryngoscopy. The patient is stabilized and then transported to the hospital. He recovered after surgery without sequelae.

(Courtesy of Dr. Peer Knacke)

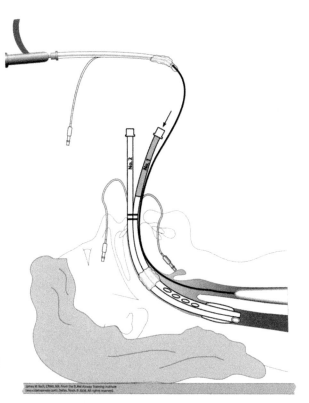

FIGURE 8-19

Exchange of the Combitube for an endotracheal tube using a flexible fiberscope. The esophageal balloon of the Combitube is lowered to allow for insertion of the flexible fiberscope and then reinflated so that ventilation can proceed while the exchange is accomplished.

Table 8-3   Limitations and Contraindications of the ETC

- As with all supraglottic devices, an esophageally placed ETC is effective only in alleviating a supraglottic airway obstruction. Glottic (eg., laryngeal spasm, massive edema, tumor, abscess, etc.) or subglottic airway obstructions require an endotracheal tube, transtracheal jet ventilation, or a surgical airway to alleviate them.[9]
- Sharp teeth can damage cuffs.[90]
- Cannot be used in a patient with a clenched jaw.[38]
- No pediatric sizes available.[38]
- Difficult to insert ETC in patients with rigid cervical collars in place.[91]
- 37F SA limited for use in patients more than 4 feet (120 cm) tall and less than 6 feet (183 cm) tall.[30]
- 41F ETC limited for use in patients more than 6 feet (183 cm) tall.[30]
- Should not be used in cases of upper airway obstruction secondary to foreign body aspiration, severe glottic edema, or epiglotitis.[38]
- Should not be used electively after ingestion of caustic substances or in patients with known esophageal disease (i.e., hiatal hernia, esophageal varices, esophagitis, etc.).[28]
- Cannot be used in patients with an intact gag reflex, regardless of level of consciousness.[28]

Summary

This chapter discussed the Combitube (ETC) versus the laryngeal mask airway (LMA) as a rescue option. Much evidence exists on the benefits of both the LMA and Combitube in resolving problems with difficult intubation and difficult ventilation.[41,42,55-59,68-71,75,92-104] Both the ETC and LMA have been available as rescue ventilation devices since the 1980s,[40,105] but both remain underutilized in emergency medicine.[106] The ETC continues to be underutilized in anesthesiology,[107] despite the long-standing recommendation by an American Society of Anesthesiologists (ASA) task force for its inclusion in the airway kit for difficult airway management and especially for CVCI situations.[3] Anesthesia practitioners are more accustomed to using the LMA rather than the ETC for difficult airway management and rescue ventilation because of the widespread use of the LMA during general anesthesia.[9,93]

However, there are good practical reasons for all practitioners to familiarize themselves with both the LMA and the ETC. Anesthesia practitioners who do not use the ETC to resolve critical airway events such as failed intubation,[4,69,99,108] difficult mask ventilation,[2,3] CMVCI,[102-104] or a crash airway situation[5,52,81,109-111] may still be required to provide anesthesia care for patients in whom the ETC has been inserted by another practitioner prior to the patient arriving in the operating room (James Michael Rich, personal observation). Reports exist of successful rescue ventilation being provided by the ETC when the LMA had failed.[103,104]

Although the standard LMA does not provide an airtight seal around the larynx beyond 20 cm H_2O or completely protect the trachea from aspiration,[9] it does provide reasonable protection against aspiration of regurgitated gastric contents, as evidenced by the much lower level of regurgitation (3.5% versus 12.4%) than occurs with BVM ventilation in conjunction with an OPA or NPA airway.[112] Furthermore, in trauma, and particularly in those patients with maxillofacial injuries, the risk of aspiration of gastric contents is likely to be less than the risk of aspiration of blood, and the cuff of the LMA has been shown to afford effective protection against the aspiration of blood arising from the oropharynx.[20]

In the esophageal position, the ETC prevents aspiration by sealing the esophagus rather than the trachea.[9] Although one study[113] reported tracheal soiling in some patients (2 of 27), all other studies[32,46,47] have reported complete airway sealing with the ETC in the esophageal position. In the tracheal position, the ETC seals the trachea like a conventional cuffed tracheal tube.

For rescue ventilation in the unfasted patient, the choice of device (ETC versus LMA—see Table 8-4) is likely to be influenced by several factors including availability and familiarity with the device, the need for a pediatric size (LMA only), the need for a device with a high level of protection against gastric regurgitation and aspiration (ETC favored), and the need to employ airway pressures in excess of 20 cm H_2O (ETC favored).

The ETC and LMA are both recommended by the Airway and Ventilation Management Group of the European Resuscitation Council[8] and the International Liaison Committee on Resuscitation (ILCOR) in collaboration with the American Heart Association.[6] The Guidelines of the American Heart Association for Advanced Cardiac Life Support classified each of them as Class IIa devices, as compared to bag-valve-mask ventilation (Class IIb).[114,115] Since 1992, the ETC has been included as an appropriate option for CMVCI situations in the American Society of Anesthesiologists Difficult Airway Algorithm (ASADAA),[39,116,117] although the current iteration (2002) of the ASADAA[3] now promotes the LMA as a "consider attempting" first-choice rescue ventilation option as opposed to the ETC, transtracheal jet ventilation, and a surgical airway. This slight word change was inspired by availability and familiarity considerations within the anesthesia community but would not be.

The ETC and LMA are both recommended by the Airway and Ventilation Management Group of the European Resuscitation Council.[8] Both devices can be stored easily on difficult airway carts[37] and ACLS carts.

Conflict of Interest Declaration

Michael Frass is patent holder of the Combitube and receives royalties from Tyco Healthcare-Nellcor. James Michael Rich is the founder and executive director of the SLAM Airway Training Institute (SATI) (www.slamairway.com) and the creator of the SLAM Universal Adult Airway Flowchart. Andrew Mason is Adviser in Pre-hospital Care to Intavent Orthofix, the distributor of the LMA in the United Kingdom and Republic of Ireland.

Table 8-4 Comparison of ETC and LMA Unique

	ETC	LMA Unique
Single-use device	Yes	Yes
Method of insertion	Blind or laryngoscope-assisted	Blind (finger, thumb, or nondigital techniques)
Suitable for use by rescuers unskilled in tracheal intubation	Yes	Yes
Ease of insertion	Easy	Easy
Skill retention	High	High
Stability of device	Excellent	Moderate (requires taping or use of Thomas tube holder during transportation)
Aspiration prevention	Excellent	Good
Reliable seal above 20 cm H_2O airway pressure	Yes	No
Training requirements	No formal training requirement by manufacturer—local protocols apply	Manufacturer recommends formal training course with 10 successful insertions into a manikin.
Available in pediatric sizes	No	Yes (sizes 1, 1½, 2, and 2½)
Available in adult sizes	Yes (Sizes 37F & 41F)	Yes (sizes 3, 4, and 5) (size 6 available in LMA Classic)
Opportunity to gain experience with device in routine anesthesia	Limited	Widespread
ASADAA recommendation for rescue ventilation	Recommended	Recommended as first-choice option
Supplier	Tyco Healthcare—Nellcor, 4280 Hacienda Drive Pleasanton, CA 94588 (800) 635-5267 www.nellcor.com	LMA North America 9360 Towne Centre Drive, Suite 200 San Diego, CA 92121 (800) 788-7999 www.LMANA.com

REVIEW QUESTIONS

1. What two devices are given Class IIa status by the American Heart Association?

2. When is elective use of the LMA contraindicated?

3. When should a rescuer proceed directly with transtracheal jet ventilation or a cricothyrotomy?

4. What problems can be caused by an overinflated LMA cuff?

5. Name at least three contraindications for the esophageal tracheal Combitube (ETC).

6. Which device, the LMA or the Combitube, can be used in pediatric patients?

CHAPTER 9

Advanced Techniques
for Difficult Intubation

James Michael Rich
Andrew M. Mason
George Beck

Chapter Objectives

After reading this chapter, you should be able to:

- List the goals and reasons for laryngoscopy and tracheal intubation.

- Discuss problems encountered with tracheal intubation.

- Describe preintubation assessment techniques for identifying a potentially difficult intubation.

- Describe the advanced techniques for managing difficult intubations.

- Identify the indications, contraindications, equipment, difficulties, and techniques for blind nasotracheal intubation.

- Describe techniques for awake intubation.

- List the available adjuncts for use in difficult intubations.

- Discuss problems related to intubation of obstetrical patients.

- Discuss problems related to intubation of obese patients.

CASE
Study _____

Medic 3 responds to a local bingo hall where someone is having difficulty breathing. They arrive to find a 67-year-old obese male sitting in a chair. He is well known to the crew members, who have transported him to the hospital on a number of occasions with heart failure. The primary survey reveals that the airway is patent, breathing is spontaneous but shallow and rapid, and radial pulses are present but rapid and weak. Oxygen is applied at 15 liters per minute via a nonrebreathing mask.

The patient is secured to the stretcher in a sitting position and is then moved to the ambulance. A cardiac monitor is attached, and an IV line is established. Vital signs reveal a blood pressure of 100/60 Hgmm a heart rate of 110 beats-per-minute, and respirations of 32 breaths per minute. The pulse oximeter shows an oxygen saturation of 88%, and auscultation of the lungs reveals crackles throughout. When the patient becomes more restless and there is a corresponding rise in his respiratory rate, spontaneous respiration is assisted with a bag-valve-mask (BVM) device fitted with an oxygen reservoir bag. Despite this treatment, the patient's condition does not improve significantly. Intubation equipment is prepared, together with a supraglottic airway device for backup.

The paramedics anticipate a difficult intubation because of the patient's obesity. He will not tolerate any reclining, so intubation has to be performed in an upright position. Pillows are used to raise the patient's shoulders into the optimal position for laryngoscopy. Etomidate is given IV to induce anesthesia, and direct laryngoscopy is attempted, but only the posterior tip of the epiglottis is visualized. A bougie is carefully advanced just posterior to the epiglottis, and the paramedic is relieved when tracheal clicking is felt and holdup is achieved. The tracheal tube is advanced over the bougie under direct laryngoscopic vision, with a 90° counterclockwise rotation of the tracheal tube just prior to advancement through the glottic opening. The bougie is removed, and correct tube position is confirmed. The tube is secured, and end-tidal carbon dioxide ($ETCO_2$) monitoring is undertaken throughout the journey. Appropriate medications are administered, and the patient's mental status and vital signs gradually improve as transport continues.

Introduction

Poor airway access, inferior glottic exposure, and inability to pass the breathing tube can create difficulties with tracheal intubation. The entire glottis, from anterior to posterior commissure (i.e., Grade 1 view), can normally be seen in only 25% of laryngoscopies; however, the unique challenges associated with the prehospital environment increase the incidence of airway difficulty and further decrease visualization of the glottis. Difficult airway situations are particularly likely in the prehospital environment due to the increased requirement for cervical-spine protection, which greatly increases the incidence of Grade 3 laryngeal views (epiglottis only). Beyond this, the prehospital environment can make it difficult to ventilate and/or intubate the patient as a result of entrapment or position of the patient. Some trapped patients may require the application of a rescue ventilation technique until they have been extricated and are in a better position for intubation.

In addition to the advanced techniques for difficult intubation that are presented in this chapter, other techniques and methods should be kept in mind when considering management of the difficult airway. These include rescue intubation techniques that are featured in the SLAM Universal Adult Airway Flowchart (SUAAF) and are discussed in Chapters 1 and 4 (that is, external laryngeal manipulation of the larynx, head-elevated laryngoscopy position, bougie-assisted intubation) and the use of fiberscopic and video-assisted devices, which are discussed in Chapter 10, along with use of the McCoy laryngoscope, which is discussed in Chapter 14.

KEY TERMS

6-D method, pp. 176, 177

acromegaly, pp. 175, 176

airway exchange catheter (AEC), p. 180

Beck airway airflow monitor (BAAM), pp. 178, 180

BURP maneuver, p. 187

cherubism, p. 175

cicatrical pemphigoid, pp. 175, 176

Cormack and Lehane laryngoscopic grades, pp. 175, 176

failed intubation, pp. 176, 178

laryngocele, pp. 175, 176

Mallampati view, pp. 176, 178

Morquio syndrome, p. 175

Quinsy and retropharyngeal abscess, pp. 175, 176

Ramsay sedation scale (RSS), pp. 177, 178

sniffing position, pp. 178, 180

subglottic web, p. 175

thalassemia, p. 175

tracheopathia osteochondroplastica, p. 175

xeroderma pigmentosum, p. 175

Overview of the Difficult Airway

A thorough analysis of the causes of difficult intubation and intubation procedures has been published by Murrin.[1] An outline of his excellent presentation can be found in Table 9-1. There are three specific reasons for problems with tracheal intubation: poor access, poor

cherubism
Painless mandibular enlargement, either with or without maxillary involvement.

tracheopathia osteochondroplastica
Benign dysplasia (abnormal growth) of the trachea and large bronchi, which gradually causes narrowing of the tracheal lumen.

subglottic web
A membrane, tissue, or tissues that extend across the lumen of the trachea.

xeroderma pigmentosum
A rare genetic disease provoked by sunlight.

thalassanemia
A group of inherited anemias that occur in Mediterranean and Southeast Asian populations.

Morquio syndrome
An inherited disease characterized by, among other things, a large head and coarse facial features, widely spaced teeth, and abnormal development of the spine. It can cause difficulty in intubation because of deformity, redundant pharyngeal mucosa, and contraindicated manipulation of the spine.

Table 9-1   Causes of Difficult Intubation and Intubation Procedures[1]

- Intubation procedures: patient positioning, use of the wrong instrument or wrong technique, inadequate muscle relaxation during direct laryngoscopy.
- Anatomical abnormalities or individual variations: short muscular neck (bull neck), receding mandible, prominent upper incisors, narrow mouth with high arched palate, limited movement of mandible, large breasts, maxillary protrusion, mandibular coronoid hyperplasia, abnormal epiglottis.
- Disease states: **cherubism, tracheopathia osteochondroplastica, subglottic web,** laryngeal edema, tracheal stenosis, **xeroderma pigmentosum, thalassemia,** mucopolysacchaarydosis, **Morquio syndrome,** scleroderma.
- Musculoskeletal problems: cervical rigidity, diffuse idiopathic skeletal hyperostosis, polyostotic fibrous dysplasia, temporomandibular joint disorders, post-temporal craniotomy, calcification of the stylohyoid ligament, pseudoxanthoma elasticum, Klippel-Feil syndrome.
- Inflammation:
  - Bacterial: gangrenous stomatits, **cicatrical pemphigoid, Quinsy and retropharyngeal abscess,** epiglottitis, leprosy, diphtheria.
  - Viral: infectious mononucleosis, croup.
  - Noninfectious inflammation: rheumatoid arthritis including instability of the cervical spine, cervical fixation, cricoarytenoid disorders; hypoplastic mandible; ankylosing spondylitis.
- Endocrine: obesity, **acromegaly,** thyroid goiter, lingual thyroid, diabetes mellitus, testicular feminization syndrome.
- Degenerative diseases: cervical spondylosis, pharyngeal pouch, **laryngocele.**
- Neoplasm: laryngeal papillomatosis, epiglottic or vallecular cysts, tumoral calcinosis.
- Occipital protuberances: occipital lipoma, decorative hairbands, hairstyle.
- Trauma: facial injuries including mandibular fractures, maxillary fractures (middle third fractures); sublingual hematoma; foreign bodies; laryngeal and trachea trauma; open injuries; closed injuries (blunt neck trauma); contusional injuries.
- Foreign bodies (e.g., tongue jewelry).

---

view of the glottis, and the inability to advance the tracheal tube (TT). The goal of laryngoscopy is to visualize the cords, but a view of the entire vocal cords is possible in only 75% of patients.[2] On the other hand, the goal of tracheal intubation is to introduce the ET tube between the cords, and difficult tracheal intubation using direct laryngoscopy may occur anywhere across the spectrum of health care.[3-11] It is reported to occur with an incidence of up to 6% in anesthesiology;[12] however, most tracheal intubations can still be performed using direct laryngoscopy, and this applies to both the hospital and the prehospital environment.

Difficult intubation occurs when multiple laryngoscopies, maneuvers, and/or blades need to be used by an experienced airway practitioner.[13] **Cormack and Lehane**[14] **laryngoscopic grades** of the airway are the standard for classifying degrees of intubation difficulty. (Figure 2-8). Grade 1 is full view of the glottis from anterior to posterior commissure; Grade 2 is partial view of the glottis; Grade 3 is epiglottis only (Grade 3a is epiglottis can be lifted and Grade 3b is epiglottis cannot be lifted from the posterior pharyngeal wall, which can limit success of bougie-assisted intubation);[15] Grade 4 is soft tissue only/no visible laryngeal anatomy. Laryngoscopic views of the airway generally associated with difficulty[14] include Cormack and Lehane Grades 3 and 4.

 PEARLS   Use of a cervical collar can increase the incidence of Grade 3 views of the larynx by up to 42%.

---

cicatrical pemphigoid
An autoimmune disease characterized by blisters and scarring of the upper airway.

Quinsy and retropharyngeal abscess
Abscess of the area between the tonsils and the pharyngeal wall.

acromegaly
A condition caused by excessive secretion by the pituitary of growth hormone. It is characterized by enlargement of the bones of the extremities and the frontal bone and jaw, with enlargement of the nose and lips, tongue, and vocal cords, and thickening of facial tissues.

laryngocele
An abnormal dilation of the larynx.

Cormack and Lehane laryngoscopic grades
A system of grading the view seen with the laryngoscope, with Grade 1 being the visualization of the entire vocal cords and Grade 4 being an inability to see any laryngeal anatomy, either the epiglottis or the cords. Grade 3 defines the difficult airway and is present when only the epiglottis is visible.

Difficult airway situations are particularly likely in the prehospital environment. The prehospital patient frequently requires cervical-spine protection, which is reported to increase the incidence of Grade 3 laryngeal views to as much as 42%.[14,16] Beyond this, the prehospital environment can make it difficult to ventilate and/or intubate the patient as a result of entrapment or the position of the patient. Some trapped patients may require the application of a rescue ventilation technique until they have been extricated and are in a better position for intubation.[6,7]

Preintubation assessment of the airway is recommended to predict a potentially difficult intubation before airway management is attempted. In the prehospital environment, this assessment should include a **6-D method**[4] (i.e., airway disproportion, airway distortion, decreased range of motion of any or all of the joints of the airway, decreased interincisor gap, decreased thyromental distance, and dental overbite) together with awareness of any environmental factors that may create difficulty, such as the patient's position and proximity to the rescuer.

According to the study by Rocke et al.,[17] compared to an uncomplicated Class I airway assessment (risk ratio of 1.0), the relative risk of experiencing a difficult tracheal intubation was as follows:[17] Class II—3.23, Class III—7.58, Class IV—11.3, short neck—5.01, protruding maxillary incisors—8.0, and receding mandible—9.71. Using the probability index and other risk factors, they showed that a combination of either a **Mallampati view** Class III or IV airway plus protruding incisors, short neck, or receding mandible meant that the probability of encountering a difficult laryngoscopy was greater than 90%. They suggested using the relative risk score to allow for better prediction of difficult tracheal intubation.

Failed intubation occurs when the trachea cannot be intubated after multiple attempts. When intubation attempts are repeated beyond three or four times, the danger of airway trauma and edema increases and may result in a critical airway event,[3,4,13] such as a cannot-mask-ventilate/cannot-intubate (CMVCI) situation. If a CMVCI event occurs, rapid intervention using a supraglottic ventilation device is usually effective in restoring ventilation and oxygenation.[3,4,13]

 If a cannot-mask-ventilate/cannot-intubate situation occurs, rapid intervention using a supraglottic device such as the Combitube or LMA is usually effective in providing effective ventilation and oxygenation.

A number of supraglottic airways are now available (Chapter 3). Supraglottic ventilation devices generally provide better ventilation and protection from aspiration than is provided by positive-pressure mask ventilation,[13] and they are often quicker and easier to insert than a tracheal tube, making them particularly suitable for the prehospital environment. The incidence of aspiration in emergency airway management using positive-pressure mask ventilation with an oropharyngeal or nasopharyngeal airway is reported to be as high as 12.4%.[18] In comparison, in one hospital-based multicenter CPR study, the incidence of aspiration with the laryngeal mask airway (LMA) was less than 1%.[19] In cases of failed intubation, if ventilation cannot be established using a supraglottic airway device, transtracheal jet ventilation[20] or a cricothyrotomy are the standard methods for providing oxygenation and avoiding disability or death.[10] Ready availability of a range of adjunctive devices is essential to prevent complications resulting from failed management of the airway.[10]

The choice of the most appropriate difficult-airway intubation technique depends on the clinical situation and the practitioner's familiarity and skill in using any particular device. Not every technique needs to be learned or mastered, but it is advantageous to be familiar with and have available more than one procedure to increase the likelihood of success because a particular technique is unlikely to work in every clinical situation.

When a difficult airway is anticipated, it is recommended that the airway be secured with the patient awake, using judicious sedation[21] unless contraindicated.[16,22] Various difficult-airway intubation techniques are recommended in the SLAM Universal Adult Airway Flowchart (Table 9-2 and on the inside front cover), and most can be performed with the patient awake while receiving a combination of intravenous sedation and/or topical local anesthesia of the airway.

Table 9-2 Techniques for Difficult Tracheal Intubation

Difficult-Airway Intubation Technique	Considerations/Requirements
Awake laryngoscopic intubation[23]	Judicious intravenous sedation[22] Topical anesthesia[22] Gentle use of the laryngoscope
Awake blind nasotracheal intubation[24]	Judicious intravenous sedation[22] Topical anesthesia[22] Spontaneous ventilation Vasoconstrictor[22] Patil intubation guide or Beck airway airflow monitor[24]
Intubating laryngeal mask airway in the awake patient	Judicious intravenous sedation[22] Topical anesthesia[22] Chandy maneuver[25] Spontaneous ventilation Patil intubation guide or Beck airway airflow monitor
Intubating laryngeal mask airway in the apneic patient	Chandy maneuver[25] Positive-pressure ventilation
Retrograde intubation[26]	Can-mask-ventilate/cannot-intubate situation Parker endotracheal tube Direct laryngoscopy
Indirect rigid fiberoptic laryngoscopy[27]	Upsher, Wu, or Bullard laryngoscope[27]
Flexible fiberoptic laryngoscopy[28]	General anesthesia Judicious intravenous sedation[22] Topical anesthesia[22] Spontaneous ventilation[28]
Lightwand intubation[27]	Should not be used in patients with pharyngeal masses or anatomic abnormalities of the upper airway[27]
Videolaryngoscopic devices[29]	GlideScope[29]
Malleable fiberoptic stylet	Shikani seeing stylet Direct laryngoscopy[30]

Used by permission of reference 4.

PEARLS

Awake intubation can be used in almost all the techniques described in this book, provided that the patient is adequately sedated.

6-D Method

Assesses airway for difficulty using 6 separate factors that each begin with the letter "D" (*d is for difficulty*): distortion, disproportion, decreased thyromental distance, decreased interincisor gap, decreased range of motion, and dental overbite.

Awake intubation can be used in almost all the techniques described in this book. Obviously, the patient cannot be wide awake with a normal level of consciousness but must be sedated to the point of what is called judicious sedation.[31] A good way to judge the depth of sedation is by using the **Ramsay sedation scale (RSS).** If judicious sedation is not contraindicated, the patient should generally be sedated to an RSS score of 3 (Tables 9-3). When indicated, this is accomplished through intravenous sedation of titrated sedatives and/or opiates[4] to the point that the patient is cooperative and tolerant of the intubation attempt, yet is still capable of following simple commands. In other words, the patient is not fully obtunded. Patients with a decreased mental status or altered level of consciousness are generally not candidates for judicious sedation. However, there is no technical reason why this type of procedure cannot be undertaken in the prehospital environment. Use of topical local anesthetics within the airway decreases the amount of sedation necessary and usually promotes a better clinical experience for both practitioner and patient. However, it is important to understand that use of topicalized local anesthesia also decreases protective airway reflexes to some extent.

Table 9-3 Ramsay Sedation Scale[32]

1—Patient is anxious and agitated or restless, or both.
2—Patient is cooperative, oriented, and tranquil.
3—Patient responds to commands only.
4—Patient exhibits brisk response to light glabellar tap or loud auditory stimulus.
5—Patient exhibits a sluggish response to light glabellar tap or loud auditory stimulus.
6—Patient exhibits no response.

Difficult-Airway Techniques

Mallampati view

The Mallampati classification system of airway views, which is different from Cormack and Lehane. The Cormack and Lehane system grades the laryngoscopic view, whereas the Mallampati system grades the view seen within the oral cavity when the patient sits upright, opens his or her mouth, and maximally protrudes the tongue.

failed intubation

When the trachea cannot be intubated after multiple attempts.

Blind Nasotracheal Intubation

Blind nasotracheal intubation (BNTI) (Figure 9-1) is often advantageous if direct visualization of the airway is difficult or impossible, such as when the mouth cannot be opened or when instrumentation might damage teeth or other structures in the oropharynx. It is also valuable when preservation of spontaneous ventilation is indicated. The right nasal passage is normally the one selected, but it is important to rule out nasopharyngeal obstruction prior to attempting the procedure. Benefits include the fact that patient need not be chemically paralyzed to perform the procedure. Additionally, patients may be supine, sitting, or in the prone position.

Methods of detecting spontaneous ventilation include listening at the proximal end of the tracheal tube; putting a narrow tube connected to a stethoscope down the tracheal tube; or using an airway whistle, such as the **Beck airway airflow monitor (BAAM)**[33] or the Patil device.[34] Airway whistles work well because the patient can be observed as the whistle signals inspiration and expiration. When using an airway whistle, the device is attached to the 15 mm connector of an appropriately sized tracheal tube that has been warmed to body temperature and lightly lubricated with water soluble lubricant. Topical anesthetic/vasoconstrictor is applied to the nares, larynx, and trachea if indicated. The clinical situation dictates the need for preoxygenation, judicious sedation, or induction of general anesthesia with the patient spontaneously breathing. The position of the patient's head is important. The **sniffing position,** with elevation of the patient's head on a pillow and the jaw thrust forward, is usually desirable.

PEARLS The gum-elastic bougie or tracheal tube introducer can be a lifesaver during difficult intubations.

Ramsay sedation scale (RSS)

A way of measuring a patient's response to sedation, involving six levels of sedation.

The patient's breathing activates the whistle, and whistling will be heard during both inspiration and expiration. The pitch and duration of the sound may serve to distinguish the particular phase of respiration, or this can be determined by observing the rise and fall of the chest/abdomen. The tube should be directed in a plane across the midline toward the opposite side so that the tip of the tube is close to the midline at the level of the larynx. The tube is then advanced within the larynx and trachea, and correct placement is accompanied by an increase in intensity of the inspiratory and expiratory whistle sounds with respiration. The tube is then advanced to a predetermined nose-to-trachea length. Deviation out of the airflow tract results in immediate diminution and/or loss of the whistle sound and indicates the need to withdraw the tube a short distance and to redirect it laterally by twisting the tube, anteriorly by extending the head or posteriorly by elevating the jaw and/or slight flexion of the neck, until the whistle sound returns. However, should cervical-spine precautions be in

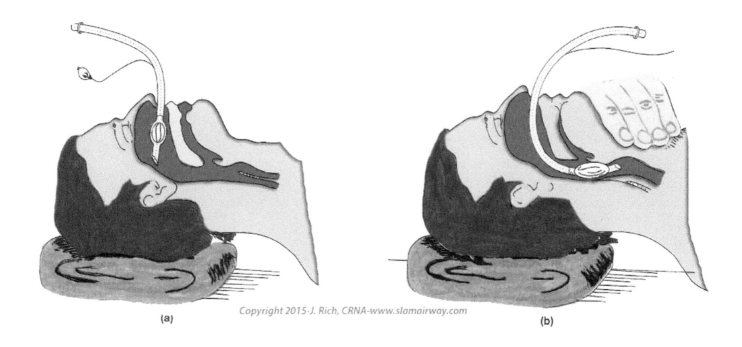

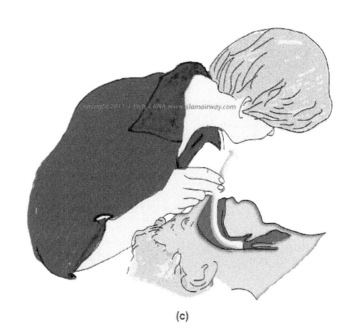

FIGURE 9-1

Nasal intubation technique. (a) Insertion of the tube straight back into the nares. (b) Insertion of the tube below the nasopharynx. (c) Listening for breath sounds.

ON TARGET When a difficult airway is anticipated, it is better to secure the airway with the patient awake, if possible, and if it is clinically appropriate.

effect, no such movement of the head or neck should be attempted. A specialized tracheal tube with a controllable tip such as the Endotrol™ tube (Figure 9-2) can be helpful in this situation. Tube insertion is repeated until it passes through the glottic opening and into the trachea.

When using a whistle, the intubator can easily hear inhalation and exhalation and, at the same time, observe the neck for lateral displacement of the tip of the tracheal tube and correlate this with any decrease in, or absence of, whistle sounds. This assists with the redirection of the tube tip into the airflow tract, larynx, and trachea. The volume of the whistling increases when the tube enters the trachea and rises to a maximum when the tube cuff is inflated. As soon as tracheal intubation is confirmed, the whistle should be removed, and postintubation management should be initiated. This should always include auscultation of breath sounds to ensure correct midtracheal tube-tip placement as well as the use of end-tidal CO_2 or an esophageal detector device.[33]

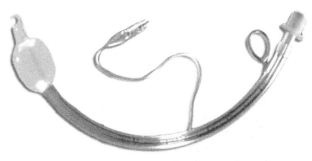

FIGURE 9-2
Pulling on the ring of the Endotrol
ETT causes the tip to move forward.

Copyright 2015-J. Rich, CRNA-www.slamairway.com

Airway Exchange Catheters

Airway exchange catheters (AECs) are long, thin, flexible hollow tubes designed for use during airway tube exchanges (Figure 9-3). Once in position, an AEC acts as both a guide for reintubation and a safety device pemitting insufflation of oxygen, end-tidal CO_2 monitoring, or jet ventilation should problems occur. Potential complications include barotrauma and perforation of the bronchi or lung parenchyma, and fiberoptic endoscopy may be considered a better and safer option for tracheal tube exchanges.

The Cook airway exchange catheter is used for uncomplicated, atraumatic endotracheal tube exchange. The removable Rapi-Fit™ adapter permits use of a ventilatory device if necessary during the exchange procedure. The through-lumen design of the catheter with distal sideports ensures adequate air flow. The blunt tip of the catheter is atraumatic to internal structures during normal careful use. Centimeter marks facilitate accurate placement with shortened endotracheal tubes. The catheter is supplied sterile in peel-open packages and is intended for one-time use.[35]

Use of an airway exchange catheter is indicated when a tracheal tube needs to be exchanged because of a torn cuff, partial occlusion, or previous incorrect sizing. It provides a much safer and more effective method of tube exchange than removing an existing tube followed by direct laryngoscopy to re-intubate the patient. In such a scenario, the airway can be lost with disastrous consequences. Use of an AEC is the safest and most rational approach to endotracheal tube exchange. One model is the Aintree intubation catheter (Cook Critical Care, Bloomington, IN), which is supplied either in a 56 cm or 83 cm length and can accommodate a 7 mm I.D. tracheal tube. It also has a longitudinal port through which oxygen can be insufflated by jet ventilation

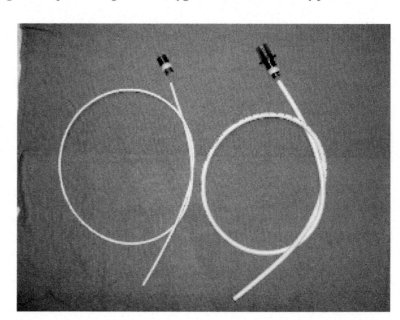

FIGURE 9-3
Pediatric and adult airway exchange catheters.

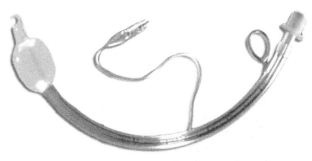

Margin glossary (left column)

Beck airway airflow monitor
Also known as BAAM or Beck whistle. A device that fits on the 15-mm connector of the ET tube and makes a whistling sound as the patient breathes in and out. The sound gets louder when the tube is closer to the glottis, rising to a maximum when the tube cuff is inflated within the trachea.

sniffing position
The position when the patient's neck is slightly flexed and the head is extended, which brings the oral, pharyngeal, and laryngeal axes into alignment.

airway exchange catheter (AEC)
A long, thin, semirigid tube designed for use during endotracheal tube exchange. The tube is hollow and permits the flow of oxygen and carbon dioxide monitoring.

or a positive-pressure manual ventilation bag. Other AECs come in a variety of lengths, from 45 cm to 83 cm, and, depending on the model, they can accommodate a tracheal tube from 3 mm I.D. up to greater than 7 mm I.D. Cook also makes an extrafirm model.

Prior to exchanging a tube, the patient is first placed on 100% oxygen and ventilated for optimal oxygenation. The tube exchanger is then lubricated and inserted into the existing tracheal tube to a depth where the tip of the exchanger is well below the vocal cords. The first tube is then removed while the exchanger is held in place. A new tube is then railroaded over the exchanger to the desired depth, and the tube exchanger is removed. The entire process requires only a few seconds to complete.

If for any reason the new tube hangs up at the laryngeal inlet, the same measures described in Chapter 4 for placement of a tracheal tube during bougie-assisted intubation should be applied. If the patient begins to desaturate during the exchange, a high-pressure oxygen line with a luer lock can be attached to the proximal end of the exchanger, and oxygen can be insufflated into the airway. Alternatively, a special 15 mm connector included with the exchanger can be attached so that a manual ventilation bag can be used for oxygenation. Although it will not provide normal tidal volumes, it will deliver sufficient oxygen to the patient and buy time until the airway exchange can be accomplished. Use of tracheal tube introducers (e.g., gum-elastic bougie, Sun Med tracheal tube introducer) are not recommended for tube exchange procedures because most do not offer a means of simultaneous oxygenation.[36]

Retrograde Intubation

A search of the literature on the subject of whether retrograde wire intubation should be retained as a procedure is inconclusive, and the method is included here for the sake of completeness. This intubation technique may be useful when the patient can be mask-ventilated but cannot be intubated by less invasive means.

When undertaking retrograde intubation, the cricothyroid membrane is first located, and a needle is then inserted through the membrane in a cephalad direction. After confirmation that the tip of the needle is in the lumen of the larynx and is not impaled in the posterior wall, a wire is threaded through the needle. The proximal tip of the wire passes upward through the airway and glottis and should eventually exit the airway at the mouth or nose. If the wire does not emerge from the mouth or the nose, it may be possible to grasp it in the pharynx using forceps (for control of the wire). The wire is then fed upward through the airway, but care should be taken not to pull the wire forcefully from the mouth or nose to avoid cutting into the airway.

When the wire has exited a sufficient distance beyond the upper airway, a tracheal tube is threaded over the wire and down into and through the glottis. To accomplish this, the wire is fixed at the skin anterior to the cricothyroid membrane with a hemostat while it is held taut in the upper airway. When resistance to advancement is encountered, the tip of the tube is at the level of the cricothyroid membrane and is prevented from further advancement by the presence of the wire. At this point, the tube should be held in position with a slight downward force. With constant application of the downward force, you can withdraw the wire carefully through the mouth or nose. As the wire exits the larynx, it should be possible to advance the tube freely into the trachea.

To prevent the tube from hanging up on the posterior cartilages, it may be advantageous to turn the tube a quarter-turn to facilitate advancement (as described above with bougie-assisted intubation). Another method of facilitating insertion is to pass a bougie down the tube before the wire is withdrawn. The bougie should drop down into the airway, and the tube can then follow the bougie infraglottically into the airway after withdrawal of the wire superiorly.

LMA Fastrach

The LMA Fastrach (LMA North America, San Diego, CA) is also known as the intubating laryngeal mask airway (iLMA) in Europe and elsewhere. It was designed especially for ventilation and intubation of patients with a difficult airway (Figure 9-4). The iLMA is inserted orally

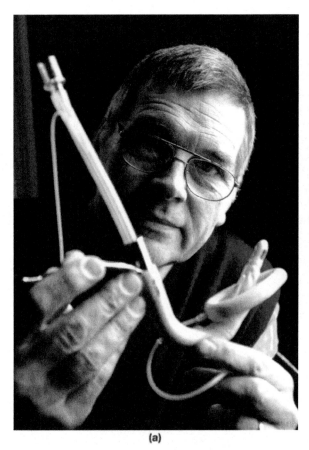

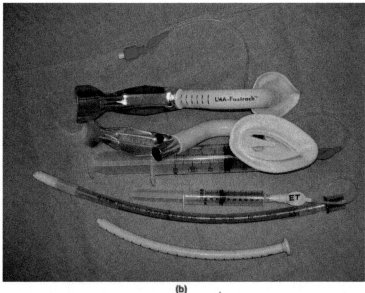

(b)

(a)

until the mask enters the hypopharynx with its tip resting in the upper esophageal sphincter. When the mask cuff is then inflated, a seal is produced around the posterior perimeter of the larynx. The LMA Fastrach (ILMA) and LMA CTrach are unique in that they provide both a means for lung ventilation and a seamless bridge to tracheal intubation without interruption of oxygenation. Both can be used for the manual ventilation of an apneic patient, or with one who is breathing spontaneously but has absent airway reflexes.

The Chandy maneuver (Figure 9-5) was developed by Chandy Verghese in the United Kingdom and significantly improves the effectiveness of the iLMA.[25] It incorporates two steps that improve lung ventilation and tracheal intubation with the iLMA. Step 1 of the Chandy maneuver facilitates positioning of the iLMA in the upper airway so that lung ventilation is maximized through the device. This is done by grasping the iLMA by the handle and moving it back and forth in the sagittal plane while observing the patient's chest excursions, tidal volume, and/or the capnographic waveform (if ventilation is being controlled manually). The iLMA is manipulated until ventilation is optimized and then maintained in this position.

If the patient is breathing spontaneously, an airway whistle (e.g., Patil intubation guide [Anesthesia Associates, San Marcos, CA] or Beck airway airflow monitor (BAAM) [Great Plains Ballistics, Lubbock, TX]) can be attached to the proximal portion of the iLMA to optimize ventilation through the iLMA (Figure 9-6). The whistle sounds with each breath the patient takes. The handle of the iLMA is then moved slowly back and forth in the sagittal plane until maximal whistling is attained. Maximal whistling indicates optimal positioning of the iLMA for ventilation. Case reports demonstrating the usefulness of this technique for both prehospital and hospital-based patients have been published (Figure 9-7).[4,7,8,34,37]

Step 2 of the Chandy maneuver involves aligning the longitudinal axis of the distal portion of the airway tube with that of the upper trachea to facilitate smooth passage of the tracheal tube into the trachea. This is achieved by lifting the handle of the iLMA at a 45° angle to the patient's chest (like a laryngoscope is lifted for tracheal intubation during direct laryngoscopy).

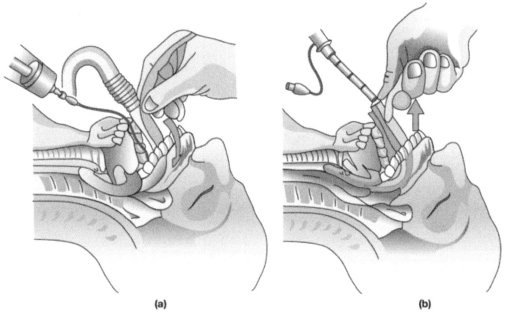

(a)

(b)

FIGURE 9-5

The Chandy maneuver. The two steps of the Chandy maneuver are performed sequentially. (a) After insertion of the LMA-Fastrach™ (LMA North America, Inc., San Diego, CA), optimal ventilation is established by slightly rotating the device in the sagittal plane, using the metal handle, until the least resistance to bag ventilation is achieved. This tilting movement helps to align the distal aperture of the device with the glottic opening. (b) Just before blind intubation, the handle of the LMA-Fastrach™ is lifted slightly (without changing the previous angle of tilt) away from the posterior pharyngeal wall. This aligns the longitudinal axis of the distal portion of the airway tube with that of the upper trachea and thus prevents the emerging tip of the endotracheal tube (ETT) from colliding with the arytenoids, which in turn facilitates the smooth passage of the ETT into the trachea.

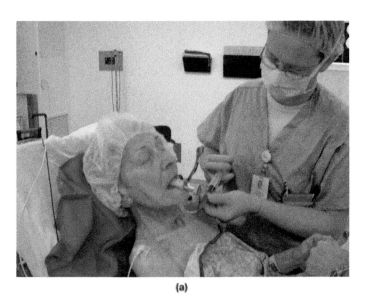

(a)

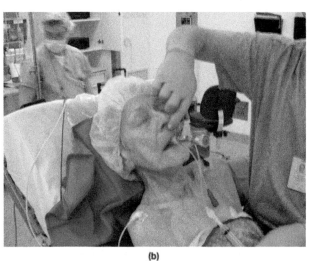

(b)

FIGURE 9-6

(a) Patil whistle attached to an LMA Fastrach. (b) Patil device attached to a tracheal tube.

(Courtesy of JM Rich, CRNA [www.slamairway.com])

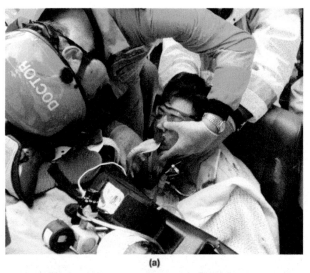

(a)

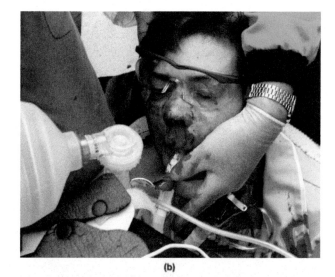

(b)

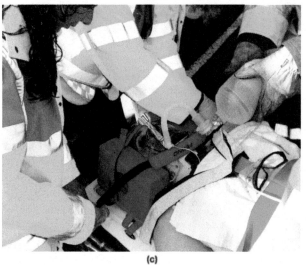

(c)

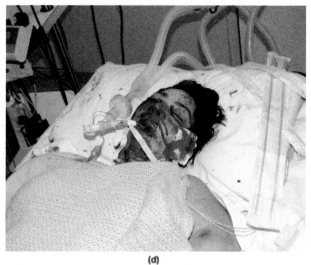

(d)

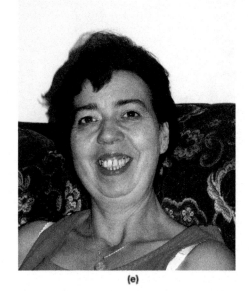

(e)

(a) After receiving preoxygenation and intravenous midazolam, the patient allows the rescuer to insert the LMA Fastrach.
(Courtesy of Dr. Andrew M. Mason)

(b) Ventilation is performed via the LMA Fastrach using a BVM device.
(Courtesy of Dr. Andrew M. Mason)

(c) After extrication, ventilation is continued via the LMA Fastrach.
(Courtesy of Dr. Andrew M. Mason)

(d) At the hospital ICU, the patient is intubated via the LMA Fastrach.
(Courtesy of Dr. Andrew M. Mason)

(e) Six months later, she is happy to be alive and doing well.
(Courtesy of Dr. Andrew M. Mason)

A special atraumatic wire-reinforced straight tracheal tube (Euromedical) is provided for use with the iLMA (Figure 9-5). The tracheal tube has a longitudinal black line (Figure 9-5) that should face the patient's nose superiorly. Proper orientation of the longitudinal line ensures that the rounded tip of the tube passes smoothly into the trachea. The tracheal tube also has a circumferential black line at a set distance from its tip equal to the length of the iLMA tube from the proximal to the distal port (Figure 9-5). At the point where the circumferential line is advanced to the proximal port of the iLMA, the distal tip of the tracheal tube is in contact with the epiglottic elevating bar (which guards the distal aperture of the iLMA) (Figure 9-5). The epiglottic elevating bar protects the distal aperture from impaction by the tip of the epiglottis during initial insertion of the device, and then raises the epiglottis so that the tracheal tube can enter the glottis unimpeded. Just before the tip of the tracheal tube contacts the epiglottic elevating bar, Step 2 of the Chandy maneuver is performed.

If the patient is breathing spontaneously, an airway whistle (Figure 9-8) attached to the proximal end of the tracheal tube sounds with each breath. As the tip of the tracheal tube enters the trachea, the volume of the whistle increases. When the cuff of the tracheal tube is inflated, the volume of the whistle increases even more, heralding the sealing of the tracheal tube within the trachea. However, tracheal intubation should always be confirmed with a

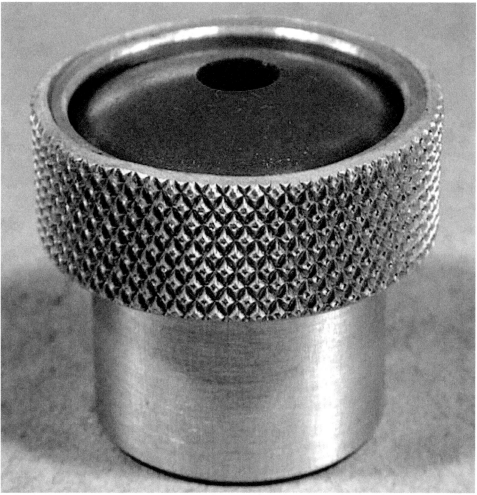

FIGURE 9-8
Patil Intubation Guide (Anesthesia Associates—San Marcos, CA)—An airway whistle is a lightweight device consisting of a diaphragm whistle and a 15 mm female port for attachment to a tracheal tube connector to magnify breath sound during blind nasotracheal and orotracheal intubation. (b) When placed on the proximal end of a tracheal tube the whistle will sound during inhalation and exhalation. The volume will increase as the distal tip of the tracheal tube passes through the vocal cords. The sound will increase maximally when the tracheal tube cuff is inflated. (Courtesy of JM Rich, CRNA [www.slamairway.com])

near-failsafe device, such as a carbon dioxide detector in patients with a perfusing cardiac rhythm or a self-inflating bulb if the patient does not have a perfusing cardiac rhythm.[38] Additionally, auscultation of bilateral breath sounds confirms that the tracheal tube is lying in a midtracheal position.

Another technique of intubating via the iLMA involves railroading the tracheal tube over a fiberscope, which is discussed in Chapter 10. When the tracheal tube is in place, the iLMA can then be removed over the tracheal tube using the dedicated stabilizing rod, or it can be left in place for short procedures with the mask deflated until it is time to extubate the trachea. The mask is then reinflated, the tracheal tube is removed, and the iLMA is left in place until the patient has recovered adequately.

Patient Groups Associated with Difficult Intubation

Various groups of patients are associated with an increased incidence of difficult intubation. These groups include, but are not limited to, patients with traumatized airway (Chapter 13), cervical spine injury (Chapter 14), the pediatric patient (Chapter 16), and the obstetrical patient (see below).

Problems with Laryngoscopy and Tracheal Intubation in the Obstetrical Patient[29,40]

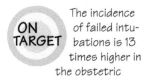

The incidence of failed intubations is 13 times higher in the obstetric patient.

Beyond the risk factors associated with difficult intubation mentioned above, other risk factors during pregnancy include weight gain and breast size. The incidence of failed tracheal intubation in general surgery patients is 1:2230 compared with 1:280 to 1:300 (an eightfold increase) in the obstetric population,[41,42] and the incidence of fatal failed tracheal intubation is 13 times higher in obstetric patients.[43] A grading of the laryngoscopic view[14] may aid in understanding the role of airway maneuvers. Cormack and Lehane[14] estimated an incidence of 1:2000 patients for a Grade 3 airway and surmised that this was the main cause for difficult or failed tracheal intubation. Failure to visualize the cords may be related to incorrect positioning, inadequate laryngoscopy, inadequate muscle relaxation, or failure to apply adequate external laryngeal pressure.

Because of pregnancy-related changes, the forces exerted during repeated tracheal intubation increase the potential for damage to the upper airway, including obstructive edema of the larynx, postobstructive pulmonary edema, pulmonary aspiration, and hypoxia.

Due to the physiologic changes of pregnancy, the obstetric patient must be treated differently with regard to critical airway events such as hypoxemia and failed intubation attempts. There should be a lower threshold for proceeding to rescue ventilation with regard to failed intubation. Only two and possibly only one failed intubation should be allowed, depending on the clinical situation, before rescue ventilation is utilized. To protect the viability of the fetus, the parturient should not be allowed to desaturate for any length of time before a Combitube or LMA is inserted.

Best Attempt at Tracheal Intubation[39]

The recommendation in case of a Grade 3 laryngoscopic view, and particularly during an emergency airway management in obstetrics, is that the second attempt at laryngoscopy should be considered the best attempt. The best attempt at tracheal intubation should:

- Be performed by a reasonably experienced endoscopist.
- Utilize the optimal sniffing position.
- Be accompanied by optimal external laryngeal manipulation.
- Allow a one-time change in laryngoscope blade type and length.

The optimal sniffing position (slight flexion of the neck and extension of the head on the neck) aligns the oral, pharyngeal, and laryngeal axes into a straight line, thus facilitating tracheal intubation.[14] To place the head and shoulders higher than the chest in a morbidly obese parturient, it is necessary to create a ramp using folded towels or blankets under the shoulders and head. Alternatively, the Troop elevation pillow (Mercury Medical, Clearwater, FL) can be used. It is shaped like a ramp and has the effect of positioning the patient so that the sternal notch and external auditory meatus are joined by an imaginary horizontal line (Figure 4-22).[44]

The use of optimal external manipulation,[45] or the BURP (backward, upward, and rightward pressure) maneuver, involves pressure on the thyroid cartilage and displacement of the larynx in three specific directions: posteriorly against the cervical vertebrae, as far superiorly as possible, and slightly laterally to the patient's right.[46] The **BURP maneuver** (Figure 4-19) improves the laryngoscopic view by at least one whole grade and reduces the incidence of failure to view any portion of the glottis from approximately 9.2% to 1.6%.[46]

In accordance with the SUAAF, useful aids for facilitating tracheal intubation include identifying the problem causing difficult visualization of the vocal cords, a change in laryngoscopic blade or handle, a smaller tracheal tube, a hockey-stick bend on the distal end of the tube, and bougie-assisted intubation (Figure 4-20).[47,48] The gum-elastic bougie has shown itself to be a lifesaver during difficult intubation in a morbidly obese patient undergoing emergency cesarean section.[47] The short-handled laryngoscope can also be helpful in the obese patient.[49] The practitioner should be aware that excessive cricoid pressure can easily obscure the glottic view, and the assistant may have to be asked to release cricoid pressure briefly in order to visualize the glottic area and vocal cords.

During emergency management of the obstetrical airway, a third attempt at tracheal intubation is really not an option. If the second or the best attempt at tracheal intubation fails, there are just two choices left, and these must be acted on immediately. If single-handed mask ventilation is easy, one option is to continue ventilation with a face mask, maintain cricoid pressure, and proceed with resuscitation or emergent delivery.[50,51] Alternatively, airway-management techniques that do not require tracheal intubation must be quickly applied. These approaches include the use of a laryngeal mask airway (LMA), Combitube, cricothyroidotomy, or transtracheal jet ventilation.[40] Following failed conventional facemask ventilation and failed tracheal intubation, the use of the LMA is primarily recommended in obstetrics.[52]

Summary

Difficulty in managing the airway can arise at any time and is particularly likely in the prehospital environment. An airway examination as well as thorough assessment of the clinical situation at the scene should always be performed. Understanding and being adept at more than one difficult-intubation technique and rescue ventilation technique can help to stave off disaster and build a bridge to successful intubation of the emergency airway patient. As mentioned previously in this book, and above all else, it must always be remembered that patients die and suffer brain death from failure to ventilate and/or oxygenate, not failure to intubate.

REVIEW QUESTIONS

1. Name three specific reasons for problems with tracheal intubation.

2. What is the primary goal laryngoscopy and tracheal intubation?

3. What are the advantages of blind nasotracheal intubation?

4. Name the adjunctive airway devices available for use with the difficult airway.

BURP maneuver

Backward, upward, rightward pressure exerted on the patient's thyroid cartilage using the thumb and forefinger. This maneuver can help to improve the view of the patient's vocal cords.

CHAPTER 10

Fiberscopic and Video-Assisted Intubation

Andrew M. Mason
Peter Krafft
Charles E. Smith
Michael A. E. Ramsay

Chapter Objectives

After reading this chapter, you should be able to:

- List the indications, contraindications, and techniques for fiberoptic intubation.

- Discuss problems and difficulties with fiberoptic intubation.

- Discuss the advantages and limitations of fiberoptic airway management.

- State the different approaches in fiberoptic airway management with awake and anesthetized patients.

- Discuss problems encountered with long-term mechanical ventilation.

- Describe the technique of tube exchange with the Combitube.

- Discuss the pros and cons of prehospital use of the LMA CTrach.

CASE Study

Life Flight 1 is sent to a rural community hospital for a trauma transfer. Their patient is a previously healthy 24-year-old male who was riding his motorcycle off-road when he lost control and struck a tree. There was no loss of consciousness but, when the ground ambulance arrived on scene, he was complaining of severe neck pain, so the paramedics transported him to the hospital emergency department with full spinal precautions in place. By the time he arrived at the hospital, he had started to complain of numbness and tingling in his arms. This quickly progressed to complete quadriplegia. Emergency CT scans revealed a burst fracture of the body of C4.

Members of the flight crew undertake a primary survey of the patient and find that he is alert but mildly agitated. Although the airway is patent, his breathing appears labored. Peripheral pulses are all present and easily palpable. Neurological examination reveals no motor function or sensation below the third cervical level, but they find no other significant injury on secondary survey.

The crew apply their monitors, which reveal a blood pressure of 98/50 mm Hg, a heart rate of 92 beats per minute, and a respiratory rate of 18 breaths per minute, with an oxygen saturation of 94%. They note that he is receiving supplemental oxygen at 4 liters per minute via nasal cannulae. There are normal bilateral breath sounds, but supraclavicular retractions and tracheal tugging are both noted, and the end-tidal carbon dioxide ($ETCO_2$) monitor shows a reading of 55 mm Hg. Respiratory distress with CO_2 retention is diagnosed, and they elect to undertake endotracheal intubation prior to transfer.

A #5 LMA CTrach is selected together with a dedicated, single-use, wire-reinforced 7.5 mm tracheal tube with an atraumatic tip. After preoxygenation by assisted mask ventilation, the patient is sedated with IV midazolam and fentanyl to the point where he briefly opens his eyes to command and continues to breathe spontaneously. Glycopyrrolate is also given IV to inhibit salivation. One of the crew takes control of the head and neck and undertakes a jaw-thrust maneuver as the anterior portion of the cervical collar is removed. Lidocaine 4% is then sprayed into the posterior pharynx. Next, the cricothyroid membrane is located, a needle cricothyrotomy is performed, and the cords and upper trachea are sprayed with 4% lidocaine.

With the head and neck held in neutral alignment, the CTrach is then inserted without difficulty, and its cuff is inflated. The patient's spontaneous ventilations are assisted with a bag-valve device, and good rise and fall of the chest is noted. The bag is then removed, and the CTrach viewer is attached to the airway and switched on. There is a Class 1 view of the entire glottis on the viewer, so the prelubricated tracheal tube is passed down the CTrach airway and between the cords under direct visual control at the first attempt. The tube cuff is inflated, and correct positioning is confirmed by capnography and chest auscultation.

After the collar has been reattached, the CTrach cuff is deflated and the device is removed from the airway, but the tracheal tube remains in situ. Correct tube position is immediately rechecked, and the patient is placed on the portable transport ventilator. Transfer to the regional spinal injuries unit is completed, where the patient undergoes successful surgical decompression of his cervical cord.

Introduction

Within the last decade, the flexible fiberoptic bronchoscope (FOB) has gained widespread acceptance as an airway management adjunct in the can-mask-ventilate/cannot-intubate situation. The FOB has been incorporated into most difficult-airway algorithms, from the American Society of Anesthesiologists difficult-airway algorithm[1] to the SLAM Universal Adult Airway Flowchart.[2,3] However, the FOB is rarely used for airway management in the prehospital setting due to technical, logistical, and training limitations. Nonetheless, new devices that incorporate aspects of the flexible fiberscope have recently been introduced to the market. These devices may have a significant impact on the management of the emergency airway in the prehospital environment due to their ease of use and the excellent view they can provide of the airway. They are not dependent upon laryngoscopy and should be able to be used in patients in whom laryngoscopy would be difficult or impossible secondary to decreased access to the patient's head or airway.

 Although FOB intubation does not lend itself well to the prehospital setting, new devices coming on the market may well result in this becoming an important tool in the future.

Overview of the Fiberoptic Bronchoscope

All fiberoptic devices are best understood when the FOB is used as a starting point. A modern FOB consists of about 10,000 glass fibers of 10 to 12 μm diameter, incorporated in an insertion cord (length: 55 to 60 cm; diameter 2.2 to 6.0 mm). This insertion cord is also equipped with one or two light guiding cables, two angulation wires to control the tip of the FOB, and a working channel (diameter greater than 2.0 mm) for suctioning of secretions. The FOB handle incorporates an eyepiece, a lever for controlling the bending motion of the tip, and a means of accessing the working channel. The bending lever controls movement of the insertion cord in a vertical axis, while flexion or extension of the wrist controls rotation of the FOB along the axis of the insertion cord. In adult patients, the inner diameter of the tracheal tube (TT) should be 1 to 2 mm larger than the outer diameter of FOB used.

FOB intubation in association with spontaneous ventilation is a well-established method for managing cooperative trauma patients with known difficult airways.[4] However, failed intubation does occur in any location where this technique is used.[5,6] Reasons for failed intubation include excessive secretions or blood in the airway, inadequate topicalization, oversedation, and laryngospasm.

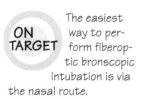

The easiest way to perform fiberoptic bronscopic intubation is via the nasal route.

The easiest way to perform FOB intubation is via the nasal route because the TT is naturally guided toward the laryngeal opening. The nasal approach is the preferred route for awake fiberoptic intubation because it is easier, better tolerated, and there is no risk of bite damage to the FOB. However, the risk of bleeding is higher than with the oral route. Also, there is a relative contraindication to nasotracheal intubation in patients with basal skull fractures that disrupt the cribriform plate of the ethmoid bone because it is said that the tube may traverse the fracture line and enter the brain. However, in a retrospective review of 82 spontaneously breathing trauma patients with facial fractures who underwent blind nasal intubation, there were no instances of intracranial penetration.[7] In the review, 83% had severe midface fractures, and 34% had cribriform plate disruption.

Prolonged mechanical ventilation via a nasotracheal tube may be associated with infectious sinusitis and pneumonia. Holzapfel et al.[8] randomly allocated 399 nasotracheally intubated patients to either a study group where there was a systematic search for evidence of sinusitis by CT scan (n = 199) or to a control group (n = 200). Patients with sinusitis in the study group (n = 80) received sinus lavage and IV antibiotics, whereas in the control group, no patient was treated for sinusitis. Ventilator-associated bronchopneumonia and mortality were significantly greater in the control group as opposed to the study group.

Thermosoftening of nasotracheal tubes in warm saline (e.g., 35 C) has been shown to improve navigability through the nasal passageways and reduce epistaxis and nasal damage during intubation.[9]

In contrast with the more direct nasal route, during oral FOB intubation, a 90° angle has to be negotiated in the oropharynx. As a result, several aids for the passage of the TT through the patient's oropharynx have been described (e.g., Ovassapian airway[10] and Williams airway[11]). These devices also act as bite blocks and displace the tongue to facilitate guiding of the fiberoptic scope and TT toward the laryngeal opening. The laryngeal mask airway (LMA) or the intubating laryngeal mask (LMA Fastrach™) can also be used to facilitate intubation using the FOB, especially in anesthetized patients.

FOB intubation can be performed in anesthetized patients, especially in can-mask-ventilate/cannot-intubate situations as an alternative to repeated attempts at laryngoscopy.[1] The major advantages of the FOB are difficult to exploit in prehospital care because they are mainly associated with awake intubation under local anesthesia with or without intravenous sedation—a technique that is probably inappropriate for the emergency prehospital setting. However, awake FOB intubation does have significant advantages because both muscle tone is preserved and the patient swallows secretions, resulting in the easier identification of landmark structures. Drugs recommended for sedation during fiberoptic airway management should be short-acting and reversible, for example, low-dose midazolam (1 to 3 mg) and/or fentanyl (50 to 100 mcg) (Table 10-1).

As with awake blind nasal intubation, local anesthesia of the upper airway decreases the amount of sedation required during awake intubation, so the nasal cavity, pharynx, and larynx should first be anesthestized. The naris is first sprayed with oxymetazoline to produce vasoconstriction of the nasal mucosa, which secondarily produces dilation of the naris. The nose can then be anesthetized by passing long, cotton-tipped applicators soaked in 4% lidocaine with epinephrine 1:200,000 along the floor of the nasal cavity. Alternatively, a local anesthetic spray can be used. Thereafter, the naris is progressively dilated using nasal trumpets soaked in 2% viscous lidocaine. These are inserted in increasingly larger diameter to anesthetize and dilate the nasal cavity (a nasal trumpet size 36Fr predicts easy passage of a 7.0 I.D. TT) (See Table 10-1).

Administration of oxygen during intubation increases the patient's SpO_2. Oral administration of local anesthetics for provision of supraglottic anesthesia can be accomplished using atomizers (oxygen flow 8 to 10 L/min; 10 mL lidocaine 4%; however, residual agent in the oropharynx must be suctioned to avoid reabsorption) or nebulizers (ultrasound nebulizers using 3 mL of lidocaine 4%). **Transtracheal anesthesia** puncture of the cricothyroid membrane and injection of lidocaine at the end of inspiration to produce anesthesia below the vocal cords and upper trachea. Nerve blocks[12] can also provide topical anesthesia, but they are seldom necessary for FOB intubation. Furthermore, those landmarks that need to be identified for successful nerve blocks are often obscured in emergency and/or trauma patients. Whatever form of topical anesthesia is used, it is important to be aware of the potential side effects and complications that can follow the rapid uptake of local anesthetics in the richly perfused tissue of the oral cavity and airway. Close attention to total drug dosage, close observation of the patient, and mandatory aspiration of the syringe prior to injection all assist in diminishing the risk of local anesthetic overdose. Topical anesthesia should be used cautiously in patients with full stomachs because they can abolish the protective airway reflexes leading to pulmonary aspiration[12] (Table 10-1).

transtracheal anesthesia
Puncture of the cricothyroid membrane and injection of 4% lidocaine 2 mL at the end of inspiration. This can produce tracheal anesthesia.

 PEARLS Topical anesthesia can abolish reflexes of the airway in patients with a full stomach, leading to aspiration. Extreme care must be taken to prevent aspiration.

Patient positioning is an important consideration prior to FOB intubation. The typical position used during direct laryngoscopy (patient lying supine with head in the sniffing position) is not the preferred position for fiberoptic access to the airway, and an approach from the front or side of the patient is often preferable. In the crashing patient, the left semilateral position may be the best.[13] Other drawbacks of FOB intubation include equipment availability, expense, durability, and training[14], which all militate against its use in prehospital care.

Use of the FOB in Special Airway Management Situations

Use of the FOB for Exchange of the Combitube

ON TARGET After several hours in place, the Combitube has to be exchanged for a definitive airway due to pressures exerted by the inflated cuffs, which might damage tissues and cause necrosis.

The esophageal-tracheal Combitube™ (Tyco Healthcare Nellcor, Pleasanton, CA) is a recommended alternative device for the management of cannot-intubate/cannot-mask-ventilate situations. When inserted blindly into the airway, the ETC enters the esophagus in more then 98% of patients, allowing supraglottic ventilation via its pharyngeal lumen. After several hours in place, however, the ETC has to be exchanged for a definitive airway. Exchange via an FOB is a very useful alternative in difficult-airway patients. The oropharyngeal balloon of the ETC is first deflated, and then the FOB loaded with a standard TT (introduced orally or nasally) is advanced toward the laryngeal opening. The patient's trachea is then intubated under direct vision. During ETC exchange, the distal cuff should be kept inflated until tracheal intubation is confirmed to prevent aspiration. Should intubation fail, the oropharyngeal balloon can be reinflated, and supraglottic ventilation resumed.

Gaitini et al. studied fiberoptic Combitube replacement without interruption of ventilatory support.[15] In 40 patients, the oropharyngeal balloon was partially deflated while the FOB was introduced posteriorly around the balloon. This technique of exchanging an alternative airway with a definitive airway, without interruption of ventilation, is of special value in patients with severe pulmonary dysfunction. Replacement was easier and was performed more quickly in spontaneously breathing patients. An alternative technique is the fiberoptically guided exchange of the ETC over a guidewire.[16]

Confirmation of Correct TT Placement

Use of the FOB is a failsafe method to confirm correct tracheal tube placement through fiberoptic visualization of the tracheal rings and carina.[17] Fiberoptic tracheoscopy not only enables accurate diagnosis of tracheal positioning but also enables the determination of correct TT insertion depth (3 to 5 cm above the carina).

Fiberoptic Intubation in Patients with Cervical-Spine Injury

As noted by Smith,[18] there is no clear consensus on the optimal method of securing the airway in patients with cervical-spine (c-spine) injuries, other than it is accepted that the head and neck must be kept in a neutral position throughout the intubation process. Traction of the cervical spine should be avoided completely during cervical immobilization because it can result in vertebral subluxation.[19] However, manual immobilization of the head and neck by a third party is necessary to prevent the intubator from causing unintentional movement of the cervical spine.[20]

Criswell et al. investigated the neurological outcome of 73 trauma patients with cervical-spine injury undergoing tracheal intubation with direct laryngoscopy and in-line axial immobilization.[21] Neurological damage induced by airway management was not observed in any patient. Nonetheless, with proper training and support, awake fiberoptic intubation is an appropriate choice for airway management in awake, cooperative patients with (unstable) cervical-spine pathologies who have no respiratory distress. Patients with head trauma or those who are unconscious or uncooperative often require rapid sequence induction and intubation with manual inline axial stabilization (MIAS).

Use of the FOB for Airway Management in Penetrating Neck Trauma

Desjardins and Varon reported that fiberoptic bronchoscopy is a valuable aid for both evaluation and intubation in penetrating neck injuries.[22] A rapid sequence fiberoptic intubation technique may be used in combative patients who otherwise do not appear difficult to intubate. In this technique, a rapid sequence anesthetic induction with in-line immobilization of the cervical spine is followed by standard laryngoscopy and insertion of a bronchoscope through the larynx to evaluate rapidly for the presence of injury or blood below the vocal cords. The bronchoscope tip is placed distal to the injury, and the endotracheal tube is then introduced over the endoscope. The cuff of the endotracheal tube should be positioned below the injury to prevent air leak and enlargement of the laceration.[22]

Table 10-1 Local Anesthesia & Sedation for Airway Management in the Awake Patient

Why It Is Important	Types of Airway Anesthesia	Drugs	Drugs (cont.)	Miscellaneous

• Allows for patient cooperation in management of the difficult airway
• Prevents hemodynamic response to laryngoscopy and endotracheal intubation
• May improve response and decrease anesthetic requirement in debilitated patients
• Useful for upper endoscopy
	Airway Blocks
	• Glossopharyngeal N.B.
	• Superior laryngeal N.B.
	• Translaryngeal Injection
	Nebulization
	• Potentially blocks the entire respiratory tract
	• Safe to administer using 4–5 mL of 4% lidocaine by nebulizer for 15–20 minutes
	Topicalization
	• Swab,
	• swish,
	• spray or
	• gargle
		Local Anesthetics Lidocaine:
		• Max Dose—400 mg (5–7 mg/kg)
		• 4% solution
		  - (spray, atomize, nebulizer, inject into trachea)
		  - Spray 1–5 mL (40-200 mg)
		• 2% solution (superior laryngeal, glossopharyngeal nerve block)
		• 2% viscous solution
		  - (swish through mouth, coat nasal trumpet/oral airway
		  - Gargle with 15 mL
		• 2% jelly or 5% ointment (apply moderate amount to:
		  - Tongue or oropharynx using tongue blade
		  - Tracheal tube shortly before use
		Cocaine:
		• Max–1–3 mg/kg (or 400 mg)
		• 1–4% solution (soak Q-tips/pledgettes for nasal application,
		• Provides vasoconstriction
		Tetracaine:
		• Max Dose 100–200 mg)
		• 2%- apply with cotton pledgetts
		• 0.5%- apply with pledgetts of inhale as nebulized 0.5% solution
		Benzocaine, Hurricane®, Topex®:
		• Apply spray to tongue/oropharynx for < 1 second
		• 1-second spray designed to deliver 60 mg
		• Toxicity observed with excessive spray
		Cetacaine®-Spray <1 sec.
		• Delivers 200 mg benzocaine/butyl amino benzoate/tetracaine residue/second
			Sedation/Analgesi a Midazolam:
			- sedation, amnesia
			- Dose-IV, 1–4 mg (.075 mg/kg)
			- S. E. - ↓ RR with high doses
			Fentanyl:
			- Analgesia
			- Dose IV 50–100 mcg (1 mcg/kg)
			- S.E.↓ RR, ↓ coughing
			Ketamine:
			- Sedation/analgesia
			- Dose-IV .5-1 mg/kg incrementally
			- S.E.- Salivation, Hallucinations
			Remifentanil:
			- Analgesia
			- Dose–IV Infusion (.05 mcg/kg/min)
			- S.E. ↓ RR, bradycardia, ↓ coughing
			Dexmedetomidine:
			- Sedation
			- IV Infusion
			- Bolus of 1 mcg/kg over 10 min. followed by infusion of 0.2–0.7 mcg/kg/hr
			- S.E. – no respiratory depression, maintains RR, slow onset
			Adjunctive Glycopyrrolate:
			Intravenous antisialogogue which facilitates drying of the mucosa to improve contact with topicalized and nebulized local anesthetics
				Tips for Success
				• Patient cooperation — enhanced by adequate explanation and preparation
				• Control secretions (Use of antisialogogue)
				• Give adequate sedation to alleviate anxiety
				• Give adquate anesthesia to ensure patient comfort
				To Avoid Complications
				• Measure/calculate all drugs
				• Suction excess volume of oral spray
				• Cautious application of L. A. in patients with sepsis or traumatized mucosa
				• Monitor carefully
				• Provide supplemental Oxygen
				Signs & Symptoms of L.A. Toxicity
				• Seizures
				• CV collapse
				• Methemoglobinemia

Developed from: Osborn I, Gooden C, Follmer J, Perez A. A Taste of Anesthesia: Improving Airway Topicalization (Brochure, Department of Anesthesiology, Mount Sinai School of Medicine, Bronx, NY, 2006. N.B.=Nevre block; L. A. = local anesthesia; RR=Respiratory Rate; S. E. = Side Effects (Courtesy of JM Rich, CRNA [www.slamaiway.com])

Use of the LMA Fastrach as a Conduit for Fiberoptic Intubation

The LMA (LMA North America, Inc., San Diego, CA) and especially the intubating laryngeal mask (LMA Fastrach™) have gained widespread attention as emergency airway management devices in cannot-intubate/cannot-ventilate situations.[23,24] Furthermore, the LMA has been incorporated into the American Society of Anesthesiologists (ASA) practice guidelines for the management of the difficult airway as the device of first choice by anesthesia practitioners in patients who cannot be ventilated by face mask.[1]

Genzwuerker et al., compared different laryngeal masks in a resuscitation model; therefore, the LMA Fastrach may be especially suitable in the prehospital setting because positioning is easy, tidal volumes are adequate, and tracheal intubation is possible through the device.[25] Blind tracheal intubation through the LMA Fastrach is possible in 76% to 96% of patients, depending on the TT type used and the extent of muscle relaxation.[26] In the remaining few patients, the LMA can be used as a conduit to facilitate guiding the FOB through the patient's glottic opening.[27] The first report on combined LMA/FOB use for difficult-airway management in a larger patient series was published by Silk et al.[28] The technique was successful in 96% (46/48). Furthermore, Kitamura et al. used the LMA for primary airway management in 128 patients with halo vests, and fiberoptic intubation via the LMA was successful in all patients.[29]

PEARLS

The LMA Fastrach may be especially suitable in the prehospital setting because positioning is easy, tidal volumes are adequate, and tracheal intubation is possible through the device.

Rigid Fiberscopes

Rigid fiberscopes offer the benefits of the FOB with the practicality of direct laryngoscopy. A number of these devices have recently been introduced to the market.

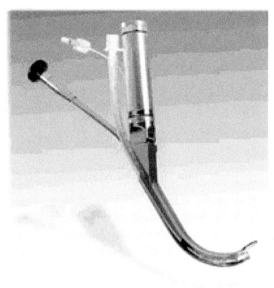

FIGURE 10-1

The UpsherScope Ultra™ is a rigid fiberoptic laryngoscope that combines a fiberoptic viewing channel with a tube-guiding blade.
(Courtesy of Mercury Medical, Clearwater, FL)

UpsherScope Ultra™

The UpsherScope Ultra™ (Mercury Medical, Clearwater, FL, Figure 10-1) is a rigid fiberoptic laryngoscope that combines a fiberoptic viewing channel with a tube-guiding blade. The scope is compatible with the full range of Upsher handles and is fully immersible and autoclavable. It allows the operator to view the tracheal tube passing between the vocal cords, and the eyepiece can also accommodate a television monitor for remote viewing. The device permits the operator to insufflate oxygen down the TT during intubation, and the tube cuff and circuit can both be tested while the tube is positioned in the scope.[30]

WuScope™

The WuScope™ (Achi Corporation, San Jose, CA, Figure 10-2) is a combination intubating device featuring a fiberoptic pathway consisting of a flexible fiberscope within a rigid tubular metal blade.[31] The tubular blade creates more viewing and intubating space in patients with a limited mouth opening, and because it is shaped to match the pharyngeal contour of the oral airway, it promotes oral access to the glottis without tongue displacement or head extension.[32] Fiberoptic laryngoscopy using the Wuscope is associated with easy glottic exposure and tracheal intubation, even in patients with anatomic factors that normally prevent adequate visualization of the vocal cords, such as cervical-spine instability, hypoplastic mandible, and protruding maxillary incisors.[33] However, a minimum of 20 mm of mouth opening is necessary to insert and manipulate the rigid Wuscope blades.

The system utilizes one handle and one fiberoptic channel that fit a number of different sizes of blade, thus increasing its versatility. The device has a separate oxygen channel to ensure a continuous stream of supplemental oxygen. The tubular blade both protects the optics from contamination and prevents redundant soft tissue from obstructing the operator's view of the larynx. During the intubation process, simultaneous suctioning is achieved by positioning a regular large-bore suction catheter within the lumen of the TT. The blade is designed to ensure that tracheal intubation is visually guided throughout the intubation process, which should be performed with the patient's head in the neutral position.

In a randomized study of the fiberoptic Wuscope versus conventional laryngoscopy in 87 patients with cervical-spine immobilization, the Wuscope was associated with lower intubation difficulty scale scores and better views of the laryngeal apertures.[32] Grade 1 views of the glottis occurred in 98% of the Wuscope patients, whereas 39% of patients in the conventional laryngoscopy group had Cormack Grade 3 or 4 views.[32] The Wuscope can also

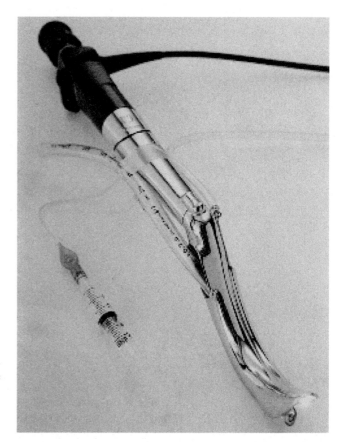

facilitate intratracheal placement of double-lumen endobronchial tubes (size 35 and 37 Fr) in patients with difficult intubation.[34] The rigid tubular blade protects the fragile tracheal cuff from tearing on the maxillary teeth. Flexible fiberoptic bronchoscopy is then perfomed to position the tube in either the left or right mainstem bronchus.

Bullard Elite™ Laryngoscope

The Bullard Elite™ Laryngoscope (Circon-ACMI, Stamford, CT) (Figure 10-3a) is an indirect fiberoptic laryngoscope with a rigid anatomically shaped blade that comes in three sizes: adult, child, and newborn/infant. The distal end of the blade consists of three components: a light bundle, an image bundle, and a hollow working channel.

The fiberoptic light bundle is illuminated via a standard battery handle and bulb, or by using a fiberoptic light source. Almost all commercially available fiberoptic light guides are compatible with the scope due to the special adapters supplied with the device. The eyepiece is also compatible with all standard surgical video camera systems. The scope is designed to facilitate visualization of the larynx without requiring alignment of the pharyngeal, laryngeal, and oral axes. The 3.7 mm hollow working channel allows suctioning of secretions, administration of oxygen, or application of local anesthetics through the proximal Luer-lock fitting (Figure10-3b). A three-way stopcock with a nipple for a suction tube line is available as an accessory, and intermittent suctioning or insufflation of oxygen through the working channel can help minimize problems with fogging and contamination of the fiberoptic tip by secretions. Intubation is facilitated by using a standard intubating stylet but, because the TT is not guided through a channel within the blade of this device, care should be taken to ensure that the tube does not impinge on the right **aryepiglottic fold** or **arytenoid cartilage**, particularly if the blade is allowed to stray away from the midline. When used with a

aryepiglottic folds
The aryepiglottic folds extend between the arytenoid cartilage and the lateral margin of the epiglottis on each side and constitute the lateral borders of the laryngeal inlet.

arytenoid cartilage
Either of two small cartilages at the posterior aspect of the larynx to which the vocal folds are attached.

(a) The Bullard Elite™ Laryngoscope is an indirect fiberoptic laryngoscope with a rigid, anatomically shaped blade that comes in three sizes: adult, child, and newborn/infant. (b) Distal end of the adult Bullard laryngoscope.

(Courtesy of Gyrus ACMI, Southborough, MA)

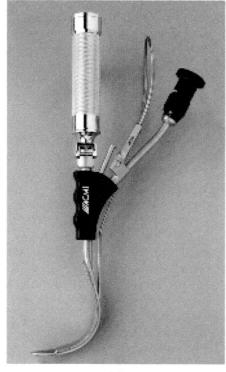

(a)

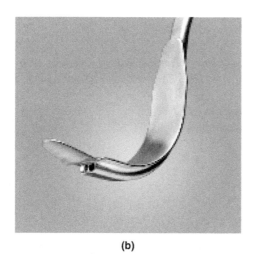

(b)

standard battery handle, the scope is easily transported throughout the hospital or to prehospital locations.

The Bullard laryngoscope is designed for oral intubation of difficult-airway patients.[35-37] The major advantage of the scope is that almost no head and neck movement is required to obtain a clear view of the vocal cords.[35,37] Also, the time to glottic visualization and intubation is faster compared with flexible fiberoptic techniques. In adult patients with simulated difficult airways (rigid cervical collar), the success rate for intubation was 88% of 40 patients with an independently styletted tube passed freehand into the trachea, and 83% of 40 patients with a multifunctional intubating stylet.[38]

In an intubation manikin head representing a Grade 3 laryngoscope view, failed intubation using the Bullard occurred in 41 of 400 attempts, with a high rate of esophageal intubations due to the tracheal tube obstructing the view of the cords during intubation.[39] Difficulty advancing the tracheal tube through the glottis also occurs usually because of right aryepiglottic fold or anterior vocal cord contact.[40]

Levitan FPS Scope™

The Levitan FPS Scope™ (Clarus Medical, Minneapolis, MN) comprises a fiberoptic channel within a malleable stylet having an atraumatic tip. The device has an integrated light source, and there is also a side port for oxygen administration. The scope was designed to mimic a traditional intubation stylet with the additional benefit of fiberoptic technology, and it allows visual confirmation of the intubation process as seen from the tip of the TT. Prior to use, the stylet is given a slight bend at the level of the proximal end of the tube cuff, but the bend angle should not exceed 35°. To prevent fogging, antifog solution is applied to the distal optics, and the stylet can also be warmed. The TT is cut so that the tip of the stylet is recessed just inside the tube bevel when the 15 mm connector is pushed up into the tube stop. Oxygen flow through the tube is set at 5 to 10 liters per minute. Both tube and stylet are lubricated prior to use, with care taken not to contaminate the distal optics. It is important to appreciate that the tip of this device must be placed under direct vision using a conventional laryngoscope. The tip is positioned beneath and away from the epiglottic edge, keeping it off the mucosa. Only then does the operator switch from a direct laryngoscopic view to a fiberoptic view. The stylet is then advanced through the glottic opening under visual control while the conventional laryngoscope is retained in place.

Shikani Optical Stylet™ (SOS)

The Shikani Optical Stylet™ (SOS) (Clarus Medical, Minneapolis, MN) is similar in construction to the Levitan FPS Scope™, except that it possesses a pistol grip and an adjustable tube stop/oxygen port, which does away with the need to cut the tube to size. It has a 10,000 pixel bundle within a malleable stylet. The tracheal tube is threaded over the stylet and locked in position, with the distal tip of the stylet slightly recessed within the tube. During insertion, the operator looks through the eyepiece instead of into the airway. It is recommended that you use a laryngoscope to facilitate insertion. When the glottis comes into view, the tube is advanced over the stylet and through the glottic inlet. The method is similar to that of the Levitan FPS Scope™.

Foley Airway Stylet Tool™ (FAST)

The FAST scope (Clarus Medical, Minneapolis, MN) is a portable, flexible fiberoptic scope that is particularly useful for guiding the tip of the TT into the trachea during intubation through the LMA Fastrach™ (intubating laryngeal mask airway [iLMA]). Tracheal intubation using the iLMA is normally a blind technique with a variable success rate, between 70% and 99%.[1] Intubation success rates can be improved significantly by utilizing the Chandy technique described in Chapter 9, but further improvement can be expected when the FAST is also used. The recent introduction of the LMA CTrach™, an advanced version of the LMA Fastrach™ with its own built-in fiberoptic channels, does away with the need for a supplementary fiberoptic device.

ViewMax™ Laryngoscope

The Viewmax™ laryngoscope (Rusch) looks very much like a conventional direct laryngoscope except that the blade incorporates a view tube with a lens system that refracts the image approximately 20° from the horizontal. This refraction allows visualization of the most anteriorly placed larynx through the eyepiece. The scope requires minimal training because the operator utilizes similar techniques to those required during conventional laryngoscopy. The difference in using this scope in contrast to conventional laryngoscopy is that the scope is inserted in the midline instead of down the right side of the tongue. The device is designed with a 3.5-inch hybrid blade, is less curved than a Macintosh and not as straight as a Miller, and is suitable for use in nearly all adults. A pediatric version of the device is also available.

McGrath Series® 5 Fully Portable Video Laryngoscope

The McGrath® Series 5 Fully Portable Video Laryngoscope (Aircraft Medical Ltd, Edinburgh, UK) is a video device that allows remote viewing of the laryngeal inlet during intubation. This highly portable scope utilizes single-use blades with a one-size-fits-all design. The full-color image is collected by an onboard miniature camera located in the Camera-Stick™ and is transferred to the compact LCD panel mounted at the top of the handle. The novel design utilizing disposable blades does away with the need for full sterilization between cases. Intubation is facilitated by means of a standard malleable stylet within the advancing TT and, as with all devices requiring this technique, care should be taken to avoid the tube tip impinging against periglottic structures. Currently there is no video-out capability with this device.

Airtraq® Optical Laryngoscope

The Airtraq® (King Systems, Noblesville, IN) is a disposable laryngoscope made largely from plastic (Figure 10-4). Designed for single use, it comes presterilized in a protective transparent pouch. The device is similar in design to the Upsherscope™, with an anatomically curved blade incorporating both a fiberoptic channel and a tube-guiding channel that is open on one side. The high-definition optical channel features a heating system controlled by microchip, which prevents fogging of the distal optics. The guide channel accommodates standard tracheal tubes up to 8.5 mm I.D. and directs the tip of the tube toward the glottic opening. The scope is powered by three built-in AAA batteries, activated by a switch at the eyepiece, that give around 1 hour of continuous use, after which time an internal microchip permanently disables the device. When first switched on, the light source blinks for up to one minute until the antifogging system has reached working temperature. The large eyepiece gives a clear magnified view of the entire intubation process. Alternatively, the rubber boot around the eyepiece can be removed and a dedicated reusable, lightweight, video-viewing head clipped into position. This optional video system

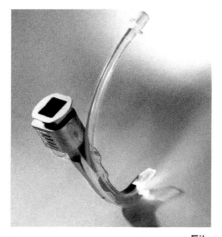

FIGURE 10-4

The Airtraq® is a disposable laryngoscope made largely from plastic.
(Courtesy of AIRTRAQ LLC with U.S. and Canada distribution by King Systems Corporation, Noblesville, IN)

allows viewing and recording of the intubation process on an external monitor or PC and is useful for teaching purposes. The Airtraq® comes in three color-coded sizes: regular (for use with TT sizes 7.5 to 8.5 mm) small (6.0 to 7.5 mm), and pediatric (4.5 to 5.5 mm). It allows the intubation of the patient in any position (e.g., seated), with the head and neck held in neutral alignment, and is suitable for patients with high Cormack and Lehane grades. The cost of each disposable unit is around $50 (U.S.).

GlideScope® Video Intubation System

The GlideScope® incorporates a laryngoscope that possesses a hybrid shape between that of a curved and straight blade (Figure 10-5). The GlideScope® Video Intubation System (Verathon Medical [Canada] ULC) is a camera laryngoscope that displays an unobstructed view of the glottis on a monitor. The reusable device is made from a durable medical-grade plastic, and a digital video camera is embedded within the blade. The camera is equipped with a proprietary antifogging system, which gives it an advantage over some other devices employing fiberoptic technology. An LED light source mounted beside the camera provides continuous illumination during the intubation process. The GlideScope® is inserted down the midline of the tongue, and a mouth opening of just 18 mm is necessary for introduction of the device. Once the epiglottis comes into view, it is lifted directly (Miller style) to reveal the laryngeal inlet, and intubation is performed while the operator views the high-resolution color image remotely on the rechargeable viewing screen. As with similar remote viewing devices, intubation is facilitated by means of a standard malleable stylet within the advancing TT or a bougie-introducer, and the same caveats apply as mentioned previously with this technique. The scope is easily detached from the video cable, and a cover plug is supplied to protect the multipin connector during sterilization. Various chemical sterilization options are available, but the manufacturer does not approve of autoclaving or exposure to temperatures in excess of 80°C. The unit has a silver-colored temperature indicator that changes to black if the unit has been exposed to excessive temperature.

The GlideScope® usually provides a Class I view of the larynx, and a large multicenter clinical trial demonstrated that successful intubation was generally achieved even when direct laryngoscopy was predicted to be moderately or considerably difficult.[41] The device is an excellent educational asset for teaching airway management and learning dynamic airway anatomy, and the manufacturer has recently developed a system for prehospital use. The device is available in a full range of sizes, with adult, pediatric, and neonatal versions.

FIGURE 10-5

Portable GlideScope System with Hardshell case. The GlideScope (Vitaid Ltd, Williamsville, NY) incorporates a laryngoscope that possesses a hybrid shape between that of a curved and straight blade. (Courtesy of Vitaid Airway Management, Williamsville, NY)

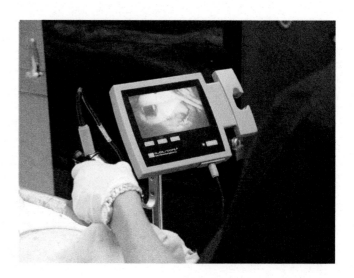

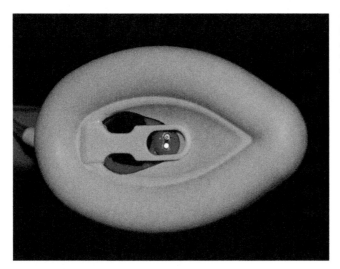

FIGURE 10-6

Fiberoptics emerging beneath fenestrated epiglottic elevating bar of the LMA CTrach™.

(Courtesy of Dr. Andrew M. Mason)

LMA CTrach™

The LMA CTrach™ (LMA North America Inc, San Diego, CA) (Figures 10-6 and 10-7) is a modified version of the intubating laryngeal mask airway (iLMA or LMA Fastrach™) described in Chapter 9. The LMA CTrach™ is unique in the field of airway management because it simultaneously functions as a secure airway in its own right, thus permitting continuous ventilation; provides a direct view of the larynx, which enables visually assisted and guided intubation; offers video-capture capability; and gives the user 100% confidence in having achieved successful intubation.

The LMA CTrach™ (ctLMA) airway possesses two integrated fiberoptic bundles that emerge distally beneath the fenestrated epiglottic elevating bar (EEB) (Figure 10-6). The bundles serve both to transmit light down to the larynx and to relay images of the intubation

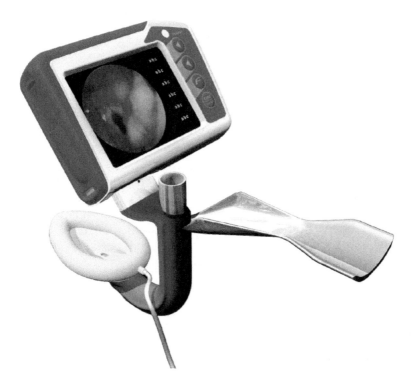

FIGURE 10-7

THE LMA CTrach™ Airway with viewer attached.

(Courtesy of The Laryngeal Mask Co. LTD., St Helier, Jersey)

Fiberscopic and Video-Assisted Intubation

process back to a wireless viewer with an 86 mm high-resolution LCD color screen. The lightweight rechargeable viewer is designed to snap onto the proximal part of the ctLMA airway by means of a magnetic latch. When the viewer is attached and switched on, real-time video images of the intubation process are visible on the screen, and the images can also be viewed on a laptop computer using the dedicated software bundled with the kit (Figure 10-7). Both video and still images can be recorded on a computer for clinical record purposes, thus providing valuable dynamic teaching material. The ctLMA airway is fully autoclavable and reusable up to 20 times. Special single-use tracheal tubes are available for use with the ctLMA (and iLMA) in I.D. sizes 6.0, 6.5, 7.0, 7.5, and 8.0 mm. These are straight wire-reinforced tubes with a removable 15 mm connector, atraumatic tip, and a low-pressure cuff.

Method of Use

The ctLMA airway is inserted in exactly the same way as the iLMA but, once in place, the entire intubation process can then be observed on the accompanying viewer and can be controlled by the operator.

Preparation

The appropriate size of the airway for the patient is first selected. The ctLMA airway comes in 3 sizes: #3 (for patients 30 to 50 kg), #4 (50 to 70 kg), and #5 (70 to 100 kg). An alternative method of sizing is to select a #3 for large children (or very small adults), #4 for adult females, and #5 for adult males. When in doubt, it is usually better to select the larger size. With the viewer attached and switched on, and by using the prefocus card supplied, you can adjust the focusing wheel to bring the image into sharp view. The viewer is then switched off and removed from the ctLMA. No further focusing should then be necessary.

Intubation

After ensuring sufficient depth of anesthesia, intubation via the ctLMA is performed in six steps, as follows:

1. The patient's head is placed in the neutral position, and the ctLMA airway is inserted, without the viewer attached, in precisely the same way as a standard iLMA.
2. The cuff of the ctLMA is then inflated with the appropriate quantity of air (cuff pressure ≤ 60 cm H_2O), and the patient is ventilated to ensure adequate oxygenation.
3. While the handle of the ctLMA is held firmly to stabilize the device, the viewer is attached onto the magnetic latch connector and switched on.
4. If necessary, the position of the ctLMA should be adjusted to bring the glottis into view. This is done by gently moving the handle back and forth in the sagittal plane. The light intensity and gain on the viewer can then be adjusted if necessary to optimize the view.
5. A prelubricated TT is inserted down the ctLMA airway tube and advanced between the vocal cords under direct vision. Smooth intubation can usually be achieved by lifting the handle of the ctLMA away from the posterior pharyngeal wall (as described in Step 2 of the Chandy maneuver—see Chapter 9). After successful intubation, the ctLMA viewer is switched off and detached.
6. The TT cuff is inflated, and intubation is confirmed by the approved method (ideally with an end-tidal CO_2 monitor in patients with a perfusing cardiac rhythm). Auscultation of the chest should also be undertaken to guard against endobronchial tube placement. The ctLMA airway can then be removed in exactly the same way as the standard LMA Fastrach, leaving the TT in place.

Summary

Since its introduction in 1966, the fiberoptic bronchoscope (FOB) has led to great advances in anesthesia and critical care medicine, although the use of the FOB in acute airway management in the emergency department began only in the 1990s. Reported success rates in the emergency room are in the 80% to 90% range, depending on experience, education, and training. In the emergency patient, we recommend awake fiberoptic intubation in the left semilateral position under adequate local anesthesia.

Use of the standard flexible fiberscope is unlikely to expand into the prehospital arena, but the growing range of compact and durable fiberoptic devices for facilitating intubation does have the potential to revolutionize prehospital emergency airway management.

PEARLS It is mandatory that the operator be absolutely proficient in the use of any chosen airway management device.

Because training is essential for safe and rapid performance of fiberoptic intubation in emergencies, residency programs must, at a minimum, include regular training with manikins. Particular indications for the use of an FOB include airway management in cervical-spine injury, the exchange of temporary for definitive airways (e.g., exchange of Combitube or laryngeal mask airway for a standard TT), the placement of double-lumen tubes, and the confirmation of correct placement of an endotracheal tube.

Battery-operated FOBs with excellent quality have started to become available, and such devices could find a place in prehospital care. In Austria, an emergency medical services helicopter is equipped with a battery-operated Olympus FOB (O.D. 5.00 mm and a working channel of 2.8 mm), and it is used for diagnostic and therapeutic purposes.[42] When paramedics are given FOB tools, it is mandatory that they be trained adequately using manikins, and preferably with either live patients in the operating room setting or with cadavers. As with any airway device, it is necessary for the paramedic to be absolutely proficient in the use of any chosen device.

REVIEW QUESTIONS

1. List three reasons for failed FOB intubation.

2. What approach is preferred for awake fiberoptic intubation?

3. What types of infection can be caused by prolonged mechanical ventilation with a nasotracheal tube?

4. Describe the steps to be taken when exchanging an ET tube for the Combitube.

5. Why is the LMA Fastrach especially suitable for prehospital use?

6. List four indications for the use of a fiberscopic device.

Lightwand Intubation

Janice A. Follmer

Chapter Objectives

After reading this chapter, you should be able to:

- Trace the concept and history of lightwand intubation.

- Describe the principle of lightwand intubation.

- Discuss applications of lightwand intubation for advanced airway practitioners in various settings.

- List the different types of available lightwand devices.

- List the major differences among the various devices.

- List indications for using the lightwand (patient selection).

- List contraindications and complications of the lightwand.

- Describe, step by step, the technique of lightwand intubation.

- List strategies for successful lightwand intubation.

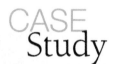

CASE
Study _____

Late one evening, Medic 8 is dispatched to a motor-vehicle collision on a rural county road. Fire department personnel at the scene report that a small passenger car has skidded on the wet road, striking a tree on the driver side. The unconscious driver is trapped in the vehicle. When the paramedics arrive, they see fire personnel attempting to ventilate the patient with a bag-valve-mask (BVM) device but with little success. The only access to the patient has been through the windshield area but, as the paramedics arrive, efforts to remove the roof of the car are successful. They find that there is no eye opening and the patient is unresponsive to painful stimuli, so they assign him a Glasgow Coma Scale score of 3. Breathing is spontaneous but the rate is a little slow, and the patient is making snoring noises. A pulse oximeter has already been attached and shows an SpO_2 reading of 88%.

After taking control of the cervical spine, an oropharyngeal airway is easily inserted, and the patient tolerates it completely. Breathing is then assisted with a BVM attached to a high-flow oxygen source. Both radial pulses are easily palpable but the rate is a little rapid. An intravenous line is established, and the patient is attached to various items of monitoring equipment. The cardiac monitor reveals sinus tachycardia with a rate of 110 beats per minute. Blood pressure is 110/72 mm Hg. Despite assisted respiration with the BVM at a rate of 12 breaths per minute, the SpO_2 reading rises only slightly to 90%, and the patient remains trapped in the vehicle.

The paramedics prepare for intubation, electing to use a lighted stylet due to limited patient access. A 7.5 mm endotracheal tube (TT) is lubricated, and the stylet is introduced down the lumen. The patient's cervical spine is manually stabilized as the lighted stylet is introduced into the mouth. The paramedic pulls the patient's tongue and jaw forward with her left hand as she advances the stylet down the center of the tongue. The rescue lights are dimmed and the tip of the stylet is seen to be illuminating the right side of the patient's neck, so she withdraws slightly and aims at the midline once again.

At the second attempt, illumination is noted in the midline just below the level of the cricoid cartilage. The tracheal tube is advanced to 21 cm as the stylet is removed. An esophageal detector bulb is attached to the TT connector and released, and it fills quickly. The BVM is attached to the tube, and ventilation is commenced. The end-tidal carbon dioxide ($ETCO_2$) monitor shows a good return of CO_2, bilateral breath sounds are found to be present, and the SpO_2 reading rises steadily to 99%.

The tracheal tube is secured, and rescue ventilations are continued throughout the remainder of the extrication, with the aim of keeping the $ETCO_2$ reading around 40 mm Hg to avoid hyperventilating the head-injured patient. After extrication onto a long spine board and transfer to the ambulance, the patient is transported to the local trauma center without further incident.

Introduction

Since the development of the laryngoscope in the nineteenth century, and the Macintosh blade in 1943, advanced airway practitioners have been searching for the airway tool that will lead to successful securing of the airway while avoiding injury. In fact, difficulty in managing the airway remains the single most important cause of anesthesia-related morbidity and mortality.[1] Many devices and modifications of devices have come and gone. Some that were initially met with skepticism, such as the LMA, have gone mainstream and become a routine part of our practice, even leading to modification of airway algorithms. It is said that necessity is the mother of invention and as long as we encounter airways that are difficult or impossible to secure, and as long as patients continue to suffer morbidity and mortality in an effort to secure their airway, whether as a prerequisite for general anesthesia or as a result of illness or trauma, the search for that perfect airway tool will continue.

This chapter introduces an alternative method for tracheal intubation utilizing **transillumination** via the lighted stylet.

transillumination
The light from a lighted stylet that can be seen externally through the tissues. If the stylet is properly placed, a bright light can be seen in the anterior neck.

KEY TERMS

airway topicalization, p. 210

arytenoid dislocation, p. 211

friable lesion, p. 210

transillumination, p. 206

History of the Lightwand

The use of the lightwand, or lighted stylet, has been reported since 1959, when Macintosh used a device to supplement the light on the laryngoscope,[2] Berman reported a similar use,[3] and Yamamura used it as an adjunct to nasal intubation.[4] Since then, numerous articles, both scientific studies as well as case reports, have been published regarding its use and usefulness. Isolated institutions and practitioners have reported employing the lighted stylet technique for many years. Rayburn reported in 1979 that the lightwand technique had been practiced for a number of years at the Brooke Army Medical Center and subsequently at Primary Children's Medical Center.[5] Early devices were modifications of those used for other purposes, such as the Flexi-lum™, an orthopedic tool. Unfortunately, complications arose, such as separation of the lightbulb from the stylet into the lung.

A few dedicated devices, both disposable plastic and reusable metal, became available, but none seemed to generate much enthusiasm. The literature on the lightwand seemed to thin, until Dr. Hung reported a new lightwand device in the *Canadian Journal of Anaesthesia* in 1995.[6] This device, known as the Trachlight™, overcame many of the shortcomings of the earlier devices. In the last five years, numerous articles have appeared—from the review article "Lighted Stylet Tracheal Intubation: A Review" by Davis et al. in *Anesthesia and Analgesia*, 2000,[7] to "Planned Lightwand Intubation in a Patient with a Known Difficult Airway" by Agro et al. in *Canadian Journal of Anaesthesia*, December 2004.[1]

At this point in time, light-guided intubations using the principle of transillumination have proven to be an effective and simple technique.[1] The Trachlight™ has been suggested as a useful option in the case of difficult or impossible laryngoscopic intubation for both anticipated and unanticipated situations.[1] As more practitioners become experienced in this technique and more research is reported, the lighted stylet may take a formal place in the difficult airway algorithm, even in the cannot-intubate/cannot-ventilate scenario. In the hands of the experienced practitioner, an attempt with the lightwand can be accomplished in seconds. The preponderance of difficult intubations that are prone to occur in the prehospital environment make the lightwand a good alternative to those who are trained and comfortable with its use.

Principle of Lightwand Intubation

Lightwand intubation is a method of tracheal intubation utilizing transillumination of the trachea as a guide. The stylet with a lighted tip is threaded into the endotracheal tube in the same manner as a standard stylet would be. Without the aid of a laryngoscope, the unit (tube with lighted stylet) is placed in the mouth and advanced toward the pharynx. The position of the tube tip can be seen from outside the throat as an illumination. When the light is bright in the median line of the throat, the tip is on the anterior pharynx, and only a further push completes the intubation.[4]

 PEARLS   A laryngoscope is not used with lightwand intubation.

The lightwand is a semirigid stylet with a light at the tip. The light is powered by a battery source in the handle. The battery may be permanently ensconced in the handle or it can be replaced. The stylet is threaded through a standard endotracheal tube. The entire unit, tube with stylet, is placed in the mouth and advanced over the tongue to the posterior pharynx, the light is switched on, ambient light is dimmed, and the glow of the light is observed midline over the neck in the cricohyoid area. The unit is then advanced until a bright light is seen above the sternal notch. The tube is then advanced over the stylet.

Correlation of the maximal transilluminated glow over the sternal notch with endotracheal tube placement at a level 5 cm from the carina was demonstrated by Stewart et al.[8] Placement is confirmed by ETCO$_2$. Placement is achieved both by observation of transillumination as well as a tactile sense.

Application of Lightwand Intubation for Advanced Airway Practitioners

The lightwand (Figure 11-1) can be used in many settings—including the prehospital setting, office setting, emergency department, intensive care unit (ICU), pediatric population, and the operating room. Securing the airway in the prehospital setting presents a myriad of situations not usually encountered in the somewhat controlled environment of the hospital. The environment may be hostile, the condition of the patient questionable as to the true extent of injury, and

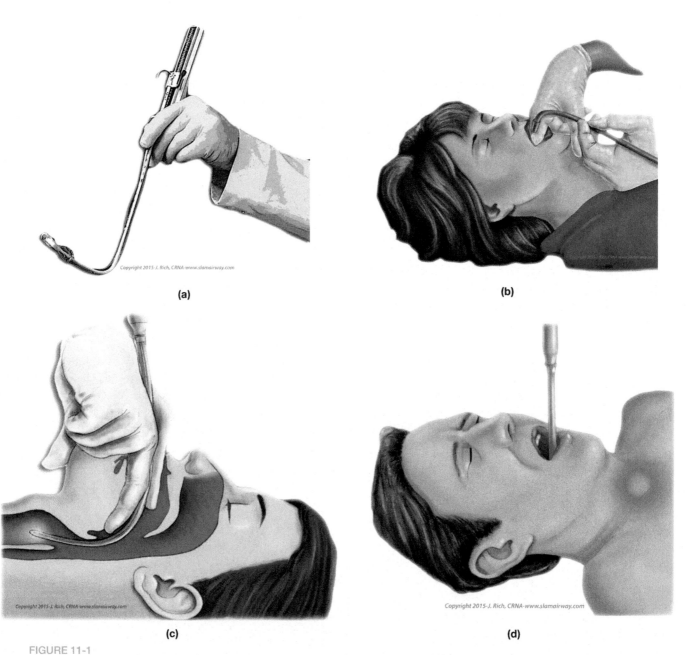

FIGURE 11-1

(a) Lighted stylet for endotracheal intubation. (b) Insertion of lighted stylet/TT. (c) Lighted stylet/TT in position. (d) Transillumination of a lighted stylet.

the presence of a difficult airway makes a bad situation even worse. Added to the scenario is the possible lack of backup personnel and equipment. The lighted stylet can be a great tool in this situation. It is small and easily portable, fits into a small mouth opening, and has even been reported to successfully secure the airway in spite of a clenched jaw.[9] It requires little if any manipulation of the cervical spine and has been reported to be perhaps superior to the iLMA in these situations.[10] It can be used in the presence of a bloody airway; however, caution must be used in suspected cases of airway disruption or a foreign body in the airway.

 Have a plan to limit ambient light when using the lighted stylet.

In 1985, Vollmer reported on the use of a lighted stylet in the prehospital setting and concluded that orotracheal intubation using a lighted stylet is an effective and safe method of emergency intubation, even in the adverse prehospital environment.[11] Ambient light in the field may make it somewhat more difficult to appreciate the transillumination, and particularly the difference in brightness of the light when the patient has a thin neck and the esophagus can transilluminate through the neck. Using a blanket or shade over the head and neck may be very helpful.

The lighted stylet can be used for infants and children as well as adults.

The use of a carbon dioxide detector for confirmation of tube placement is paramount. Practicing with the lighted stylet in the field in nontraumatized easy airways helps the prehospital practitioner successfully apply the technique when faced with the difficult airway.

The lightwand can also be used in the face-to-face position in the field.

Lighted stylet intubation can be done with the cervical spine immobilized.

Pediatric Population

The differences between the adult and pediatric airways have been well described.[13] In addition to the anatomic differences, infants and children have high oxygen consumption relative to reserves and desaturate much quicker, leaving little time for airway manipulation. Few if any children and certainly no infant can be expected to cooperate for awake intubation or tracheostomy.

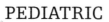

PEDIATRIC
NOTE
The Trachlight device has a child and infant stylet for use in the pediatric population.

The lighted stylet has been demonstrated to be a valuable tool in the pediatric population.[15] In addition to the child with a normal airway, the lightwand has been reported to be useful in children with facial anomalies, a small mouth opening, an abnormal upper airway, restriction of movement, and cervical-spine immobilization.[14,15-18]

It has been used in the austere environment of the medical relief mission,[16] making corrective surgery possible. This technique is applicable to all advanced airway practitioners caring for the pediatric population whether in the field, ICU, emergency department or operating room (OR). In addition, the lighted stylet has been successfully employed as a tool to confirm proper endotracheal tube placement in premature and term infants,[19] thus reducing the need for radiologic exam and exposure.

Table 11-1	Four Models of Lightwand			
Device	Handle	Battery	Stylet	
Trachlight™	Detachable	Replaceable 3 AAA	Three sizes; retractable inner wire; reusable 10 times	
Vital Light	Detachable	Encased	One size; disposable	
Aaron Medical	Fused	Encased	One size; disposable	
Metropolitan Medical	Fused	Replaceable	Entire unit available in adult and pediatric size; metal; reusable	

Lightwand Combined with Other Techniques

The lightwand has been paired with intubating LMA;[20-23] retrograde intubation;[24] fiberoptic bronchoscope;[25] difficult tracheostomy;[26] modified blind nasal intubation;[28,29] and the iLMA in supine, right, and left lateral positions.[29]

Types of Lightwands

All devices are stylets with a light at the tip, powered by a battery. Some are disposable; some are reusable. Some have a detachable handle; some stylets are fused to the handle. Some have replaceable batteries in the handle; some have batteries encased in the handle. Some stylets have a retractable semirigid wire; others are one piece. Some have one size stylet; others have interchangeable stylets of different sizes. See Table 11-1 for commercially available devices.

Patient Selection

airway topicalization
Use of a topical agent, such as 4% lidocaine spray, to anesthetize the oropharynx in preparation for awake intubation.

friable lesion
An injury, wound, or other disruption of local tissue that might easily be punctured.

Almost anyone requiring endotracheal intubation can be a candidate for lightwand intubation. However, patients with known or suspected lesions of the pharynx or trachea may not be the best candidates. Suspected disruption of the airway in trauma patients is a contraindication. Careful, gentle advancement of the lightwand unit is paramount. Familiarity and experience with the technique determines patient selection to some degree. For example, a patient presenting for emergency appendectomy (full stomach—not elective) with small mouth and cervical-spine immobility is not the case for the inexperienced lightwand practitioner. However, the experienced practitioner may feel very comfortable securing the airway with a lighted stylet.

Circumstances that make use of the laryngoscope blade difficult—such as small mouth opening, large protruding teeth, inability to extend neck, deliberate avoidance of extension, or presence of restrictive devices—lend themselves to use of the lightwand. Circumstances that make use of the fiberoptic scope difficult, such as a bloody airway or extreme neck flexion, can be overcome with use of the lightwand.

In comparing lightwand and fiberoptic techniques to secure the airway in awake patients with cervical-spine injuries, Saha et al. found the lighted stylet technique to be significantly faster.[31] This technique can be utilized in asleep or awake patients. If using it in awake patients, follow standard protocols for **airway topicalization.**

Contraindications and Complications

There are no absolute contraindications for use of the lightwand. Relative contraindications include any situation in which blind passage of the device might worsen the situation, such as known vascular or **friable lesions** of the airway, or traumatic disruption of the airway.

Reported complications include loss of the lightbulb from the stylet in an early device,[31] desheathing of the plastic tip of a Vital Signs lightwand that has not been lubricated,[32] **arytenoid dislocation**[33] (which a subsequent retrospective study determined to be no more common than in classic intubation with laryngoscope).[34] Common sense dictates that careful handling and gentle manipulation goes far in avoiding unnecessary trauma to the airway. The experience and comfort level of the advanced airway practitioner with the technique determine which airways can be safely secured utilizing the lighted stylet.

Description of Technique

arytenoid dislocation
Complete separation of the arytenoid cartilage from the cricoarytenoid joint. It usually results from severe laryngeal trauma and can be caused by attempts at intubation or removal of an ET tube with the cuff inflated.

1. Prepare stylet. Place a drop of lubricant at the proximal inlet of the endotracheal tube. Pass the lighted stylet through the lubricated proximal end of the tracheal tube until the distal tip of the lighted stylet rests at the distal end of the tracheal tube. Bend the distal end of the unit (stylet and tube) to suit the morphology of the individual airway but with a maximum angle of 80° to 90°.[35] Less of an angle is required in airways having a shorter thyromental distance.[36]

2. Position the patient with his or her head in the sniffing position, if possible. Have the stretcher or table as low as possible. You want to be above and slightly over the patient. Place your nondominant hand in the patient's mouth off to the left side and on the interior surface of the jaw. Lift the jaw upward. This lifts the epiglottis. With your dominant hand, slide the endotracheal tube with the threaded stylet into the patient's mouth midline, gliding along the tongue. As you approach the posterior pharynx, switch the light on. (In devices without a switch control, the light will be on already.) Dim the ambient light and look for a bright glow on the patient's neck in the cricohyoid area. The light should be in the midline. If it is not, withdraw the device and re-advance. Once the device is off to one side, it is probably caught in the vallecula, and it is almost impossible to bring it to the midline without first withdrawing it.

3. Once the glow is seen midline in the cricohyoid area, advance slightly. Look for an even brighter glow, and advance the endotracheal tube over the stylet. With devices utilizing a movable inner stylet, the inner stylet can be withdrawn slightly at this point. The endotracheal tube should advance freely. If resistance is encountered in spite of withdrawing the inner stylet, gently manipulate or rock the tube. If resistance persists, do not apply force. Withdraw. Try lessening the angle of bend. Do not force. This is a gentle, almost effortless technique. Once the tube is advanced, check for $ETCO_2$.

Summary

Intubation with the lighted stylet is a simple, versatile, relatively inexpensive, easily mastered technique. In the December 2004 issue of the *Canadian Journal of Anesthesia*, Inoue reported on a five-year experience with 1,500 consecutive intubations with a less than 0.5% failure rate and no serious adverse effects.[36] The technique is widely applicable to many situations and environments. The equipment is small, sturdy, portable, and easy to maintain. Use of the lighted stylet has been reported in the literature since 1957, and recent innovations in equipment have sparked renewed interest and publications. The technique of lighted stylet intubation is a valuable addition to the skills of all advanced airway practitioners and well within their reach. It just requires practice.

Familiarize yourself with the device you will actually be using. Arrange to practice on manikins. Get access to the operating room and normal, easy-airway patients. Devise a system to use in the field to minimize ambient light, at least over the head and neck. And remember to start with easier airways that need intubation but are not in crisis.

REVIEW QUESTIONS

1. Is a laryngoscope required for lighted stylet intubation?

2. Can lighted stylets be used in pediatric patients?

3. What must you be able to visualize while performing lighted stylet intubation?

4. From what positions can the practitioner approach the patient to perform a lighted stylet intubation?

5. Can lighted stylet intubation be used in bright sunlight?

CHAPTER 12

Cricothyrotomy

Alexandre F. Migala
Dave Nigel Nanan
James Michael Rich

Chapter Objectives

After reading this chapter, you should be able to:

- Discuss the technique of cricothyrotomy in its historical context.

- Describe the indications and application of cricothyrotomy in emergency airway management.

- Contrast cricothyrotomy with other rescue ventilation techniques.

- Describe the cricothyrotomy technique utilizing available kits.

- Describe the techniques of surgical cricothyrotomy.

- Discuss complications associated with the use of cricothyrotomy.

- Establish guidelines for training based on the available literature and equipment.

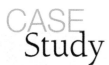

CASE
Study _____

Life Flight 2 is called to respond to a male who has been shot in the face. After landing, they approach the ground ambulance to find ground paramedics attempting to ventilate the patient with a bag-valve-mask (BVM) device. There is a large amount of blood coming from the oropharynx. The ground paramedics report that the patient was sitting in his car when an SUV drew alongside. A passerby heard a shot and saw the patient slump forward at the wheel. The ground crew members say that the patient was responsive only to painful stimuli when they arrived, so they undertook rapid extrication of the patient from his car while maintaining spinal precautions. When they placed him on his back, they noted gurgling respirations due to blood in the airway. In addition to bagging the patient and regular suctioning of his airway, the ground paramedics report that they have attempted direct laryngoscopy but found that blood was obscuring the view. They also have tried to insert an esophageal-tracheal Combitube without success.

Primary assessment reveals extensive oral trauma, and the paramedics from Life Flight 2 realize that they are faced with a cannot-ventilate/cannot-intubate situation. They quickly open their airway bag and locate their surgical airway kit. They remove the anterior portion of the cervical collar while maintaining manual inline axial stabilization (MIAS). The area is cleaned with povidone-iodine solution, and the anatomical landmarks of the anterior neck are identified. With the larynx stabilized between thumb and middle finger, a midline incision is made in the skin extending from the inferior portion of the thyroid cartilage to the cricoid cartilage below. The wound edges are stretched apart, the cricothyroid membrane is identified, and a horizontal incision is made through the membrane with a short-blade scalpel. A curved hemostat is inserted through the incision and dilated horizontally. A 7.0 mm tracheal tube is then fed in a caudal direction through the opening as far as the proximal end of its cuff. The cuff is then inflated, and bag ventilation is commenced via the tube. End-tidal carbon dioxide is detected, and the presence of bilateral breath sounds is confirmed. The anterior portion of the cervical collar is replaced, and the tube is carefully secured. The patient is then transferred to the aircraft and flown to the local trauma center.

Introduction

The technique of **cricothyroidotomy** involves the creation of access to the airway via the cricothyroid membrane, an easily identifiable, superficial structure located on the anterior larynx between the thyroid and cricoid cartilages. Because this membrane can be identified using surface markings on the anterior neck, it is possible to apply this technique despite variation in human anatomy. The understanding of the anatomy of this membrane is also pivotal to other airway techniques, including **transtracheal jet ventilation, retrograde intubation,** and the injection of local anesthetic agents for fiberoptic intubation. In addition, the cricoid cartilage, to which this membrane is attached, is utilized for cricoid pressure and airway protection during rapid sequence endotracheal intubation.

As an emergency intervention, cricothyrotomy is generally reserved for the cannot-ventilate/cannot-intubate (CVCI) situation as described in the cricothyrotomy pathway of the SLAM Universal Adult Airway Flowchart.[1]

KEY TERMS

barotrauma, p. 233

cricothyroidotomy, p. 214

cricothyrotomy, p. 214

neoplasm, p. 219

pneumocyst, p. 222

pneumomediastinum, p. 233

retrograde intubation, p. 214

Seldinger technique, p. 215

stomal granulation, pp. 227, 228

tracheo-esophageal malacia, pp. 227, 228

tracheo-innominate fistula, p. 234

tracheotomy, pp. 214, 215

transtracheal jet ventilation, p. 214

trismus, p.219

Overview of Surgical Airways

It is important to distinguish between a **cricothyrotomy** and a **tracheotomy.** The cricothyrotomy technique requires access via the cricothyroid membrane. A tracheotomy occurs at a lower level and involves dissection to the level of the tracheal rings, with subsequent division and introduction of an airway device.

By convention, any device designed for the specific purpose of cricothyrotomy is referred to as an airway catheter. This is in contrast to a tracheotomy or tracheostomy tube, which is designed for use in a tracheotomy technique. To add to the potential confusion, however, these devices may be interchangeable with the use of tracheostomy tubes for emergency surgical cricothyrotomy.

Historically, the cricothyrotomy technique evolved following the standardized use of tracheotomy for emergency airway access in the modern era. Cricothyrotomy may also be performed using available commercial kits that provide packaged components for the performance of this technique. If these are not available, a surgical cricothyrotomy can be done utilizing equipment usually available in an emergency medical setting.

Needle cricothyrotomy can also be performed for transtracheal jet ventilation and retrograde wire intubation. The objective of transtracheal jet ventilation is the insufflation of oxygen, not ventilation with the elimination of carbon dioxide. The objective of retrograde wire intubation is to provide a method in which the patient can be intubated, with the wire used for guidance if the vocal cords cannot be visualized.

History

Surgical access to the airway is among the earliest described surgical procedures. It was referenced in the medical literature of Egypt and India over 3,000 years ago.[2] Indeed, there are similarities between the age-old techniques and modern-day practice. Galen (129 to c. 199 A.D.) described a technique for emergency airway access that involved excision of the cricoid cartilage and cricothyroid membrane. He recommended the use of a vertical incision as opposed to a horizontal incision (the latter requires more accurate placement and does not allow for extension superiorly or inferiorly).

In 1546, Antonio Musa Brasavola performed the first tracheotomy, which was referred to as a bronchotomy. In 1626, an Italian surgeon, Sanctorio Sanctorius, performed the first percutaneous tracheotomy.[3] Heister, in 1718, introduced a technique he identified as a tracheostomy, but it was essentially the same technique originally introduced by Brasavola over 150 years earlier.

Although recognized earlier as an area to be used for access to the airway, the cricothyroid membrane, as an access route, fell into disrepute following the work of Chevalier Jackson Sr. He published the standardized technique for the open surgical tracheotomy in the first two decades of the twentieth century. He demonstrated the subsequent development of laryngeal stenosis through his long-term follow-up reports on patients who had received surgical airways.[4,5]

Laryngeal (subglottic) stenosis is regarded as a serious consequence of airway trauma and surgery. It is associated with significant morbidity and mortality secondary to a decrease in airway patency and an increase in resistance to airflow. What was not recognized at the time was the influence of airway infection on the subsequent development of laryngeal stenosis. It is now understood that airway infection can lead to a higher incidence of subglottic stenosis. Therefore, this initially resulted in the acceptance of formal tracheotomy as the only safe technique for a surgical airway. The incision was placed low, in the tracheal rings. This proved to be an essentially flawed assumption that was dismissed when the issue of cricothyroidotomy was revisited in the late 1970s and challenged the professional dogma of the low tracheotomy.

Subsequently, the literature demonstrated the safety of surgical airway access through the cricothyroid membrane and avoidance of incision through the cricoid or thyroid cartilage. This began with a large patient series published by Brantigan and Grow in 1976.[6,7] They reported on this as an elective technique. Evaluation of this procedure has continued, along with multiple small descriptive studies of its application to the emergency airway. Its use, however, has not been without debate and controversy.

In 1969, Toye and Weinstein described the technique of percutaneous cricothyroidotomy, a precursor to the modern **Seldinger technique.**[8]

Applied Anatomy

The cricothyroid membrane or ligament is located between the inferior border of the thyroid cartilage and the superior border of the cricoid cartilage (Figure 12-1). It is derived from the fibroelastic membrane of the larynx, being its inferior portion, and connects the thyroid, cricoid, and posterior cartilages of the larynx. It is approximately 10 mm in vertical dimension and 22 mm in horizontal dimension.

 PEARLS Practice locating the cricothyroid membrane on many different people, males and females, including those with short necks and obese necks. You should be able to find and palpate the membrane with your eyes closed or in the dark.

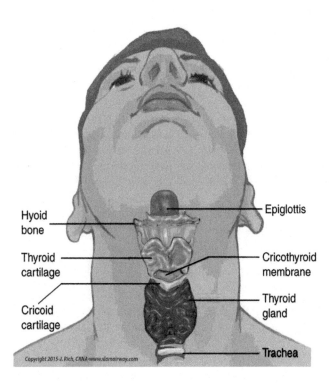

FIGURE 12-1
Anatomical landmarks for cricothyrotomy.

Labels on figure:
Hyoid bone
Thyroid cartilage
Cricoid cartilage
Epiglottis
Cricothyroid membrane
Thyroid gland
Trachea

Copyright 2015-J. Rich, CRNA-www.slamairway.com

Two well-defined segments can be identified: first, the median cricothyroid ligament with its broad base connected to the cricoid cartilage and extending upward to a narrow insertion on the thyroid cartilage; and second, the smaller lateral cricothyroid ligaments. It is important to recognize from this description that it is not a flat continuous structure. (You may wish to refer back to Chapter 2, Figure 2-3.)

The membrane is composed of yellow elastic tissue that characteristically does not calcify with age, unless previously traumatized or incised. Calcification, when present, may lead to failure of cricothyrotomy, so it is quite beneficial that this membrane does not calcify with age under normal physiologic conditions.

Identification of this membrane can be performed from above by first locating the hyoid bone, the laryngeal prominence at the notch of the thyroid cartilage (i.e., Adam's apple) and then sliding the palpating finger downward until a depression is encountered on the thyroid cartilage. In general, the laryngeal prominence is generally easier to palpate in males than in females. Palpation of the laryngeal prominence in females is generally more challenging, which can increase the placement of cricothyrotomy.

Performance of cricothyrotomy examination includes palpation and identification of the cricoid cartilage over its entire anterior surface. From below, placing the little finger in the suprasternal notch, then laying the hand on the anterior neck can help in estimating the position of the cricoid cartilage. The position of the cricothyroid membrane should generally coincide with one's index finger. This is a useful maneuver if the anterior anatomy of the neck is poorly defined (e.g., as in extreme obesity). Frequent elective practice in the palpation of the cricothyroid membrane and the surrounding anatomy should improve the skill required in locating the cricoid cartilage when an emergency situation occurs. Superficial to the membrane lies the skin, the anterior cervical fascia, and generally a small quantity of subcutaneous tissue.

An error that may occur during this procedure is cannulation of the thyrohyoid membrane, which would incorrectly place the cannula above the glottis.[9] Therefore, it is imperative that the hyoid bone be identified along with the notch of the thyroid cartilage and the thyrohyoid ligament that lies above the thyroid cartilage. Another error that may occur is cannulation of the airway through the first or second tracheal ring.[10] Only through correct identification of the thyroid cartilage, cricoid cartilage, and cricothyroid ligament can cannulation occur accurately. Structures to be avoided include the vocal cords, which lie approximately

1 cm superior to the cricothyroid membrane. The vocal cords are rarely damaged during the procedure unless landmarks are misjudged.

In close relation to the cricothyroid membrane lie the superior cricothyroid vessels that cross the superior portion of the membrane. Therefore, to avoid hemorrhage, the safest point of incision is the lower third of the membrane. Not to be overlooked, the middle thyroid veins and the anterior jugular veins lie just lateral to the membrane.

Confining dissection to the midline and placing the initial incision in the vertical midline position should assist in avoiding blood vessels that may produce hemorrhage during this procedure. This approach also avoids the pyramidal lobe of the thyroid gland. The thyroid gland itself lies in close relation to the cricothyroid membrane and is highly vascular. Laterally, the lobes can be avoided by careful attention to detail, placing the incision in the midline of the membrane, with the thyroid isthmus inferior and therefore not encountered. In contrast, note that with a low tracheotomy, the isthmus of the thyroid gland may need to be divided and suture ligated for an approach to the tracheal rings to be possible.

Many authors recommend the transverse or horizontal incision. Surgical literature emphasizes the transverse incision, whether from dogma or practicality, because Langer's line (a surgical incision point) lies transversely across the neck. Incising through this line can provide better cosmetic healing; however, in the emergency situation, establishing the airway takes priority over cosmetics. The practitioner's clinical situation must always be considered; therefore, safety and expediency always take priority over any cosmetic considerations. Posterior to the larynx, the esophagus may be traumatized with too deep an incision or overaggressive placement of a cannulation device. Far laterally, and usually out of reach, are the internal carotid arteries and jugular veins.

As a general rule, this technique should not be performed in children younger than 10 years of age due to difficulty in identifying landmarks in the immature larynx and the variation that occurs in immature laryngeal anatomy. Most important is the fact that the cricoid is the narrowest part of the pediatric airway, so a cannula placed via the cricothyroid ligament encounters this region, which can create difficulty in cannulation with the subsequent production of subglottic edema. A low tracheotomy is therefore considered preferable for this age group.

Cricothyrotomy for the Non-Surgically Trained Practitioner

Lack of surgical training is a cause of anxiety when considering cricothyrotomy. This anxiety can be overcome only by a thorough understanding of the applied anatomy of the cricothyroid membrane and surrounding structures; knowledge of the available equipment; and training on simulators, animal models, and cadaver specimens, together with sound clinical judgment and knowledge of the indications for this procedure and outcome if this procedure is not performed. Any reluctance about performing a cricothyrotomy must be weighed against the considerable risk of not establishing an airway, with attendant hypoxia and death.

Unlike surgeons trained in the procedure and who generally operate on an elective basis, prehospital practitioners may be required to perform the technique of cricothyrotomy in a far less controlled environment. Prior to 1995, only 80% of American anesthesiology residency training programs provided instruction in cricothyrotomy, of which 60% consisted of lectures only.[11] A survey in 2001 revealed that only 30% of anesthesiologists reported skill in performing a cricothyrotomy.[12] A subsequent survey in 2003 revealed that only 49% of anesthesiology residency training programs offered cricothyrotomy as part of an airway management rotation.[13] Cricothyrotomy is recognized as a required skill for emergency medicine physicians.[14] On the average, only two cricothyrotomies are performed by any emergency medicine resident prior to graduation.[15] Wong et al. demonstrated a proficiency curve with repetitive performance of the percutaneous dilational cricothyrotomy on manikins. They noted that at least four attempts were required to achieve a plateau for maintenance of consistent skill and success.[16]

In the extreme clinical situation, emergency airway access may have to be established with inadequate lighting or instruments and on patients who exhibit trauma, hemorrhage, respiratory distress, or cardiovascular instability. It is fair to say, therefore, that the demands on the provider who is attempting to establish a cricothyrotomy are considerable. The situation requiring a cricothyrotomy only compounds the stress and pressure associated with performing the procedure. However, the requirement to establish an airway in the patient outweighs the consequences of not performing the procedure. Securing the airway is of utmost importance before further treatment can proceed. Expedient establishment of an airway is therefore of paramount necessity.

Indications

Overview

It is only with practice that cricothyrotomy can be considered an option for emergency airway management. Swanson and Fosnocht[17] showed how the establishment of an airway education program resulted in decreased rates in the use of cricothyrotomy. Additionally, rescue ventilation techniques now exist that can obviate the need for a cricothyrotomy, and an adjunctive ventilation device should be tried while simultaneously preparing for placement of a criothyrotomy. Recommended supraglottic airway devices include the Combitube and laryngeal mask airway, but this does not preclude use of other devices approved by the Food and Drug Administration that have not yet received an American Heart Association Class IIa classification.[1,18] However, if a supraglottic airway fails to provide ventilation (e.g., glottic and/or infraglottic obstruction, airway disruption),[1,18] the final choice for treatment is placement of a cricothyrotomy.

The condition in which a patient cannot be intubated or ventilated (by any means) is one of the most demanding scenarios in airway management and can be the end result of multiple anatomical and pathophysiological factors. In this situation, the surgical airway has a definite role.

A surgical airway option may result from the development of airway obstruction and the inability to intubate, or it may be considered as an initial approach to the airway where intubation or placement of a rescue ventilation device is not an option or considered hazardous. Here, as in many difficult airway scenarios, anticipation and preparation are paramount. At a minimum, this includes the identification of trained personnel along with preparation and availability of equipment necessary for the procedure.

It is also important to note that a cricothyrotomy is generally not useful for airway obstruction at or below the level of the cricothyroid membrane. Therefore, with lower intrathoracic injury, access to the airway may need to be redefined based on the level of anatomic obstruction. Beyond this, specialized techniques such as endobronchial intubation may be required.

Trauma and Foreign Body

A traumatized airway at any level may cause ventilation to be obstructed. In addition, distortion of airway anatomy complicated by airway hemorrhage may make direct laryngoscopy or fiberoptic techniques inapplicable. Such distortion may be significant enough to cause immediate airway compromise and thus diminish the success of either intubation or ventilation.

Specific to the necessity for a surgical airway are massive facial trauma, base of skull fracture with failed endotracheal intubation (it is contraindicated to attempt a blind nasal intubation due to the possibility of introducing a foreign body into the cranium),[19] expanding hematoma of the neck resulting from vascular injury, and penetrating or blunt neck trauma as well as known unstable cervical-spine fracture.[20] Facial fractures may be able to be treated with adjunctive supraglottic[21-23] devices but may warrant a surgical airway due to hemorrhage into the airway or displacement and distortion of the facial bones. A needle cricothyrotomy is the recommended cricothyrotomy airway for the pediatric patient, but its use in children ranging from 3 to 12 years—at which the surgical cricothyrotomy is recommended—is still in debate. A recommended guideline exists that if the cricothyroid membrane is palpable, then cricothyrotomy by an experienced practitioner may be considered.[19,24,25] Direct laryngotracheal trauma, blunt or penetrating, with injury to the laryngeal cartilages may require a surgical airway if the injury is above the level of the cricothyroid membrane. Any trauma below this level requires specialized techniques for airway management.

PEDIATRIC
NOTE

Surgical cricothyroidotomy should not be used in children younger than 10 years of age; however, needle cricothyrotomy may be used in children 3 to 12 years old if the cricothyroid membrane can be palpated.

A variety of foreign bodies may be inhaled and produce airway obstruction. In this situation, the principle of airway disruption applies to the presence of a foreign body in the airway. If the level of obstruction is above the cricothyroid membrane, cricothyrotomy is indicated to relieve such obstruction. Therefore, it is important to establish the anatomical location of airway disruption and/or foreign body prior to consideration of a surgical airway.

Infection

Among the oldest indications for a surgical airway are head and neck infections, producing either airway obstruction or predisposing to a difficult intubation. These may have various implications, depending on the level of the obstruction or disruption. Those involving the floor of the mouth and submandibular and sublingual spaces restrict visualization for direct laryngoscopy. This may produce a critical airway event such as difficult intubation or cannot-mask-ventilate/cannot-intubate (CMVCI). If this cannot be overcome with rescue ventilation, a cricothyrotomy is indicated.[1,18] A parapharyngeal space infection can compromise the airway with the potential for rupture into the airway during direct laryngoscopy. Supraglottic infections, presenting with hoarseness and stridor, have the potential for airway obstruction. A surgical airway should be considered when treating airway obstruction caused by these infections.

Severely limited opening of the mouth can preclude use of rescue ventilation devices.[26] Limited airway access through the oral cavity that stems from limited mouth opening for whatever reason may require placement of a surgical airway. Conditions creating this situation may include but are not limited to those producing decreased range of motion of the temperomandibular joint (e.g., **trismus**, condylar fracture of the mandible, head and neck tumor).

Neoplasm

A **neoplasm** or a variety of neoplastic conditions, benign or malignant, may involve the airway either as extrinsic lesions encroaching on the airway or as intrinsic lesions within the airway. Any of these may produce difficult ventilation, difficult laryngoscopy, or failed intubation. A neoplasm may produce rapid and unanticipated airway obstruction. If the tumor is malignant, it is important that the operator be aware that friable or vascular tumors may hemorrhage and limit both intubation and ventilation. This can necessitate placement of a cricothyrotomy or other surgical airway.

Other situations that warrant consideration of a cricothyrotomy include, but are limited to, clenched teeth (which may respond to muscle relaxants) and caustic or thermal injury to the airway. In this situation, an empiric cricothyrotomy may be indicated to protect the airway from deterioration during transport, especially in the face of failed oral or nasal intubation or the inability to perform a rescue ventilation.[27]

trismus
Contraction of the muscles in the jaw.

neoplasm
A growth or tumor. It may be benign or malignant.

Contraindications

Understanding any intervention or procedure requires that the operator know not only when a particular technique is indicated but also when it is contraindicated. Contraindications may be divided into absolute and relative, and depend on the clinical situation.

Tracheal transection is an absolute contraindication to cricothyrotomy because an incision may sever the cervical fascia, which may be the only structure holding the trachea in position. Loss of it would result in a catastrophic retraction of the distal stump of the trachea into the mediastinum.[20,25] Other absolute contraindications include laryngeotracheal separation,[20] penetrating neck trauma in the upper Zone 2 or Zone 3 of the neck when associated with an expanding hematoma,[20] and a fractured larynx or other significant damage to the cricoid cartilage or larynx.[25]

Relative contraindications may be ignored depending on the urgency of the situation. Relative contraindications include children below the age of five years (or if the cricothyroid membrane cannot be identified), bleeding diathesis, massive neck edema, and acute laryngeal disease.[25]

ON TARGET

Tracheal transection is an absolute contraindication to cricothyrotomy.

Technique

Cricothyroid Needle Puncture

Cricothyroid needle puncture involves the percutaneous puncture of the cricothyroid membrane by a needle or catheter. Once percutaneous access to the larynx is confirmed and depending on the clinical situation, the operator can proceed using any one of several percutaneous techniques. These include, but are not limited to, transtracheal jet ventilation (TTJV) or a more secure cricothyrotomy airway using a percutaneous Seldinger technique or other effective method.

Needle cricothyrotomy entails appropriate identification of the cricothyroid membrane and stabilization of the trachea with the nondominant hand using the thumb and index finger along its lateral margins. A 10-, 12-, 13-, 14- or 16-gauge intravenous catheter attached to a syringe that is partially filled with saline or water is advanced percutaneously at a 45° angle through the skin overlying the cricothyroid membrane in a caudad (toward the lung) direction while continuously aspirating. The aspiration of bubbles indicates that the larynx has been entered. The needle should then be advanced several millimeters further to ensure placement of the needle tip well within the laryngeal lumen. The catheter can then be advanced off the needle as the needle is withdrawn.

It is recommended that the fluid-filled syringe be attached once again to the catheter and bubbles aspirated to confirm correct placement of the catheter. After that, the catheter should be held in place constantly by hand to avoid losing the catheter once insufflation of oxygen is begun or another maneuver is attempted through the catheter. Dislodgement or kinking of the catheter is a serious complication that curtails further attempts to oxygenate or ventilate the patient.

Transtracheal Jet Ventilation (TTJV)

TTJV uses high-frequency jet ventilation or oxygen insufflation through a resuscitation bag via the cricothyrotomy catheter.[28] In actuality, TTJV should be called translaryngeal jet ventilation (TLJV) because it provides oxygen insufflation at the level of the larynx (not the trachea). Even though it is a misnomer, TTJV will probably remain the accepted terminology for this technique.

TTJV can be lifesaving because it promotes oxygenation. However, it does not facilitate elimination of carbon dioxide and therefore does not provide adequate lung ventilation and thus should be used only as a temporary bridge until a definitive airway can be established.

The advent of rescue ventilation devices such as the Combitube and LMA has greatly diminished the need for TTJV (and cricothyrotomy in general) in recent years.[1,18] Because the technique is rarely used, it is recommended that a prepared commercial kit be available that is specially designed for this procedure. One such kit has a large catheter embedded with metal that is unlikely to kink and is easy to grasp (e.g., ENK oxygen flow modulator,

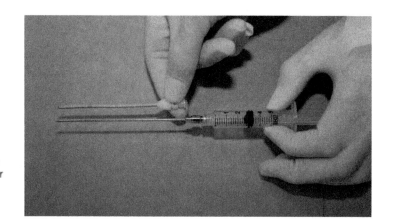

FIGURE 12-2
ENK cricothyrotomy needle
with a kint-resistant catheter
by Cook Critical Care.
(Courtesy of JM Rich, CRNA
[www.slamairway.com])

Cook Critical Care, Bloomington, IN) (Figure 12-2). Additionally, caution should be used when utilizing a pressurized oxygen source to include high-pressure tubing and a down-regulator to limit the maximum pressure. The jet ventilation source should provide between 45 and 60 pounds per square inch (psi). Some wall sources and aircraft provide direct pressure in excess of 100 psi, which could result in a disastrous outcome.

Several techniques have described the equipment for attempted ventilation via a needle cricothyrotomy. A common method is the attachment of either a 3-cc syringe to the catheter, which then connects to a 7.5 endotracheal tube connector (Figure 12-3a), or attachment of the connector from a 3.0 endotracheal tube directly to the catheter (Figure 12-3b). Another technique involves using a portion of intravenous tubing to connect the catheter to a 2.5 endotracheal tube connector and thus permit greater flexibility at the airway connection during transport.[29] The concern with this technique is the increased airway resistance caused by the small-caliber tubing that is used.

Most authors recommend ventilation with a high-pressure source (45 to 60 psi) for one second followed by passive exhalation for four seconds before repeating the cycle. One TTJV catheter is available that does not require high-pressure jet ventilation (Table 12-1 and

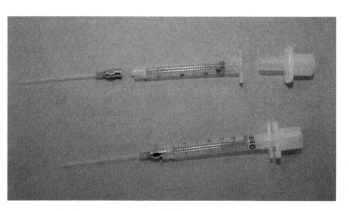

(a)

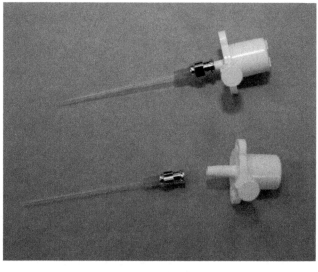

(b)

FIGURE 12-3

Quick-build cricothyrotomy kit from off-the-shelf products. (a) A 14 gauge catheter, 3 cc syringe, and a 15 mm connector from a 7.0 endotracheal tube. (b) A 14 gauge catheter and 15 mm connector from a 3.0 endotracheal tube.

(Courtesy of JM Rich, CRNA [www.slamairway.com])

Table 12-1   Transtracheal Catheter Ventilation Without Jet Ventilation

The ENK oxygen flow modulator is designed for transtracheal catheter ventilation when used with a needle cricothyroidotomy. Needle cricothyroidotomy and transtracheal catheter ventilation are temporary measures that are designed to facilitate oxygenation until such a time as endotracheal intubation or a surgical airway can be established.

Purpose

To provide a patent airway to the patient who is in respiratory or cardiac arrest or has a complete airway obstruction.

Indications

The adult* patient who is in respiratory or cardiac arrest or has a complete airway obstruction where conventional methods to establish an airway have been unsuccessful. This includes orotracheal intubation, nasotracheal intubation, esophageal tracheal airway device intubation, bag/valve/mask ventilation, and standard methods for correction of airway obstructions.

*CAUTION: Needle cricothyroidotomy should not be attempted in patients less than 5 years of age unless authorized by a base station physician.

Contraindications

1. When other BLS or ALS adjuncts can successfully maintain the airway.
2. When landmarks cannot be clearly identified.
3. Transection of the trachea distal to the cricothyroid site.
4. Relative contraindications may exist such as known tracheal disease, cancer, lower airway obstruction. However, this is a procedure of last resort; thus, consider the benefit versus the risk.

Equipment

- 10–14 gauge reinforced style catheter (minimum of 2½" long)
- 5 cc syringe
- Betadine swabs
- Normal saline
- Twill tape
- Tape
- Oxygen flow modulator
- Oxygen source (15–30 liters per minute flow capacity)

Complications

- Subcutaneous emphysema
- Tracheal mucosal injury
- Mediastinal emphysema
- Bending of catheter
- Hemorrhage
- **Pneumocyst**
- Esophageal or mediastinal puncture
- Aspiration
- Barotrauma
- Thyroid perforation

Used by permission of Cook Critical Care, Bloomington, IN.

pneumocyst
A pocket of air in the tissues.

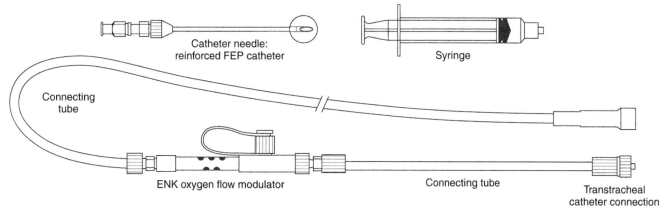

Catheter needle: reinforced FEP catheter

Syringe

Connecting tube

ENK oxygen flow modulator

Connecting tube

Transtracheal catheter connection

FIGURE 12-4

ENK oxygen flow modulator system by Cook Critical Care, Bloomington, IN. Procedure: Low pressure system. (Cook Critical Care, 1-800-457-4500) Oxygen flow modulator regulates the flow of oxygen and thus the rate of insufflation and exhalation according to the oxygen liter flow being used and how many holes are covered at any one time. (Cook Critical Care, 1-800-457-4500) Sequential instructions for use include: (1) Attach oxygen flow modulator to oxygen source. (2) Place the patient in a recumbent or semirecumbent position with neck slightly extended. (No extension if the patient needs c-spine precautions.) (3) Identify cricothyroid membrane. (4) Prepare the patient's neck with betadine swab. (5) Stabilize the larynx with the thumb and middle finger and place the index finger over the cricothyroid membrane. (6) Attach the transtracheal airway catheter to a 5 cc syringe filled with 2 cc of normal saline. Insert the catheter at a 45° angle directed inferiorly through the cricothyroid membrane. (7) Cannulate the trachea through the cricothyroid membrane and advance the transtracheal airway catheter until aspiration of air is noted in the syringe. (8) Remove the needle while firmly holding the catheter in place. (9) Secure the catheter in place with twill tape, reinforced with adhesive tape. (10) Attach the Luer lock of the oxygen flow modulator to the transtracheal airway catheter. (11) Select an oxygen flow of at least 15 up to 30 liters per minute. (12) Cover all vent holes of the oxygen flow modulator using thumb and forefinger for one second and release all vent holes for two seconds. Continue oxygenation cycle as above. (13) Auscultate the patient's chest and the upper abdomen for breath sounds to confirm pulmonary inflation and exhalation. Note: ETCO$_2$ device cannot be used with flow modulator.
(Photo courtesy of Cook Critical Care Inc., Bloomington, IN)

Figure 12-4). At a minimum, an appropriately sized oral airway should be inserted into the patient's mouth to ensure optimal upper airway patency in the event that exhalation of expired gases is possible through the upper airway. However, another method that can be employed to facilitate the exhalation phase is placement of a second catheter alongside the first catheter within the cricothyroid membrane. The sequence then is as follows: obstruct one catheter with your thumb, then administer oxygen for one second, and finally uncover the second catheter and permit exhalation via both catheters. This technique is also recommended if there is a significant airway obstruction above the cricothyroid membrane that precludes adequate passive exhalation through the upper airway. The rescuer should be prepared for the development of some degree of subcutaneous emphysema given the pressure of the gradients involved.

 In a cannot-ventilate-by-any-means/cannot-intubate situation, consider using needle cricothyrotomy immediately as a temporary method of oxygenation while preparations are made to perform definitive surgical cricothyrotomy. Remember, the unventilated patient will soon be either brain-injured or dead.

Current recommendations are that TTJV be used only briefly as a temporizing measure to oxygenate the patient until a definitive airway can be established. Due to the inability to ventilate optimally during TTJV, the duration of its use is limited by the resulting accumulation of carbon dioxide. Using a 15 liter/minute oxygen source attached to a one-liter self-inflating bag, a 7-0 endotracheal tube connector, and either a 13-gauge or 16-gauge catheter achieved a tidal volume of 500 cc between 1.8 to 5 seconds, respectively.[30] This might prove sufficient for a small-framed individual, providing a respiratory rate of 12 breaths per minute. Although this requires further study, it is a consideration for the prehospital provider with prolonged transport times should rescue ventilation devices be unavailable or ineffective.

Many authors describe the technique for TTJV and the necessity of a high-pressure oxygen source. One of these authors[31] provides recommendations for the pediatric patient, including the ventilation pressures necessary during TTJV. Butler's recommendations are to employ only bag-valve-mask-generated pressure on children less than five years of age, 20 to 30 psi for children between five and 12 years of age, and 50 psi for children older than 12 years of age.[31]

Retrograde intubation starts as a cricothyrotomy technique and involves use of a cricothyroid needle puncture similar to that discussed above, with the exception that the needle is oriented cephalad in contradistinction to the caudad position. However, this is a technique employed only to facilitate tracheal intubation over a wire that exits either through the mouth or the nose. Above all, it should be used only in the patient who can be mask-ventilated (thus maintaining oxygenation during the procedure) but cannot be intubated (Chapter 9).

Percutaneous Dilational Cricothyrotomy: Seldinger Technique

Percutaneous dilational cricothyrotomy (PDC) involves placement of an airway catheter through the cricothyroid member that can be used for lung ventilation. It can be performed either electively or as an emergency procedure. First, the patient should be positioned with a roll under the shoulders, unless spinal injury is suspected. If the patient is awake, local anesthetic skin infiltration should be administered. Antiseptic skin preparation should also be used for infection control. Note that hyperextension of the neck is not normally required for cricothyrotomy.

Beyond this juncture, the technique of PDC as well as its inherent sequential steps depends on the device selected for use. Several kits are commercially available and fall into two groups: those that employ a wire and use the Seldinger technique (Cook-Melker) (Figure 12-5), and

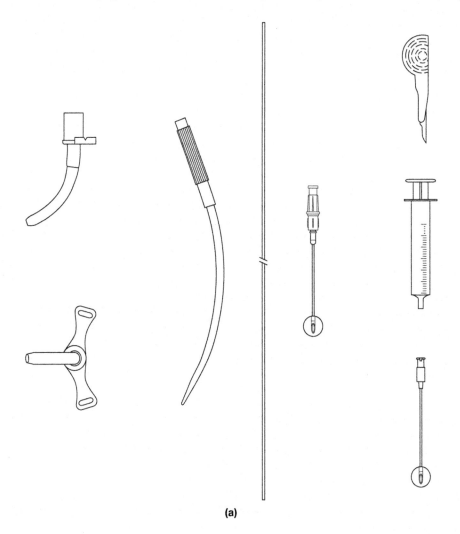

(a)

FIGURE 12-5

(a) Melker emergency cricothyrotomy catheter system.

(Courtesy of Cook Critical Care Inc., Bloomington, IN)

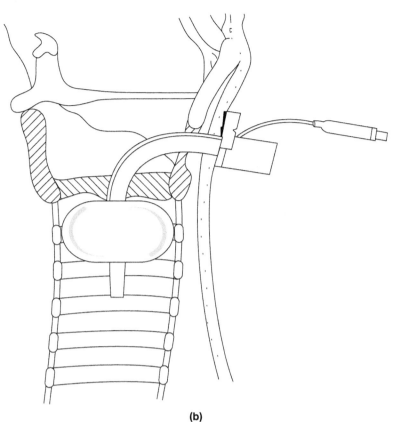

(b)

FIGURE 12-5
(continued)
(b) Melker emergency cuffed cricrothyrotomy catheter.
(Courtesy of Cook Critical Care Inc., Bloomington, IN)

those that involve the introduction of an airway device over a needle, nylon introducer, or sharp introducer like QuickTrach (Figure 12-6), Nu-Trake (Figure 12-7), Portex Emergency Cricothyroidotomy Kit, Pertrach, or Patil (Figure 12-8). Whichever technique is selected for use, it is important that the instructions of the manufacturer be uniformly applied.

The Seldinger technique has certain advantages when used by non-surgically trained providers because it utilizes a familiar method that is used universally for placement of central intravenous catheters. With this technique, the airway device or catheter is inserted over a dilator through which a guide wire is passed. The Cook-Melker (Figure 12-5) is a commercially available kit that facilitates rapid placement of a cuffed or non-cuffed cricothyrotomy airway catheter and is available in a variety of sizes. However, the technique can be similarly performed utilizing equipment that is generally available in most emergency settings (e.g., needles, wires, scalpels) as long as prior planning and staff training are accomplished before hand. The primary benefit of this technique is the practitioner's technical familiarity in previously using the Seldinger technique to obtain vascular access.

Non-Seldinger Percutaneous Techniques: Pertrach, QuickTrach, Nu-Trake, and Patil Emergency Cricothyrotomy Catheter

The QuickTrach (Figure 12-6) and Nu-Trake (Figure 12-7) are similar in design; they are single-step devices that generally require no additional equipment. Once the cricothyroid membrane is identified, the needle/trocar is used to puncture the skin and enter the larynx, whereupon the entire system is advanced into position. This is followed by the withdrawal of the needle/trocar core, which leaves only the airway shell in place.

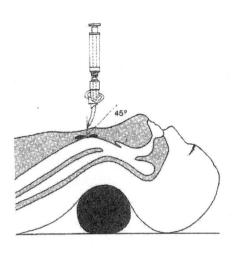

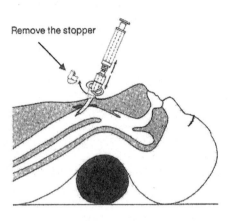

Remove the stopper

FIGURE 12-6
The Rusch QuickTrach allows quick and safe access for ventilation in the presence of acute respiratory distress with upper airway obstruction. See the manufacturer's instructions for complete information.
(Courtesy of Rusch and Teleflex Medical, Research Triangle Park, NC)

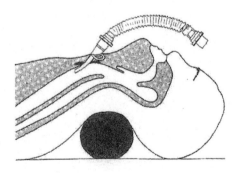

PEARLS A three-way test for correct placement of the needle is: first, a "pop" is felt as the needle and catheter puncture the membrane; second, air bubbles are aspirated into the syringe; and third, a wire placed through the needle and catheter can be freely moved back and forth in the trachea, ensuring that the tip of the needle has not gone into the posterior wall of the larynx.

Complications can occur regardless of the type of technique utilized (Table 12-2). Abbrecht et al. studied the complications of various commercially available cricothyroid catheters and reported their clinical observations.[32] There was a linear correlation between

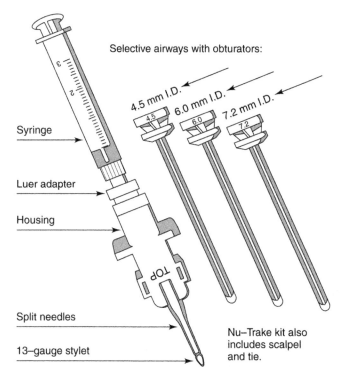

Selective airways with obturators:

4.5 mm I.D.   6.0 mm I.D.   7.2 mm I.D.

Syringe

Luer adapter

Housing

Split needles

13–gauge stylet

Nu–Trake kit also includes scalpel and tie.

FIGURE 12-7

(a) Components of the Portex Nu-Trake Perecutaneous dilational cricothyrotomy patented system provides a 4.5, 6.0, and a 7.2 mm I.D. airway within seconds. The integral 15 mm connection allows for immediate ventilation. A suction catheter can be introduced through the Nu-Trake® airways. Nu-Trake® Device; 3 mL Syringe; #11 Blade Scalpel; 4.5 mm I.D. Airway; 6.0 mm I.D. Airway; 7.2 mm I.D. Airway. (b) Sterile, portable kit. Procedure: patient's head is hyperextended, if possible, and the cricothyroid membrane identified; palpate. (c) Pinch 1 cm of skin, and insert the sharp tip of the knife blade through the skin. Cut in an outward motion. (d) The needle should puncture the membrane just beyond the entry at approximately the same angles as the lower edge of the housing. Aspirate; easy-moving spring obturator denotes tracheal entrance. (e) The stylet and syringe are removed as a unit by twisting the Luer adapter counterclockwise and lifting out. (f) The blunt needle is gently moved further into the trachea until the housing rests on the overlying skin. A freely rocking motion confirms proper depth of insertion. (g) In all cases, begin with the smallest airway (4.5 mm), and insert the airway and obturator together *pushing with the thenar eminence* resting against the cap of the obturator. Airway and obturator are *pushed* (not squeezed) downward into the needle, which is divided lengthwise and spreads apart to accommodate them. (h) The obturator is removed, leaving a clear passage for air to reach the lungs. If the airway size requires a change, this can be easily performed by leaving the housing and needle guide in place, while removal and insertion of airways are made. Ties are threaded through the brackets on the sides of the housing. (i) System in operation: bag valve or universal (15 mm) adapter may be fitted to the top of the housing. Expansion of lungs can also be started by mouth-to-mouth respiration, with fingers closing off the vents in the housing. (j) Use the enclosed cloth tie to secure the airway.
(Illustration courtesy of Smiths Medical, Weston, MA)

the device diameter and insertion force. An increase in puncture force was associated with an increase in the incidence of complications. Posterior tracheal wall complications occurred more frequently with curved penetrating devices. Of note was the fact that complications were minimized by using a small pilot needle to guide the large cannula during intubation. Last, the use of lubricant to decrease skin adherence to the instruments introduced was less effective when the device used had a large change in diameter. These findings amplify the need for common sense when using such techniques and additionally emphasize the need

Table 12-2 Complications Associated with Cricothyrotomy

Immediate	Intermediate	Delayed/Long Term
Bleeding	Subglottic stenosis	Tracheal granulation
Pneumothorax	Tracheo-esophageal fistula	Persistent wound
Pneumomediastinum	Vocal cord dysfunction	Lower airway injury
Subcutaneous emphysema	**Stomal granulations**	Vocal cord dysfunction
Difficult cannulation	Accidental decannulation	**Tracheo-esophageal malacia**
Incorrect tube placement	Tracheal edema	Dysphonia
Damage to recurrent laryngeal artery	Acute respiratory failure secondary to decannulation	Hemorrhage from tracheo-innominate fistula
Damage to thyroid gland	Infection	Infection
Esophageal perforation		
Damage to cricoid cartilage		
Aspiration		

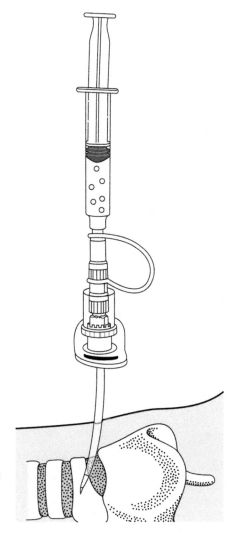

FIGURE 12-8
Patil emergency cricothyrotomy catheter set consists of a scalpel, dilator, and airway catheter. It has a metal beveled needle loaded coaxially inside the dilator.
(Courtesy of Cook Critical Care Inc., Bloomington, IN)

for applying safety concerns. A small needle has less resistance and advances readily, while a larger needle has greater resistance, requires more force for insertion, and may be more difficult to control once the skin is punctured.

Another study compared four commercially available emergency kits and measured successful placement and ventilation of the patient within an established time limit. The Quick-Trach and Cook-Melker set were 100% successful using the study's criteria, while an unacceptably high failure rate was identified with the Transtracheal Airway Catheter with ENK-Flow Modulator" as well as Patil's airway.[33]

The Portex Emergency Cricothyroidotomy Kit (PECT) and the Pertrach are both unique in design as devices for PDC. The PECT utilizes new technology that provides a visual feedback mechanism to alert the operator whenever the needle is in contact with something (e.g., posterior wall of the laryngeal aperature). The Pertrach is unique because it has a breakaway needle and utilizes a pseudo-Seldinger technique. The initial technique of identifying the landmarks and puncturing the skin with a needle attached to a syringe partially filled with normal saline or water and aspirating air bubbles to identify entry into the larynx has been previously described.

One of the unique features of the Pertrach is that the needle used is bivalved with so-called butterfly wings to permit the needle to be snapped apart and removed on placement of a pseudo-wire-guided dilator/cricothyrotomy device. As with any prepared or commercially available kit, the Pertrach kit requires prior practice using airway manikins, cadavers, or animal models prior to using it for the first time in an emergency situation. It comes with a single needle that can be snapped prematurely if care is not taken when attaching it to the syringe or during the skin puncture. Previous training using the Pertrach should reduce early snapping of the needle. Another feature to be addressed during Pertrach training is that the pseudo-wire-guided dilator may not be sufficiently long enough for some extremely edematous or obese necks. A final concern is cuff rupture, which can happen when the butterfly needle is snapped. The snap-away needle fragments have the potential to puncture the cuff occasionally on the Pertrach tube. Special breakaway needles are available from the manufacturer for practice.

Surgical Cricothyroidotomy: The Rapid Four-Step Technique

This technique can be performed electively or emergently in what is referred to as an open cricothyroidotomy. It does not require the use of a manufactured kit (Figure 12-9). The fundamental principles remain the same, with the difference being that a scalpel is used to create access, and a tracheostomy or endotracheal tube is used for cannulation of the airway and ventilation.

In 1996, Brofeldt and Panacek introduced the rapid four-step technique (RFST) for cricothyrotomy (Figure 12-10). They reported that it could be completed within 30 seconds without use of suction or additional lighting while using a #20 scalpel, a tracheal hook with a large radius, and a cuffed tracheostomy tube. The steps are (1) palpation of the cricothyroid membrane via external landmarks, (2) stab incision (transversely or horizontally) through both the skin and cricothyroid membrane, (3) inferior (or caudal) traction with the tracheal hook, and (4) tube insertion.[34] This technique was further modified by Davis et al. with the recommendation of using a bear claw (miniature tissue retractor) instead of the tracheal hook, with a reported reduction in intubation time of 18 seconds.[35] Unfortunately, the bear claw is not readily available in most prehospital settings or emergency departments. Comparing their four-step technique to the standard cricothyrotomy, the authors reported that, although the four-step technique was performed faster than the standard surgical approach (which required an average of 43 seconds versus 134 seconds) there was a trend toward major complications (3 of 32 attempts versus 1 of 32 attempts).[36]

Davis et al. compared the rapid four-step technique with the standard surgical cricothyrotomy in 1999, finding a complication rate of 16.7% with the rapid four-step technique and 0% with the standard approach. The most common complication was cricoid cartilage fracture[37] (a serious complication).

Several critical issues must be considered when utilizing this method. Because the entire technique for accessing the airway involves a single stab with a #20 scalpel, caution should be taken to prevent stabbing the trachea so deeply as to cause esophageal injury. Also, care should be exercised in the placement and advancement of the endotracheal tube to avoid withdrawing or repositioning the tube in such a way that the cuff of the TT is punctured with the tracheal hook.

Surgical Cricothyroidotomy: Traditional Approach

The traditional approach entails appropriate identification of the cricothyroid membrane and stabilizing the trachea with the nondominant hand using the thumb and index finger along its lateral margins. If time permits, local anesthetic with epinephrine may be administered for analgesia and hemostasis. Make a 3-cm midline longitudinal incision over the skin that is superficial to the cricothyroid membrane. Identify the cricothyroid membrane and make a 1-cm transverse incision across the caudal or inferior portion of the cricothyroid membrane. Insert a tracheal hook and pull traction upward and in a cephalad (toward the head) direction to stabilize the trachea. Insert either a Trousseau dilator or hemostat into the slit to enlarge it (horizontally). Insert the tracheostomy or endotracheal tube carefully into the hole in a dorsal (posterior, toward the spine) direction and then direct it caudally (toward the feet) once it is in the laryngeal lumen using a malleable stylet. Then inflate the cuff, remove the malleable stylet, ventilate and confirm positioning of the tube.

ON TARGET It is absolutely necessary to correctly identify the thyroid cartilage, cricoid cartilage, and cricothyroid ligament before attempting a surgical airway maneuver.

ON TARGET The tracheal hook is an instrument not normally found on ambulances. Therefore, its use requires planning and advance preparation.

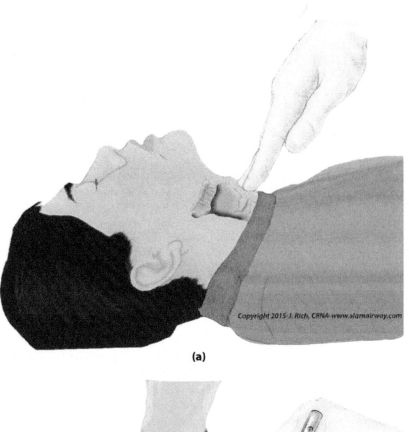

(a)

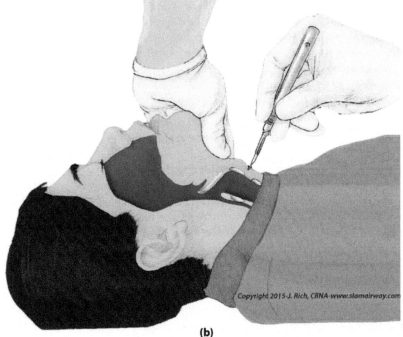

Copyright 2015-J. Rich, CRNA-www.slamairway.com

(b)

FIGURE 12-9

Open Cricothyrotomy Method (a) Begin the open cricothyrotomy method by locating the cricothyroid membrane. (b) Then stabilize the larynx and make a 1- to 2-cm skin incision over the cricothyroid membrane.

Some authors describe and advocate flipping the scalpel blade after making the incision through the cricothyroid membrane and using the handle by turning it 90° to identify and secure the airway until a cricothyrotomy or endotracheal tube can be inserted. Caution should be taken if this approach is used because the now-contaminated scalpel blade is oriented toward the rescuers, which could cause inadvertent injury to the operator or assistants. Using a hemostat (spread horizontally) to open, visually identifying appropriate placement, and securing the airway until the tube is placed is a viable consideration. Another

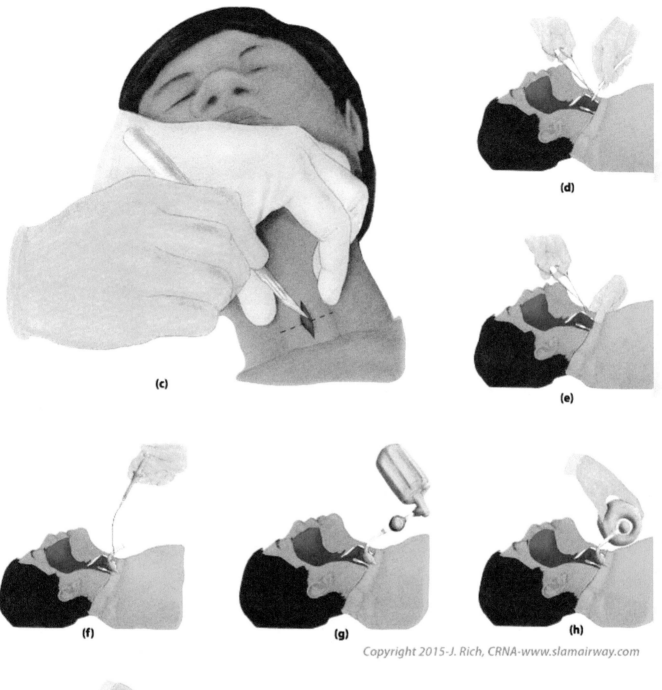

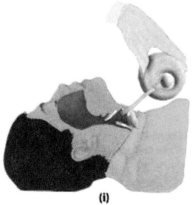

FIGURE 12-9
(*continued*)
(c) Make a 1-cm horizontal incision through the cricothyroid membrane. (d) Using a curved hemostat, spread the membrane incision open. (e) Insert a TT (6.0 or 7.0) or Shiley (6.0 or 8.0). (f) Inflate the cuff. (g) Confirm placement. (h) Ventilate. (i) Secure the tube, reconfirm placement, and evaluate the patient.

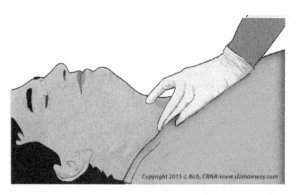

Step 1: Palpation

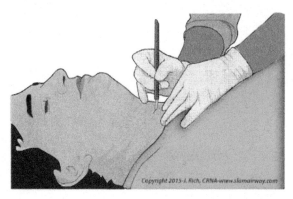

Step 2: Incision

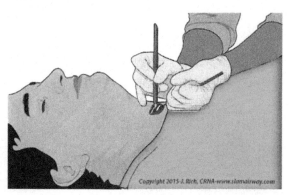

Step 3: Traction

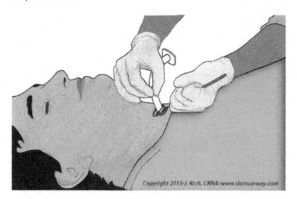

Step 4: Intubation

Rapid four-step technique.

option is to place a gum-elastic bougie alongside the scalpel, prior to removing the scalpel after the incision, and use it in a modified Seldinger technique. This secures patency of the airway and prevents loss of the surgical planes as the tube is passed over the bougie into the laryngeal incision. Additionally, use of the gum-elastic bougie may reduce the potential risk of perforating the cuff on the cricothyrotomy or endotracheal tube during placement, as might occur while passing it through the open hemostat.

Schaumann et al. compared the performance of the Seldinger technique with the standard surgical cricothyrotomy by 21 physicians.[38] Despite no significant difference in time to begin the procedure or finding the landmarks, the time to tracheal puncture and initial ventilation were significantly longer using the standard surgical technique. No statistical difference was found in the success rate of tracheal cannulation via the cricothyroid membrane (88% versus 84%). However, 4% of the cannulae were misplaced subcutaneously using the Seldinger technique, while none were misplaced using the standard surgical method.

In contrast, the standard surgical technique resulted in an incidence of 6% complications involving punctures of the thyroid vessels. The Seldinger technique resulted in no such injuries.[38] Each method definitely has its own benefits and risks that must be considered before performing the procedure.

Managing a difficult airway in the prehospital setting can be a more difficult and time sensitive issue than in a hospital setting, where more resources and staff are available. A study evaluating the performance of surgical cricothyrotomies by paramedics in the field found it to be used in as high as 9.8% of cases. These included situations with clenched teeth (trismus) or significant amounts of blood and vomit in the airway, which precluded orotracheal or nasotracheal intubation. The success rate was 94% (47/50 cases).[39] Major complications occurred in only two cases when dislodgement of the endotracheal tube occurred. Numerous studies demonstrate the effectiveness of surgical and PDC technique as a quick and viable option that can be applied by trained practitioners when neither tracheal intubation or rescue ventilation is possible.

Complications of Cricothyrotomy

Immediate

The most disastrous complication is failure to establish an airway. Hemorrhage is the most common complication encountered with a cricothyrotomy. If the horizontal incision is used through the skin, lacerating the pyramidal lobe of the thyroid can occur, also resulting in significant additional bleeding. Air leak and **barotrauma** can occur immediately upon establishing the airway or at anytime during its use and can present as pneumothorax; **pneumomediastinum;** or, more frequently, subcutaneous emphysema. The development of subcutaneous emphysema after transtracheal jet insufflation is not uncommon. Every effort should be made to confirm and document correct placement of the airway catheter prior to proceeding with ventilation. Also, damage to the recurrent laryngeal nerve or trauma to the pyramidal lobe of the thyroid may occur more commonly with the horizontal incision in comparison with the use of a vertical approach. Other immediate complications include damage to the vocal cords, esophageal perforation, and aspiration.

Intermediate

Respiratory distress secondary to obstruction or displacement of the airway as well as lower airway trauma or hypoxemia secondary to overzealous suctioning has been reported.[40] Injury to the vocal cords, either temporary or chronic,[41] may result from traumatic placement of the endotracheal tube during retrograde wire intubation or transtracheal jet insufflation, or traumatic placement of the airway after inappropriate identification of landmarks.

An abnormal passage-way or "tube" between the trachea and the in-nominate artery, result-ing in hemorrhage into the trachea or into the surrounding tissues.

Long-Term

Development of granulation tissue is a long-term complication of cricothyrotomy, after the endotracheal tube has been present for a prolonged period of time or even after its removal. [40] Bleeding, though usually minimal, can develop at any time but can be massive from development of a **tracheo-innominate fistula**.[40,42] Other long-term complications include voice changes (occurring in up to 50% cases), vocal-cord dysfunction,[43,44] infection, dysphagia, subglottic stenosis, tracheo-esophageal fistula, tracheomalacia, and persistent stoma.[42]

Much has been published with respect to complications, comparing one technique to that of another. One large series of 655 cases reported a 6.1% incidence of largely correctable complications.[6] Another study reported an 8.6% incidence of complications, with the most common being hemorrhage and damage to the cricoid cartilage.[45]

Practitioner-Specific Considerations

Training in surgical airway procedures can be a challenge given the fact that most students will never be allowed to participate in such a procedure in the hospital setting. Therefore, other means of training must be used. Manikins such as the Laerdal Airway-Man can be used, but they are limited in value because they lack the feel of a real patient. Practicing on cadavers is optimal but can be limited by the cost and availability of cadaver labs. One solution that works well and is relatively inexpensive is to practice using pig laryngeal-tracheal segments, which can be obtained from commercial packing houses.

When teaching needle cricothyrotomy and surgical cricothyrotomy, a good way to start is to have students first identify the cricothyroid membrane on themselves and then on several other students. Ask them to close their eyes and find the landmarks by touch. Then have the students don gloves and gowns and examine the pig trachea segments. Use at least one segment per student. The instructor should point out the anatomical landmarks using a specimen as a model.

Point out the epiglottis, arytenoid cartilages, false vocal cords, true vocal cords, and esophagus. Point out the cartilage rings in the trachea and let the students feel them with their fingers. Ask them to put their fingers into the esophagus and feel its soft, muscular structure as opposed to the more rigid trachea. This is also a good time to point out that the rings do not extend to the posterior of the tracheal wall, the wall that is lying against the esophagus. It is easy for students to see how an esophageal perforation might occur with an aggressive technique. Also, the instructor can use this opportunity to show the students how the bougie feels as it clicks along the tracheal rings. Finally, show students how to palpate the cricothyroid membrane. There is usually some glandular tissue left, so they can see how easy it would be to lacerate thyroid tissue and that it would bleed profusely.

Demonstrate needle cricothyrotomy first and allow the students to perform the operation. Pair the students, with one student firmly holding the pig specimen for the other. It is important to stress safety. After percutaneous needle procedures have been done, it is time to do the surgical procedure. The instructor should demonstrate the method first, describing each step as it is taken. Safety is of the utmost importance here, and the instructor must have enough helpers to monitor each pair of students to be sure that nobody is cut.

Each pair of students should be provided with a scalpel, hemostat, or a tracheal hook, and a bougie if possible. The students should practice the procedure with each of those adjuncts if possible. Students will readily learn the procedure and will appreciate the feel of the tissues as the technique is performed. Always point out that the pig segments do not have the overlying skin attached, and that therefore there will be more tissue to dissect in a human patient. However, they can learn to retract the tissues overlying the membrane with thumb and first finger, and they will see that this helps to minimize the tissue thickness as well as to move glandular tissue to the side.

Selection of Equipment

As the old airway adage states, "You can never use a blade too large or a tube too small to establish an airway." Given this statement, there are several considerations in the selection of the cricothyrotomy techniques and kits. Several of the prepared percutaneous dilational cricothyrotomy kits are available in only two sizes, one for children (internal diameter 2 mm) and one for adults (internal diameter 4 mm). While this may be sufficient for oxygenating and ventilating a small-frame individual, the oxygen requirements of a larger-frame individual in extremis may encourage consideration of using a gum-elastic bougie after several minutes of oxygenating and ventilating to exchange the tube for a larger-diameter endotracheal tube. This can be accomplished by cutting a standard endotracheal tube just proximal (above) the inflation tubing for the cuff and replacing the hub of the tube on the newly created end. By shortening the tube, the risk of inadvertent displacement or manipulation is reduced while providing a more physiologic airway. This larger tube may be replaced with a more definitive airway in the more controlled environment of the hospital.

As mentioned before, the environment in which one performs a surgical cricothyroidotomy may affect the decision about which technique to use and which incision to use. Having one's fingers straddling the cricothyroid membrane to stabilize it while attempting a transverse or horizontal incision in a moving vehicle or aircraft significantly increases the potential of accidentally lacerating one's own finger if bumps, turns, or turbulence are suddenly encountered. The percutaneous dilational cricothyroidotomy or the vertical, or longitudinal, incision may be considered more appropriate in the prehospital environment and in a world of deadly communicable blood-borne pathogens. Always be careful and pay attention to detail.

Summary

Techniques and apparatus for the safe and effective performance of cricothyrotomy for airway access have evolved from the outcome studies of this technique. We can look forward to a wider acceptance of this technique, as well application in not just the operating room or emergency department, but also in the prehospital setting.[44,45]

It is better to be completely familiar with a few methods of establishing an airway than to be vaguely familiar with many. In other words, be good at what you do. The non-surgically prepared practitioner must be intimately familiar with direct laryngoscopy and tracheal intubation, and rescue ventilation and a cricothyrotomy technique with which he or she has practiced and is immediately available as an option. As stated previously, it is only with practice and competence that cricothyrotomy can be considered as a final option for emergency airway management. Remember, the condition in which a patient cannot be intubated or ventilated is one of the most demanding and dreaded scenarios in airway management and can be the end result of multiple factors that may or may not be in your control. Here, the surgical airway has a definite role.

REVIEW QUESTIONS

1. Describe the anatomy of the larynx so that you can locate the thyroid and cricoid cartilages and the cricothyroid membrane.

2. List two complications of surgical airways.

3. Describe the techniques for percutaneous needle cricothyrotomy.

4. Describe the techniques for surgical cricothyrotomy.

5. Which surgical approach is best for emergency medical services (EMS) field work?

CHAPTER 13

The Traumatized Airway

Micha Y. Shamir
Edgar J. Pierre

Chapter Objectives

After reading this chapter, you should be able to:

- Discuss principles of airway management in the trauma patient.

- Describe injuries and injury patterns to airway and related structures.

- List major concerns with injuries to the airway and related structures.

- Recognize the signs and symptoms of the traumatized airway.

- Explain the timing and proper methods for definitive airway control in the presence of a traumatized airway.

CASE Study

Medic 14 is dispatched to a hockey rink for a medical emergency. They arrive on scene to find a group of people frantically directing them to the bleacher area. There they find a 30-year-old male sitting upright with his hands clamped on his thighs. Bystanders state the patient was playing hockey when a slapshot puck hit him in the throat. They say that the player instantly fell to the ground grabbing at his throat, and a 911 call was made as he was being assisted off the ice. The primary survey reveals that the patient's airway is open, breathing is labored with stridorous noises clearly audible, and the radial pulse is strong and regular. There is obvious bruising and some tenderness of the neck just below the larynx, but no other injury is identified. Cervical-spine precautions are taken, and high-flow oxygen is administered via a nonrebreathing mask. Monitors are applied and show sinus tachycardia with a rate of 110 beats per minute, a blood pressure of 148/90 mm Hg, a respiratory rate of 28 breaths per minute, and an oxygen saturation level of 95%.

The paramedics are very concerned about the possibility of loss of the airway, so they decide to perform early rapid sequence intubation. The equipment is prepared as an intravenous line is established. The patient is given 20 mg of etomidate and 150 mg of succinylcholine. With the onset of muscle relaxation, the patient is reclined with control of the cervical spine. Direct laryngoscopy is performed, and a good view of the larynx is obtained. An 8.0 mm endotracheal tracheal tube (TT) is passed between the cords, but it meets with firm resistance just 2 cm below the glottic opening. The tube is removed, and a 7.0 mm TT tried. Once again, the tube will not advance more than 2 cm below the glottic opening.

The patient's oxygen saturation is seen to be 93%, so a third intubation attempt is made. A bougie is introduced through the glottic opening and is advanced with tracheal clicking until hold up at 28 cm. The 7.0 mm tracheal tube is then advanced over the bougie under direct laryngoscopy. Some resistance is felt at 17 cm, but the tube then passes down to 23 cm at the incisors. The bougie is removed, and correct tube placement is confirmed. Postintubation management is initiated, and the patient is secured to the backboard. Transport is completed to the nearest trauma center, where a tracheal ring fracture is diagnosed. The patient survives the incident with no long-term sequelae.

Introduction

The immediate care of the trauma patient should be devoted to obtaining basic information about the individual's physical condition: stable, unstable, dying, or dead. The primary survey involves rapid evaluation and stabilization of the functions that are crucial to survival: airway patency (A), breathing (B), circulation (C) with hemorrhage control, brief neurological exam (disability, D) and complete removal of the patient's clothing (exposure, E). When assessing the airway, it is prudent to determine whether there is an immediate need for intubation.

Airway trauma (direct injury to the face or neck) can be caused by blunt, penetrating, and thermal mechanisms of injury. Thermal injuries are discussed separately in Chapter 15.

The goal of airway intervention is to relieve or prevent airway obstruction and to secure the unprotected airway from aspiration. Bleeding, secretions, tissue edema, and debris might interfere with the identification of the airway anatomy that is already distorted. In addition, the stomach is assumed to be full and the cervical spine unstable. Consequently, intubating the traumatized airway is the ultimate test to the provider's technical skills, ability to improvise, and familiarity with equipment. Successful control of the traumatized airway therefore mandates anticipatory knowledge of hazards.

The algorithm developed by the American Society of Anesthesiologists Task Force on Difficult Airway Management is only generally applicable. In cases of severe trauma, the crisis approach to management often precludes continuing with nonsurgical methods of airway ventilation, and a definitive airway is usually achieved by surgical cricothyroidotomy within the first moments of patient care.

This chapter will review the injuries, explain the hazards, and discuss various options to achieve airway control.

Le Fort's fracture

Réné Le Fort, a French physician, described three different types of facial fractures: Le Fort I, a transverse fracture of the body of the maxilla just under the nasal septum; Le Fort II, a fracture of the central maxilla and palate, wherein the nose and its structures are displaced; and Le Fort III, a fracture in which the whole facial skeleton separates from the skull. Le Fort IV, not one of Le Fort's original classifications, involves the frontal bone as well as the facial skeleton. These serious injuries usually require aggressive airway management.

KEY TERMS

cribriform plate, p. 238   Le Fort's fracture, p. 238

Facial and Pharyngeal Trauma

Mechanisms of Injury

Most upper airway injuries are secondary to direct blunt or penetrating trauma (knife or gunshot). Patients with blunt or penetrating injury of the midface, mandible, or oral cavity are at risk of upper airway obstruction and consequent anoxic brain damage or death. The most common fractures involve the mandible and midface maxilla, or **Le Fort's fracture.**

Fragmentation of bone and teeth and disruption of adjacent soft tissues characterize severe injuries of the mandible. Tears of the floor of the mouth can extend to the pharynx, tonsil, submaxillary triangle, and hyoid bone.

Midface fractures or Le Fort fractures of the maxilla present difficult clinical problems. Motion of the maxilla independent of the remainder of the face indicates a Le Fort I fracture. In addition, the Le Fort II fracture can extend through the orbital rim, medial orbital wall, ethmoid sinuses, and nose. Injury of the ethmoid sinus roof or **cribriform plate** may result in cereberal spinal fluid (CSF) rhinorrhea, meningitis, and or temporary or permanent loss of smell. Le Fort III fracture is a transverse fracture above the malar bone and through the

cribriform plate

The sievelike bone that forms part of the braincase at the roof of the nasal cavity. The sievelike holes allow axons of the olfactory nerves to connect with the neurons of the olfactory bulbs.

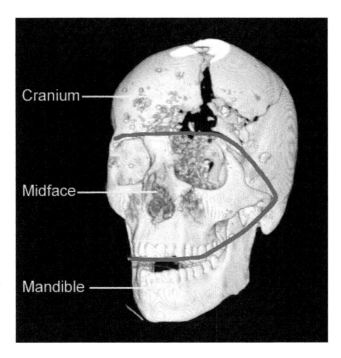

FIGURE 13-1

Facial zones in penetrating trauma. Substraction three-dimensional CT reconstruction of gunshot injury to the forehead.

(Courtesy of Hadassah University Hospital, Jerusalem, Israel)

orbits. It is characterized by complete separation of the maxilla from the craniofacial skeleton, epistaxis, and a flat dish-face deformity.[1]

Penetrating trauma to the face can be described by a number of facial zones divisions. The simplest one divides the face to midface and mandibular zones (Figure 13-1). Practically all stab wounds and most gunshot wounds (71%) are to the midface zone.[2]

Coexisting Injuries

Spine injury coexists in 0 to 4% of the patients suffering facial trauma.[3] It is the most serious coexisting injury because it complicates airway management. (No hyperextension of the head is allowed during laryngoscopy because it might cause spinal-cord transection in the presence of unstable vertebral fracture.) Life-threatening hypovolemia is uncommon as a result of isolated facial trauma, occurring only in 1% to 4% of the patients.[4] Tears in the dura occur in 25% of all Le Fort II and III fractures, along with leakage of cerebrospinal fluid.[1] Other injuries of immediate concern regarding the airway are head and vascular injuries.[2]

Diagnosis

Most facial injuries are obvious because they are associated with bleeding, edema, erythema, and facial distortion. Because assessment of the airway is urgent, it should be almost entirely clinical without diagnostic studies. Important findings in the clinical evaluation to note include reduced air movement through the mouth and nares, snoring, drooling, use of accessory respiratory muscles, refusal to assume the supine posture, anxiety, and inability to phonate.

In a minority of cases, mainly isolated facial blunt trauma, edema and erythema might not appear in the very early stages. In this case, bony crepitus (a grating or crackling sound or sensation produced by the fractured ends of a bone moving against each other) on palpation should alert for facial injury.

Trauma is a dynamic process, especially in the acute phase, including insidious airway obstruction (as edema and hematoma propagates). The importance of regular reassessment of the patient's ABCs cannot be overemphasized to prevent late diagnosis of lethal airway obstruction.

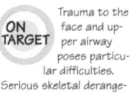

Trauma to the face and upper airway poses particular difficulties. Serious skeletal derangements may be masked by apparently minor soft-tissue damage. Failure to identify an injury to the face can lead to insidious airway obstruction secondary to swelling and hematoma.

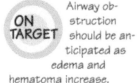

Airway obstruction should be anticipated as edema and hematoma increase.

PEARLS Do not force patients with traumatized airways into a recumbent position which may lead to rapid airway obstruction or collapse. The awake patient will usually assume a position that facilitates airway patency and respiration.

Airway Control

Airway management should begin with an assessment of the need and urgency for definitive airway control. Intraoral hemorrhage, pharyngeal erythema, and change in voice are all indications for early intubation. Penetrating mandibular injuries often require early intervention.[2] Bilateral mandibular fractures and pharyngeal hemorrhage may lead to upper airway obstruction, particularly in a supine patient. These patients initially may be able to maintain a patent airway by positioning themselves forward so that broken bones and lacerated tissue fall forward, relieving any obstruction. They should be allowed to maintain this position until the trauma team is ready to definitively manage their airway.[1,4]

PEARLS Intraoral hemorrhage, pharyngeal erythema, and change in voice are all indications for early intubation.

<table>
<tr><td>

ON TARGET RSI with cervical in-line immobilization is the preferred method of intubation in the trauma patient. Both the LMA and Combitube enable reasonable airway protection and ventilation as a rescue ventilation solution until hospital arrival.

</td><td>

If the clinical situation permits, it is generally better to postpone intubation until hospital arrival. The presence of experienced practitioners in the controlled and well-equipped environment of the hospital can greatly increase the success of controlling and securing the traumatized airway.[4] An oral or nasopharyngeal airway may be required to temporarily maintain a patent airway until tracheal intubation can be performed at the hospital.[4] Usually facial injuries present as a difficult-intubation issue rather than as an impossible-intubation issue. Patients with jaw and zygomatic arch injuries often have trismus. Although the trismus will resolve with the administration of neuromuscular blocking agents, pre-induction assessment of airway anatomy may be difficult.[1]

Rapid sequence intubation with cervical in-line immobilization is the preferred method of intubation in the trauma patient (see Chapter 14). Both maxillary and mandibular fractures will probably make mask ventilation more difficult. On the other hand, mandibular fractures make intubation easier because of loss of skeletal resistance to direct laryngoscopy.

Le Fort II and III fractures mandate oral intubation because of the intranasal damage. In the case of mandibular or Le Fort I fractures, if no trismus or mechanical problem exists, routine rapid sequence tracheal intubation is the technique of choice.[1,4] If it is judged that direct laryngoscopy may be difficult, then any technique that preserves spontaneous ventilation should be used, such as awake fiberoptic, retrograde, and laryngeal mask-guided intubation.[4-7]

The use of blind nasal intubation in the presence of facial trauma is controversial. The source of disagreement is multiple case reports of nasogastric tubes placed intracranially in the presence of base of skull fracture.[8] Cephalic placement of an endotracheal tube is rare (two cases) because the tube is much less flexible.[8,9] No significant complications were identified in a retrospective evaluation of blind nasal intubation of 82 patients suffering facial fractures.[9] This issue is well summarized in an editorial statement: "Rapid sequence induction is the cornerstone of modern emergency airway management. Nasotracheal intubation is not contraindicated in the presence of severe maxillofacial or skull injuries providing a proper technique is utilized."[10]

The options for emergency nonsurgical airway ventilation after failed intubation following anesthetic induction include transtracheal jet ventilation, laryngeal mask ventilation (LMA), or esophageal-tracheal Combitube (ETC) ventilation.[4-7] LMA and ETC insertions require less experience and therefore carry higher success rate. Both LMA and ETC enable reasonable airway protection and ventilation as a rescue ventilation solution until hospital arrival. Extra care should be taken while inserting an LMA because the semiconscious patient might injure the provider's fingers with consequent blood-borne viruses hazard.[11]

</td></tr>
</table>

Precious time may be wasted in the struggle to intubate while the patient's respiratory status and intracranial pressure deteriorates, and therefore cricothyroidotomy is a useful alternative. The Israeli Defense Forces Medical Corps reports that this procedure has an almost 90% success rate even in inexperienced hands.[12] Perhaps early cricothyroidotomy, rather than repeated multiple attempts to intubate, would result in less hypoxia and improved patient outcome. Emergency tracheotomy is not considered an appropriate method for establishing emergency definitive airway because the procedure takes a long time and carries significant rate of complications.

Definitive Treatment

The definitive diagnosis of injury extent is made using plane x-rays or computed tomography. Definitive treatment is rarely urgent once the airway is safe. Methods for definitive treatment are beyond the scope of this chapter.

Neck Injuries

The neck is a very narrow corridor containing multiple structures (main airway and digestive conduits, cervical spinal cord, and nerves and blood vessels). Because all these components are vital to life, injury to the neck carries a high rate of mortality and morbidity.[13] Obstructive injury to the airway is the second most common cause of death associated with trauma to the head and neck.[14] Mild to moderate trauma may cause tissue edema, hematoma, or mucosal tears. Severe injuries can result in disruption of the airway, neurovascular bundle, and visceral rupture.[15] Fortunately injuries to the cervical aerodigestive tract are uncommon, ranging from 1.2% in blunt trauma to 10.2% in penetrating injuries to the neck.[16]

The most important injuries in the neck include:

- Disruption of tracheal continuity (partial/total).
- Fractures of larynx/cricoid obstructing the airway.
- Major arterial/venous bleeding leading to hemorrhagic shock or hematoma formation compressing and obstructing the airway.
- Cervical-spine injury causing apnea or neurogenic shock.
- Perforation of esophagus.

Mechanisms of Injury

Penetrating neck trauma can be caused by gunshot, knife, or other foreign bodies. These injuries are usually described according to the entrance site as one of three zones of the neck (Figure 13-2). Zone I extends from the clavicles to the cricoid cartilage and carries high mortality. In addition to neck organs, it contains upper thoracic lung and blood vessels. Zone II lies between the cricoid and the mandibular angle. It contains major cervical arteries and veins as well as extrathoracic air and food tracts. It is the most frequently injured area, and mortality is less because of easy surgical access. Zone III comprises the area between the base of the skull and the angle of the mandible. This area is also difficult to approach surgically.[17]

A different classification divides the neck into anterolateral or posterior portion divided by the sternocleidomastoid muscle. Naturally, injury to the anterolateral part is more dangerous because of the proximity to the trachea, larynx, and cervical vessels.[17]

Blunt laryngotracheal injury may be caused by three mechanisms. The first is direct: vehicular dashboard, human assault (such as strangulation), sports injury (ball, baseball bat, etc.), fall from height, and hanging. The second is deceleration: car collisions and falls can exert shearing injuries to fixed organs such as the cricoid cartilage or tracheal carina. The third mechanism is increased pressure: sudden anteroposterior chest compression against closed glottis can cause abrupt increase in intrathoracic pressure. The result can be linear rupture of the posterior membranous trachea.[13,18]

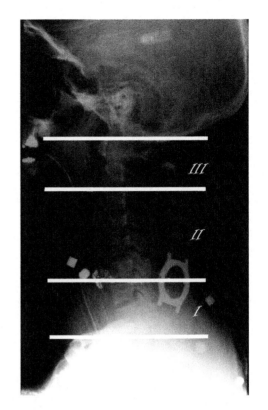

FIGURE 13-2

Penetrating neck injury zones. Zone I—from clavicle to cricoid; Zone II—from cricoid to mandibular angle; Zone III—from mandibular angle to the base of the skull.

(Lateral cervical x-ray of a suicide bombing victim. Jerusalem, November 21, 2002. Courtesy of Hadassah University Hospital, Jerusalem, Israel)

Coexisting Injuries

Penetrating neck injuries are obvious and dramatic, so attention might be distracted from other coexisting life-threatening injuries such as head or chest trauma.[19] On the contrary, blunt neck trauma is associated with other, more overt injuries at a rate as high as 50% or more. These injuries might mask potentially lethal neck injury because they are more common and obvious (spine and maxillofacial fractures, chest trauma, and closed-head injuries).[13]

Diagnosis

The diagnosis of penetrating neck trauma is usually simple because the injury is overt and obvious (Figure 13-3). On the contrary, diagnosis of blunt neck trauma that is not associated with such obvious tissue manifestations depends on a high index of suspicion.[14] Clinical examination remains the most reliable sign of laryngotracheal injury. The only hard diagnostic sign to airway trauma is air leaking through the neck wound. Other signs and symptoms include subcutaneous emphysema, dyspnea, hemoptysis, hoarseness, stridor, and crepitance on palpation.[18,19] Soft-tissue swelling is responsible for the sensation of choking, dyspnea, dysphagia, hoarseness, and stridor experienced by these patients.[15] Transcervical gunshot wounds evidenced radiographically or by the existence of entrance and contralateral exit wounds carry high risk for major vascular or visceral damage.[20] Crepitus on palpation of the cricoid/tracheal cartilages is of the utmost importance in diagnostic airway injury.

The quality of the victim's voice (i.e., hoarseness) is important. A hoarse voice indicates major airway injury until proven otherwise. This finding should never be overlooked unless the patient is alert and can verify the existence of hoarseness prior to the injury. Information from emergency medical service (EMS) providers documenting the development of hoarseness should immediately alert the practitioner to the presence of an airway injury.

As mentioned previously, there is no way to overemphasize the importance of regular reassessment of the patient's ABCs. Trauma is a dynamic disease, and therefore insidious airway obstruction should be the assumption as edema and hematoma increases.

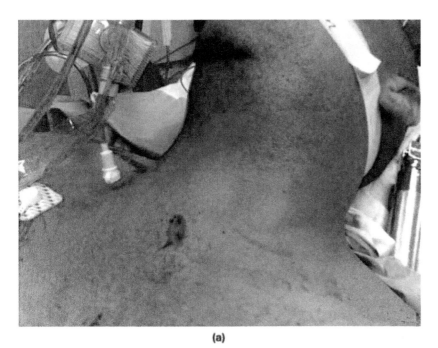

(a)

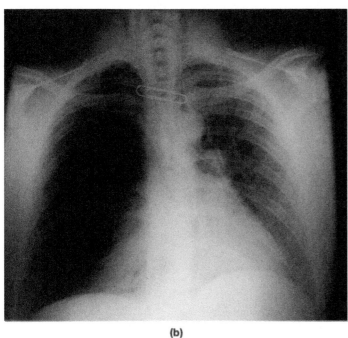

(b)

FIGURE 13-3

(a) Stab wound to the anterior neck.

(Courtesy of Micha Y. Shamir, MD, Hadassah Medical Center, Jerusalem, Israel)

(b) Chest x-ray of the patient demonstrating total right lung collapse secondary to pneumothorax. Paper clip demonstrates skin stab site.

(Courtesy of Micha Y. Shamir, MD, Hadassah Medical Center, Jerusalem, Israel)

Airway Control

The most urgent priority in penetrating and blunt neck trauma is securing the airway. The end result should be an endotracheal tube with an inflated sealing cuff positioned entirely distal to a laryngotracheal perforation. Nevertheless, intubation of the trachea might be extremely difficult because pharyngeal or neck hematoma might obscure the vocal cords or distort the anatomy. Blind passage of the endotracheal tube is dangerous because it might follow or cause a false route or complete a partially transected airway.[18,20] The obvious conclusion is to avoid tracheal intubation at the scene or emergency department (as long as the patient is stable).

The more common neck injuries (stab wounds and low-velocity gunshots) usually do not mandate prehospital or emergency department intubation. Intubation should be performed in the operating room by the most experienced available anesthesia provider with the proper equipment and availability to perform surgical interventions. On the contrary, high-velocity gunshot bullets and severe blunt neck injuries often mandate urgent airway control at the scene.[18]

Rapid sequence orotracheal intubation, laryngeal mask airway, and esophageal obturator are contraindicated in patients suspected of having laryngotracheal discontinuation. If rapid sequence orotracheal intubation is necessary (combative patient, for example), concomitant preparation for fiberoptic confirmation of the proper tube position is mandatory as well as continuing preparations for the establishment of a surgical airway (cricothyroidotomy) establishment. Emergency tracheotomy is not considered an appropriate method for establishing an emergency definitive airway because the procedure is lengthy and carries significant rate of complications.

The unstable patient with a slashed throat (Figure 13-4) can be intubated through the incision as a life-saving act.[21] For prehospital personnel, cricothyroidotomy is practically the only appropriate alternative if artificial airway establishment cannot be delayed until arrival at the hospital.

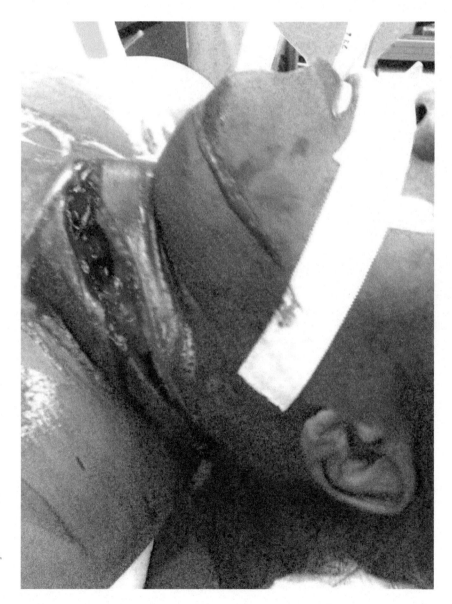

FIGURE 13-4

Slashed neck. The patient's respirations were stable, and therefore he was intubated orally.

(Courtesy of Micha Y. Shamir, MD, Hadassah Medical Center, Jerusalem, Israel)

In the past, cricothyroidotomy or tracheotomy were the procedure of choice even in the hospital.[13] Recent literature allows for orotracheal intubation providing it is done under direct vision of a bronchoscope, thus ensuring that the entire path of the tube is intraluminar. Using a bronchoscope is also helpful in placing the entirety of the sealing cuff distal to the perforation in the trachea.[16,17] However, bronchoscopy is not available in the prehospital setting.

Cervical Hematoma

Signs for vascular injuries are hematoma (Figure 13-5), hypotension, and persistent bleeding.[15] The hematoma can be limited without jeopardizing the airway. On the other hand, bleeding and edema may gradually enlarge, especially in patients taking anticoagulants. In this case, a critical point may abruptly be reached in which the airway is obstructed and the patient deteriorates.[15] It is reasonable to postpone tracheal intubation until arrival at the hospital because of the inability to predict the clinical course and the possibility of a difficult tracheal intubation (bulging hematoma and soft tissue swelling). Nevertheless, close monitoring of the patient and evaluation of the size of the hematoma is crucial. Preventive intubation should be done if the hematoma enlarges or if the patient shows progressive signs of

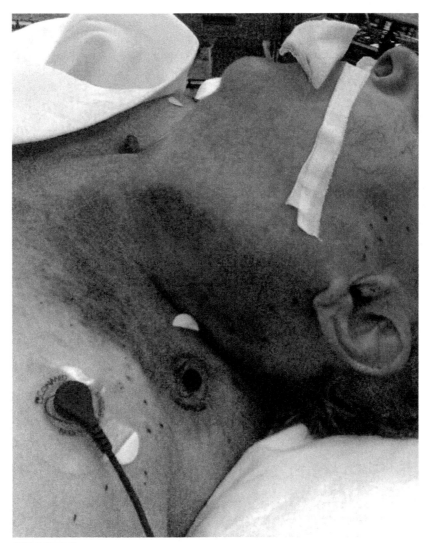

FIGURE 13-5

Cervical hematoma. Notice the bluish periphery of the hematoma, indicating ongoing subcutaneous dissection of blood. Also notice the anterior neck bulging that might compress and/or displace the larynx and trachea.
(Courtesy of Micha Y. Shamir, MD, Hadassah Medical Center, Jerusalem, Israel)

airway compromise. A low threshold for intubation is advocated if the evacuation time is long or if the provider's skills are limited (less experience mandates intubation before anatomy significantly distorts). In the field, emergency-department and operating-room difficult intubation should be anticipated, and the technique should be planned accordingly.

Definitive Treatment

Once the airway is secured, a meticulous diagnostic workup must be started to verify the exact location of injury and choose the appropriate surgical intervention. Paramedics can assist by reporting their observations in detail to the trauma team. In the hospital, this includes fiberoptic examination of the pharynx, larynx, trachea, and esophagus. Other modalities can include chest and neck radiographs, computed tomography, angiography, and contrast swallow fluoroscopy. The detailed surgical treatment, conservative or invasive, is beyond the scope of this chapter.

Summary

Penetrating neck trauma is usually obvious, but blunt trauma mandates a high index of suspicion to recognize its existence. Comprehensive understanding of injury is mandatory to plan the best timing and method to secure the airway. If the airway is stable, it is advised that airway control is carried out on arrival at the hospital and in the operating room by the most experienced anesthesia provider available with the a surgical airway. If any doubt exists as to the clinician's ability to secure the airway, it is better to use a technique that maintains spontaneous ventilation.

REVIEW QUESTIONS

1. What is the goal of airway intervention in the traumatized airway?

2. What are the most common fractures involving the face?

3. Describe the injuries in each of Le Fort's type fractures.

4. How often does cervical-spine injury accompany facial trauma?

5. What is the major concern with blunt trauma to the neck?

6. When are rapid sequence orotracheal intubation, laryngeal mask airway, and esophageal obturator contraindicated?

CHAPTER 14

The Cervical-Spine-Injured Patient

Charles E. Smith
Darko Vodopich

Chapter Objectives

After reading this chapter, you should be able to:

- Describe the incidence of and risk factors for cervical-spine (c-spine) injury.
- Describe the presenting symptoms and signs of c-spine injury.
- Discuss prehospital spinal immobilization and clearance criteria.
- Discuss the impact of spinal immobilization on airway management.
- Discuss outcome studies of airway management techniques in patients with c-spine injuries.
- Identify and implement strategies for managing the airway in patients with known or suspected c-spine injury.

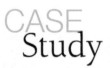

CASE Study

Medic 14 responded to a call for an injured person at a dance club. They arrived to find a 20-year-old female who was dancing in the club when she was hit in the neck with an unknown object and fell limp to the floor. Employees at the club found the patient lying on the dance floor unconscious and bleeding from the head.

The paramedic's primary evaluation found the patient's airway open, breathing was spontaneous but shallow and irregular, and peripheral pulses were present with regular rate. Cervical-spine precautions were undertaken as oxygen was applied via a nonrebreathing mask. Secondary evaluation revealed a small laceration to the back of her head. There was also a large deformity noted to the back of the patient's neck around her third cervical vertebrae. Her lungs were clear, but suprasternal muscle use was noted. Neurological exam revealed the patient would open her eyes to verbal stimuli, her verbal response was confused, and she exhibited no extremity motor response to any stimuli. The paramedics noticed she would follow with her eyes and was licking her lips, but she would not move her extremities.

The patient was secured to the spine board and loaded into the ambulance. Full monitors were applied, which revealed sinus tachycardia with a rate of 108, blood pressure of 92/40, respiratory rate of 8, with oxygen saturations of 94%. An intravenous line was established.

During transport, the patient's respiratory status declined. The need for intubation was identified. Concerned about a spinal-cord injury, the paramedic prepared for nasal intubation. Neosynephine was administered to both nares, and a nasal trumpet was covered with lidocaine jelly and placed into her right nare. A 7.0 Endotrol tube was lubricated, and a whistle tip was applied to the adapter. Versed 4 mg was administered IV.

The nasal trumpet was removed as the tracheal tube was introduced into the right nare with the bevel against the septum. It was slowly advanced while the paramedic listened to the whistle with respirations. The paramedic's second hand was placed over the patient's mouth as he advanced to the point of maximum whistle. He then quickly advanced the tracheal tube on inspiration. A louder whistle was established as the cuff was inflated. Tracheal tube position was confirmed with bilateral breath sounds and good color change in the CO_2 detector. The tube was secured while ventilations were assisted. The patient was delivered to the emergency department without incident.

Introduction

Cervical-spine (c-spine) injuries continue to be a major health problem. Major trauma is associated with a 2% to 6% risk of cervical-spine injury. This chapter discusses the approach to airway management and tracheal intubation in patients with known or suspected c-spine injuries.

KEY TERMS

anterior atlanto-axial dislocation, pp. 250, 251

antisialagogue agent, p. 255

atlanto-occipital dislocation, pp. 250, 251

bilateral facet dislocation. p. 250

clay shoveler's fracture, pp. 250, 251

flexion teardrop fracture, p. 250

hangman's fracture of C2, pp. 250, 252

Jefferson fracture, pp. 250, 253

odontoid fracture with lateral displacement, pp. 250, 251

ovassapian airway, p. 255

posterior atlanto-axial dislocation, pp. 250, 252

posterior neural arch fracture, pp. 250, 252

subluxation, p. 250

transverse process fracture, pp. 250, 252

wedge fracture, p. 250

Overview

The c-spine supports the head and permits a wide range of motion in three dimensions (flexion/extension, lateral bending, axial rotation) without damaging the spinal cord.[1] The normal lateral and upper structural relationships (Figures 14-1 and 14-2) promote a wide range

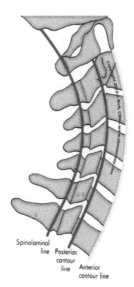

FIGURE 14-1

Normal lateral c-spine structural relationships.
(From Hockberger RS, Kirshenbaum KJ, Davis PE. Spinal injuries. In *Emergency Medicine*, Fourth Edition. Mosby, St Louis. Editor-in-Chief: Rosen P. 1998, pp 462–505, with permission.)

Spinolaminal line   Posterior contour line   Anterior contour line

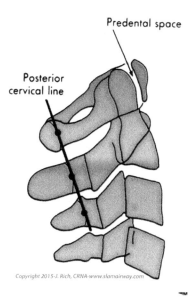

Predental space

Posterior
cervical line

Copyright 2015-J. Rich, CRNA-www.slamairway.com

FIGURE 14-2

Normal upper c-spine structural relationships on the lateral view.
(From Hockberger RS, Kirshenbaum KJ, Davis PE. Spinal injuries. In *Emergency Medicine*, Fourth Edition. Mosby, St Louis. Editor-in-Chief: Rosen P. 1998, pp 462–505, with permission.)

of c-spine motion, but they make the c-spine the most vulnerable region to injury, with approximately 55% of spinal injuries occurring in the cervical region.[2] The incidence of c-spine injuries following blunt trauma is 2% to 9% (Table 14-1).

There are approximately 10,000 new cases of spinal injury each year in the United States, and the majority of victims are young men between the ages of 15 and 35 years.[12] The annual cost to society has been estimated at $5 billion due to the tremendous multisystemic implications of these injuries, including social, medical, surgical, and rehabilitative complications.[12,13] Approximately 10% of patients with c-spine fractures have a second, noncontiguous vertebral column fracture.[14] Preserving and restoring neurologic function is the cornerstone of treatment. Strategies include optimization of oxygenation, cord perfusion, use of methylprednisolone, and spinal-cord decompression.

Diagnosis

C-spine injury is diagnosed based on mechanism of injury and symptoms and signs (Tables 14-2 and 14-3). The majority of c-spine injuries occur as a result of motor-vehicle collision (MVC). In one study of 133 patients with c-spine injuries, 64% were due to MVCs; 19%,

Table 14-1	Incidence of C-Spine Injuries	
Population	**Incidence (%)**	**Reference**
Trauma, $n = 1,823$	5.0	Baculis, 1987[3]
Trauma, $n = 9,044$	4.3	Criswell, 1994[4]
Trauma, $n = 987$	6.1	Wright, 1992[5]
Trauma, $n = 6,500$	3.2	Domeir, 1999[6]
Trauma, $n = 7,518$	2.2	Scannell, 1993[7]
Trauma, $n = 749$	2.4	Cadoux, 1987[8]
Facial fractures, $n = 582$	1.0	Beirne, 1995[9]
Head trauma, $n = 886$	3.2	Nefield, 1988[10]
Head, face, and clavicular trauma, $n = 5,021$	4.5	Williams, 1992[11]

Table 14-2 Symptoms and Signs of Cervical-Spine Injury[12,15,16]

- Neck pain, palpation tenderness, deformity
- Paresthesias, tingling
- Diaphragmatic breathing
- Hypoventilation
- Neurogenic shock with hypotension and bradycardia
- Spinal shock with flaccidity and loss of reflexes
- Absent rectal tone
- Sensory and motor abnormalities (inability to perceive pain below level of lesion may mask serious injury elsewhere)
- Priapism

Table 14-3 Mechanism of Injury and Resultant Type of Fracture or Injury[12]

- Flexion
- **Wedge fracture, flexion teardrop fracture, subluxation, bilateral facet dislocation, atlanto-occipital dislocation, anterior atlanto-axial dislocation, odontoid fracture with lateral displacement, clay shoveler's fracture, transverse process fracture**
- Flexion rotation
- Unilateral facet dislocation, rotary atlanto-axial dislocation
- Extension
- **Posterior neural arch fracture (C1), hangman's fracture of C2, posterior atlanto-axial dislocation,** extension teardrop fracture avulsion
- Vertical compression (axial loading)
- Burst fracture of vertebral body, **Jefferson fracture (C1)**

wedge fracture
A vertebral compression fracture occurring anteriorly (front) or laterally (side).

flexion teardrop fracture
The most severe fracture of the cervical spine, usually occurring at C5-6, often caused by a dive into shallow water. Characterized by complete instability of the cervical spine, often resulting in quadriplegia. On x-ray, identified by a teardrop-shaped bone fragment that is separated from the vertebral body.

subluxation
Dislocation of vertebrae.

bilateral facet dislocation
An unstable flexion injury involving the articular joints between and posterior to adjacent vertebral bodies. The integrity of all the spinal ligaments as well as the intervertebral disc and facet joint capsules is lost. With complete dislocation, the inferior articular facets of the body above lie anterior to the superior facets of the body below.

falls; 7%, assault; 5%, diving; and 5%, sports (Figure 14-3).[17] In the study, 81% of injuries involved the subaxial segments C3–C7, and the remainder involved the occipito-atlantal and atlanto-axial segments (Figure 14-4).[17]

One-third of patients with upper c-spine injuries die at the scene from high cervical quadriplegia.[2] The majority of patients with injuries at this level who survive are neurologically intact on admission. With injuries at C-3 or below, there is a high incidence of neurologic deficit. If the upper or middle cervical cord is injured, the diaphragm may be paralyzed because of involvement of the C-3 to C-5 segments, which innervate the diaphragm via the phrenic nerve. With lower cervical-cord injuries, paralysis of the intercostal muscles can result in hypoventilation. Sensory deficits can mask potentially serious injuries below the level.

Clearing the C-Spine Before Intubation

One of the greatest worries is the failure to diagnose a c-spine injury in a neurologically intact patient.[1] Field clearance of the spine is becoming more prevalent, and studies show that patients can safely be cleared by using specific criteria.[2] The general rule is that c-spine precautions are needed after blunt trauma in patients with one or more of the following: spine pain or palpation tenderness, any neurologic abnormality or symptoms, altered level of consciousness, or suspected intoxication.

Dislocation of the base of the occiput and the arch of the atlas (C1), involving complete disruption of all ligaments between the occiput and the atlas. This injury usually causes immediate death from stretching of the brainstem, which causes respiratory arrest. Cervical traction is completely contraindicated in this injury because it can cause further stretching or dissection of the brainstem.

Displacement of the atlas from the axial spine.

The odontoid, also called the dens, is a toothlike bony process extending upward from the atlas. This fracture is usually stable but may become unstable.

A fracture of the spinous process (the posterior prominence that can be palpated on the back) resulting from abrupt flexion of the neck or a blow to the neck or the back of the head, causing forced flexion of the neck, usually occurring at C-7-T1.

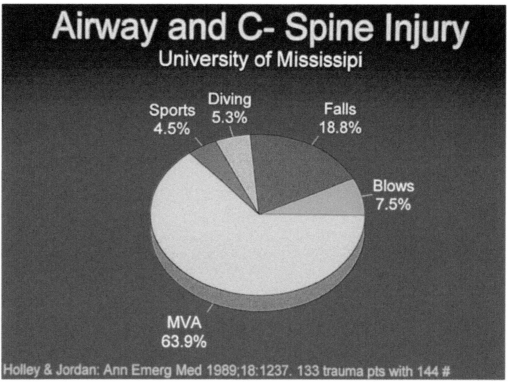

FIGURE 14-3

Mechanism of injury in 133 adult patients requiring operative repair of traumatic, unstable cervical-spine fractures.

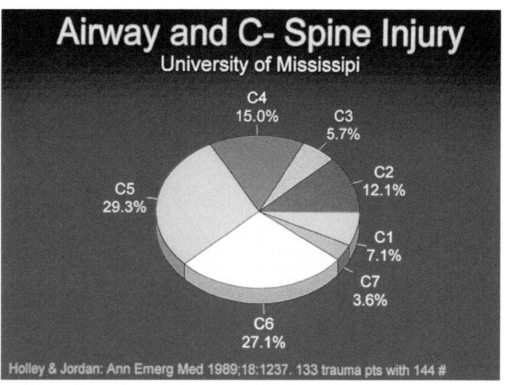

FIGURE 14-4

Fracture site incidence in 133 adult patients with 144 fractures who underwent operative repair of their traumatic cervical-spine fractures.

transverse process fracture

A fracture of the bony protrusions extending out from each side of the vertebral column at about a 45° angle. It is usually stable. The most common transverse process fractures are in the lower thoracic and lumbar spine.

Lateral, anteroposterior view, and open-mouth odontoid views should be obtained. On the lateral view, the base of the skull, all 7 cervical vertebrae, and T1 vertebrae must be visualized in order to avoid missing fractures or fracture dislocations in the lower c-spine (Figure 3-7).[12,18,19] The open-mouth odontoid view should show the entire odontoid process and the left and right C-1, C-2 articulations. All patients with penetrating trauma to the c-spine region need films. In a large prospective multi-center study of over 34,000 emergency patients with blunt trauma, serious c-spine abnormalities were found in approximately 2% of patients with 1 or more criteria for diagnostic imaging.[20] Conversely, c-spine abnormalities were found in only 1 of 4309 patients with no criteria for imaging, and that patient did not suffer neurological sequelae. The sensitivity of clinical criteria in identifying blunt trauma patients with c-spine injuries was 99% with a negative predictive value of 99.8%. Specificity was 12.9% and the positive predictive value was 2.7%.[20]

PEARLS Trauma patients who are awake and alert and who have no mental status changes, no neck pain, no distracting pain, and no neurological deficits (e.g., ETOH/drug ingestion) may be considered clinically to have a stable c-spine.

posterior neural arch fracture

A hyperextension injury wherein the posterior neural arch of C1 is compressed between the occiput and the spinous process of C2. The posterior arch of C1 is thin, and this compression causes it to break.

hangman's fracture of C2

Named for the fracture that occurs with hanging, now it usually results from hyperextension in trauma such as motor-vehicle collisions. May be stable or unstable, depending on whether the fracture extends through the pedicles and results in facet dislocation.

The recommendations by the Eastern Association for the Surgery of Trauma[21,22] are followed at the author's institution:

- Trauma patients who are alert and awake, and who have no mental status changes, no neck pain, no distracting pain, and no neurologic deficits may be considered clinically to have a stable c-spine.
- All other trauma patients receive spinal precautions in the field, followed by the following three c-spine x-rays once the patient is in the hospital: lateral view revealing the base of the occiput to the upper border of the first thoracic vertebrae, anteroposterior view revealing the spinous processes of the second cervical through the first thoracic vertebra, and an open mouth odontoid view revealing the lateral masses of the first cervical vertebra and entire odontoid process. Axial CT scans with sagittal reconstruction are obtained for any questionable level of injury, or through the lower c-spine if this area cannot be visualized on plain radiographs. Before removing immobilization devices, all x-rays are read by a physician with expertise in interpreting these studies.
- If the patient has a neurologic deficit, he or she receives immediate subspecialty consultation.
- If the patient has an altered level of consciousness due to a traumatic brain injury or due to other causes that are considered likely to leave the patient unable to complain of neck pain or neurologic deficits for 24 or more hours after the injury, he or she may be considered to have a stable c-spine if adequate x-rays (CT supplementation as necessary) and thin-cut axial CT images through C1 and C2 are read as normal by an experienced physician.

Airway Management

posterior atlanto-axial dislocation

A rare injury in which the posterior atlas is dislocated onto the axis without fracture of the odontoid process.

For airway management in the c-spine-injured patient, the principles of ATLS™ are followed.[2] Measures to establish a patent airway should be instituted while protecting the c-spine. Life-threatening injuries are identified and attended to while minimizing any movement of the spinal column. New neurologic deficits occur 7.5 times more frequently with an unrecognized injury, and up to 10% of c-spine-injured patients suffer a new neurological deficit if not immobilized.[23] At least 5% of spinal and spinal-cord trauma patients experience the onset of neurologic symptoms or worsening of preexisting symptoms after reaching the

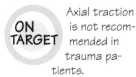

emergency department due to ischemia or progression of edema.[2] Therefore, the head and neck are immobilized during all airway maneuvers if there is any suspicion of injury, and supplemental oxygen is provided. Basic airway maneuvers to ensure oxygenation and ventilation are done prior to tracheal intubation. Indications for intubation include requirements for surgery and general anesthesia, respiratory distress, airway protection, shock, and tracheal toilet.

The relative risk of airway maneuvers in a patient with an unstable c-spine depends on both direct and indirect factors. Direct factors include type of injury, anatomic location of injury, and severity of structural compromise. Indirect factors consist of cardiovascular instability; shock; degree of respiratory compromise; and the presence of other injuries such as head, maxillofacial, abdomen, aorta, and pelvic trauma.

Overzealous chin-lift maneuvers, jaw-thrust, and conventional laryngoscopy can all cause movement of the unprotected c-spine.[15] Head extension is contraindicated in the patient with known or possible c-spine instability. Similarly, inadequate airway anesthesia during awake intubation may cause vigorous coughing, retching, and vomiting when the endotracheal tube is manipulated into the pharynx and larynx, which in turn can cause dangerous patient movement. The vast majority of cervical motion during glottic visualization and intubation with a Macintosh blade is produced at the occipito-atlantal and atlanto-axial joints.[24] The subaxial cervical segments are only minimally displaced.[24]

Methods for Preventing C-Spine Motion During Tracheal Intubation

Soft and hard collars are of minimal to no value in preventing c-spine motion during direct laryngoscopy, especially motion of the upper c-spine.[1] The collars also limit mouth opening. Manual in-line axial stabilization (MIAS) reduces movement to some degree. Axial traction also reduces occipital-C1 extension but can distract attention from a complete injury or augment translational motion at the injury segment.[1] For these reasons, axial traction is not recommended.

Approaches to Tracheal Intubation

A variety of approaches and devices have been described, including blind nasotracheal intubation, flexible fiberoptic bronchoscopy, conventional laryngoscopy, McCoy laryngoscope, rigid fiberoptic intubation (Bullard, Wuscope), gum-elastic bougie, lighted stylets, iLMA, retrograde technique, and cricothyroidotomy (Table 14-4).

The goal is to establish tracheal intubation without causing further injury to the spinal cord.[16,27] Patients with head trauma or those who are unconscious or uncooperative often require rapid sequence induction and intubation with MIAS.[27,28] Failed intubation usually necessitates a cricothyrotomy.

There are no clear guidelines for the optimal method to secure the airway in patients with c-spine injuries, with the exception that the head and neck must be kept in a neutral position throughout the intubation procedure.[15,29] At the author's institution, prevention of head and neck movement and stabilization of the spine during oral intubation are often obtained with MIAS (Figure 14-5).[19] The collar is removed to facilitate mouth opening.

All stabilization methods make conventional direct laryngoscopy more difficult.[30,31] For example, Nolan et al.[32] showed that MIAS of the c-spine resulted in a 22% incidence of Grade III views in which the vocal cords were not seen, although the epiglottis was visualized. MIAS reduced the optimal view of the larynx in 45% of patients (Table 14-5).

Intubation via conventional laryngoscopy may be impossible with halo-fixation.[1] Anything that limits extension of the upper c-spine and flexion below C2 makes glottic visualization during direct laryngoscopy more difficult.

The Cervical-Spine-Injured Patient 253

Table 14-4 Selected Retrospective Studies of Airway Management Techniques and Outcome in Patients with Cervical-Spine Injuries Requiring Endotracheal Intubation

Number of Patients and Year of Study	Techniques	New Neurologic Deficit
n = 454; 1992[25]	165 patients needed intubation (36%): awake flexible fiberoptic—76; awake blind nasal—53; awake direct laryngoscopy—36	11 patients total (2.4%): nonintubated—7; intubated—4; before intubation—2; several hrs after normal postintubation exam—2
n = 393; 1994[4]	104 needed intubation: RSI—73; blind nasal—18; flexible fiberoptic—11; cricothyrotomy for failed intubation—2	No new deficit (95% confidence interval 0 to 4%)
n = 150; 1991[26]	All needed intubation for surgical stabilization: GA and direct laryngoscopy—67; GA, other technique—14; awake flexible fiberoptic—37; awake direct laryngoscopy—22; awake lighted stylet—8	2 patients (1.3%): 1 radiculopathy, resolved after 72 hrs; 1 quadraplegia—surgical wire passed through cord
n = 60; 1992[5]	53 had unstable injuries: oral intubation—26; nasal intubation—25; cricothyrotomy—2	1 patient (1.8%) after nasal intubation
n = 168; 1993[7]	81 needed intubation, all with RSI	None; 4 had improvement in deficit after intubation

Abbreviations: RSI = rapid sequence intubation; GA = general anesthesia.

Nonurgent Cases

In nonurgent cases such as c-spine fusion, the patient in a halo vest, awake flexible fiberoptic intubation is a fast, safe, and reliable technique with a very low failure rate, provided that the operator has all the equipment, training, and skills necessary to perform the technique (Chapter 10).[36,37] Awake intubation allows evaluation of the patient's neurologic status after intubation or after positioning, before inducing general anesthesia. Sufficient

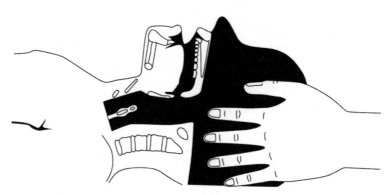

FIGURE 14-5
Manual in-line axial stabilization (MIAS) is applied by holding the sides of the neck and the mastoid processes and exerting downward pressure, thus preventing movement of the head and neck during intubation.
(From Smith, CE. Cervical spine injury and tracheal intubation: a never-ending conflict. Trauma Care 2000; 10(1)20–26. Used with permission from International TraumaCare (ITACCS).)

Table 14-5 Incidence of Difficult Direct Laryngoscopy by Experienced Anesthesiologists During General Anesthesia and Complete Neuromuscular Blockade: Effect of C-Spine Precautions

Type of Precaution	Incidence of Grade III and IV Views (%)	Reference
MIAS	14	Hastings, 1994[30]
MIAS	22	Heath, 1994[31]
MIAS	39	Smith, 1999[33]
Rigid collar	26	Gabbott, 1996[34]
MIAS and cricoid pressure	22	Nolan, 1993[32]
MIAS and cricoid pressure	34	Laurent, 1996[35]
Rigid collar with tape and sandbags	66	Heath, 1994[31]

Abbreviation: MIAS = manual in-line axial stabilization. Grade 3 view = only epiglottis visible, glottis cannot be seen. Grade 4 view = only hard palate visualized, epiglottis and glottis cannot be seen.

antisialagogue agent
An agent that diminishes or prevents the flow of saliva.

ovassapian airway
The fiberoptic intubating airway.

airway anesthesia, conscious sedation (e.g., midazolam, fentanyl, dexmedetomidine), an **antisialagogue agent,** and a topical vasoconstrictor (if the nasal route is chosen) are essential elements of awake fiberoptic intubation. An antifog solution should also be used to ensure optimal illumination through the fiberscope. Two suction devices should be available—one for the fiberscope and another for the Yankauer. A silicone spray or other lubricant is recommended to ensure easy advancement of the tracheal tube over the fiberscope. The **ovassapian airway** is particularly useful as a guide for flexible fiberoptic orotracheal intubation.

Although not widely used in the field now because of cost, there are several new versions of fiberscopes that may become available soon, making fiberoptic field intubations more feasible. Rigid fiberoptic laryngoscopy with anatomically shaped blades (e.g., Bullard laryngoscope[38-40] and Wuscope[33,41,42]) are also reliable techniques to visualize the glottis and intubate the trachea. Unlike conventional laryngoscopy, the Bullard and Wuscope devices do not require head and neck movement to obtain a Grade 1 view of the vocal cords. The WuScope is composed of a rigid blade portion and a flexible fiberscope (Chapter 10). The rigid blade is anatomically shaped to match the pharyngeal contour of the oral airway, thus allowing oral access to the glottis without tongue displacement or head extension. The tubular blade of the WuScope creates more viewing and intubating space and permits oral intubation in patients with limited mouth opening. At least 20 mm of mouth opening, however, is necessary to insert and manipulate the rigid fiberoptic blades. The WuScope also has a separate channel for providing supplemental oxygen.

Rigid fiberoptic laryngoscopy using the Wuscope was associated with easy glottic exposure and tracheal intubation in patients with c-spine instability.[41] In a randomized study of fiberoptic Wuscope versus conventional laryngoscopy in 87 patients with c-spine immobilization, the Wuscope was associated with Grade 1 views of the glottis in 98% of the patients, whereas 39% of patients in the conventional laryngoscopy group had Cormack Grade 3 or 4 views.[41] The Wuscope can also be used for the placement of double-lumen endotracheal tubes (sizes 35 Fr and 37 Fr) or Univent bronchial blocking tubes in patients with c-spine instability who require one-lung ventilation.[43]

The laryngeal mask airway (LMA) can provide a rapid clear airway in fasted patients with c-spine injuries presenting for elective surgeries. The LMA can also be used as an aid to flexible fiberoptic intubation and as a bridging maneuver in the case of failed intubation. The intubating LMA (iLMA) allows "blind" placement of an endotracheal tube of up to 8.0 mm I.D. However, the iLMA exerts greater pressures against the cervical vertebrae than do other intubation techniques (e.g., flexible fiberoptic) and can produce posterior displacement of the c-spine.[44] Moreover, the rigid iLMA tube compresses the posterior pharynx and has resulted in severe pharyngeal edema in patients undergoing anterior c-spine fixation.[45] The lightwand has also been used successfully in patients with c-spine disorders and had a higher success rate compared with the iLMA (97% versus 73%).[46]

Urgent and Emergent Cases

Conventional laryngoscopy is a faster means to secure the airway than most other techniques. RSI with conventional laryngoscopy has not been shown to increase the risk of c-spine injuries as long as the head and neck are kept in a neutral position throughout the intubation procedure.[4] With RSI, it is advisable to remove the rigid cervical collar after applying MIAS because the collar restricts mouth opening[47] and impedes the performance of cricoid pressure or external laryngeal manipulation. Anesthesia may be induced with thiopental, etomidate, ketamine, midazolam, or propofol.[48] Induction agents may need to be given in reduced dosages to prevent hypotension and myocardial depression, which might jeopardize spinal cord perfusion. Neuromuscular relaxants such as succinylcholine, vecuronium, or rocuronium can be used.[33] Proliferation of extrajunctional acetylcholine receptors requires at least 24 to 48 hours after denervation injury.[27,48] Thus, succinylcholine-induced hyperkalemia is unlikely to occur in the acute setting.

When using conventional laryngoscopy, the operator must be prepared for a higher incidence of Grade 3 laryngeal views. External laryngeal manipulation or backward pressure on the thyroid cartilage applied by the operator's right hand often improves the view at laryngoscopy.[49,50] The simple maneuver of having the assistant ease up or release previously applied cricoid pressure during RSI under direct laryngoscope vision may alleviate airway distortion and permit rapid insertion of the tube through the vocal cords.[51] The benefit of rapidly inserting the tracheal tube and inflating the cuff outweighs the potential risk of aspiration during the brief time that the cricoid pressure is not being applied.

The McCoy Corazelli London or Heine CL flex tip laryngoscope blade has a hinged blade tip that is controlled by a lever attached to the blade (Figure 14-6). This laryngo-

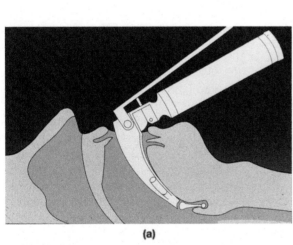
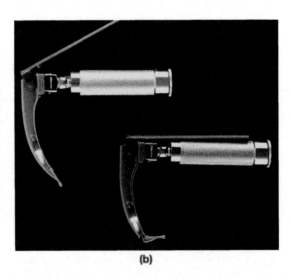

(a) (b)

FIGURE 14-6

(a) The McCoy laryngoscope blade has a hinged blade tip that is controlled by a lever attached to the blade. The tip of the blade adjusts through 70° by squeezing the lever, which allows the epiglottis to be elevated to expose the glottic opening without requiring excessive lifting force or c-spine movement.
(Courtesy of Dr. Charles E. Smith)
(b) How activation of the lever flexes the blade tip, which stretches the hyoepiglottic ligament within the valleculae, thus further lifting the epiglottis and improving the laryngeal view.
(Courtesy of Dr. Charles E. Smith)

scope blade, which attaches to a standard laryngoscope handle, allows the epiglottis to be elevated without requiring excessive lifting force and significantly improves the view at laryngoscopy in patients with c-spine immobilization.[34,35,52] Use of the McCoy laryngoscope is invaluable for improving the laryngeal view and facilitating intubation in adult patients with difficult airway anatomy. Of particular note is the very short learning curve for using this blade.

The gum-elastic bougie is used to facilitate tracheal intubation in patients with c-spine immobilization whenever a Grade 3 view is encountered.[32] (See also Chapter 5 for rapid sequence intubation.) While performing direct laryngoscopy and maintaining adequate laryngoscopic force to keep the epiglottis in full view, the bougie is introduced by the operator and gently advanced anteriorly under the epiglottis and into the trachea. With the operator still maintaining laryngoscopic force, a second operator then inserts the endotracheal tube over the bougie. Occasionally, the tube may need to be rotated 90° to facilitate its passage through the glottis. It is relatively easy to insert a bougie through the glottic opening when only the epiglottis (Grade 3 view) or posterior aspect of the glottis (Grade 2 view) can be visualized. Tracheal placement is then confirmed using end-tidal carbon dioxide (ETCO$_2$).

PEARLS   External laryngeal manipulation (BURP) can convert *Cormack and Lehane* Grade 3 view to a Grade 4 view.

Depending on skills, experience, and other factors, urgent and emergency tracheal intubation can also be performed using a variety of techniques including, but not limited to, rigid fiberoptic laryngoscopy (e.g., Wuscope, Bullard), flexible fiberoptic, and lighted stylets.[19] Cricothyrotomy is appropriate when emergency tracheal intubation is required and other techniques have failed or the pharynx is obscured by copious amounts of blood or vomitus.[53] The LMA or Combitube are recommended as nondefinitive airways when tracheal intubation has failed and there is difficulty with bag-mask ventilation.

Summary

Major trauma is associated with a 2% to 6% risk of c-spine injury. Motor-vehicle collisions account for the majority of these injuries. C-spine x-rays are indicated for all trauma patients who have midline neck pain, palpation tenderness, neurologic abnormality referable to the c-spine, altered level of consciousness, or suspected intoxication. No imaging modality is accurate 100% of the time, although most injuries can be detected with a three-view spine series and CT supplementation. Manual in-line axial stabilization is an effective technique to prevent c-spine movement during intubation but may result in an increased incidence of difficulty with vocal cord exposure using conventional laryngoscopy. Moreover, rigid cervical collars restrict mouth opening and further decrease the chance of seeing the laryngeal inlet using direct laryngoscopy.

There are no prospective studies documenting that any intubation technique is either safe or dangerous provided that immobilization precautions are maintained. Awake intubation techniques permit neurologic evaluation after intubation. Intubation after induction of general anesthesia and neuromuscular blockade provides excellent intubating conditions, especially in patients who are not cooperative or who cannot be adequately sedated. The optimal method of intubation ultimately depends on the patient's condition, the degree of cooperation, the urgency of the situation, and the skills of the airway operator.

REVIEW QUESTIONS

1. What percentage of spinal injuries are to the cervical spine?

2. At what level of the c-spine can injury cause disruption of all the muscles used in respiration?

3. List four indicators for field immobilization of the c-spine.

4. When is axial traction recommended in the field?

5. How does manual in-line axial stabilization (MIAS) affect the ability to intubate in the field?

6. List several techniques and devices that can be used to achieve airway control and ventilation in the spine-injured patient.

Burns and
Inhalation Injuries

Gary F. Purdue
Brett D. Arnoldo
John L. Hunt

Gary F. Purdue
Brett D. Arnoldo
John L. Hunt

Chapter Objectives

After reading this chapter, you should be able to:

* Recognize the different types of airway injury specifically associated with burns.

* Describe the treatment modalities most appropriate for each type of injury.

* Apply the treatment modalities unique to the burn patient.

* Recognize the need for a surgical airway and be aware of its limitations in both adults and children.

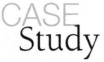

CASE
Study _____

Fire department personnel respond to an apartment fire, where they find a woman unconscious in her smoke-filled bedroom. The victim is immediately removed to safety, and oxygen is administered by face mask pending the arrival of the paramedics. When the Medic unit arrives, they find a 60-year-old female lying on the ground receiving oxygen. The paramedics begin treatment by opening her airway using a jaw-thrust manever. As they do so, they notice sooty deposits in and around her mouth and nose.

The patient is tachypneic, with a respiratory rate of 32 breaths per minute and, on auscultation of her chest, moist crackles are audible throughout both lungs. Neurological assessment reveals no eye opening, but the patient is making incomprehensible moaning sounds and withdrawing from pain, so they assign her a Glasgow Coma Scale score of 7.

While monitors are being applied, the paramedics decide to assist spontaneous respirations with a bag-valve-mask (BVM) fitted with an oxygen reservoir. Monitors reveal a blood pressure of 180/90 mm Hg, sinus tachycardia at a rate of 120 beats per minute, and an oxygen saturation level of 100%. Aware that carbon monoxide poisoning gives falsely high SpO$_2$ readings, and also suspecting inhalation injury to the respiratory tract, the paramedics prepare for intubation. An intravenous line is established, and the patient is given 5 mg of diazepam and 200 mcg of fentanyl IV. Cricoid pressure is applied as the medications take affect.

Direct laryngoscopy is performed, and the larynx is clearly identified. The laryngoscopist notices carbon particles in the hypopharynx and sees that edema is beginning to form around the glottic opening. A 7.0 mm endotracheal tube is advanced between the vocal cords, and correct placement of the tube is confirmed using an end-tidal carbon dioxide ($ETCO_2$) monitor and chest auscultation. Postintubation management is initiated, and the patient is transported to the regional burn center.

Introduction

The patient with burn or inhalation injury often presents problems not seen in other patient categories.

Hypoxic Injury

Hypoxia is the most common cause of death at the fire scene and is most often associated with burns sustained in a closed-space environment. The resulting altered level of consciousness is additive to that of intoxication with drugs or alcohol. The "lucky" survivor of a fatal structure fire is at special risk of hypoxic injury. Significant injury should be suspected in patients who are removed from a closed-space fire by others (such as firefighters) because such a situation implies a depressed level of consciousness or severity of injury such that the patient is unable to extricate him- or herself, with subsequent prolonged exposure. The heart and brain are the organs most sensitive to hypoxic injury. Thus, a first arterial blood gas showing a metabolic acidosis that is not corrected by hyperventilation (pH < 7.4 associated with a pCO_2 < 40) is one marker of this injury and portends future neurologic dysfunction if the patient survives.[1]

Carbon Monoxide Poisoning

Exposure to carbon monoxide, one of the products of incomplete combustion, is a difficult clinical diagnosis to make because the classic findings of cherry red mucosa, nausea, and headaches are usually absent in the hypoxic, smoke-stained burn patient. Hemoglobin has approximately 210 times the affinity for carbon monoxide than it has for oxygen and shifts the oxygen-hemoglobin disassociation curve to the left. Calculated saturations and pulse oximetry are inaccurate monitors of physiologic homeostasis in the presence of elevated carboxyhemoglobin (COHb). Normal levels of COHb are <5 mg/dL and <10 for smokers, with higher levels being seen in highway and tollbooth workers and those chronically exposed to automobile exhaust. An elevated COHb indicates potential for an inhalation injury, while normal COHb levels do not rule out smoke inhalation. Carboxyhemoglobin levels are only very poorly related, however, to severity of a concomitant inhalation injury, mortality, and ultimate neurologic outcome. The half-life of COHb is four hours while breathing room air, decreasing after about 40 minutes on 100% oxygen. Treatment is administration of high-flow oxygen via nonrebreathing mask in the field, followed by endotracheal intubation as indicated by the patient's clinical status. The goal of therapy is to decrease COHb to less than 20 mg/dL. Treatment of carbon monoxide poisoning with hyperbaric oxygen has been shown to decrease neurologic sequelae at 6 and 12 months postinjury in nonburned patients.[2,3] However, in patients with significant burns, hyperbaric oxygen treatment increased both morbidity and mortality.[4] Exchange transfusions have no useful role.

Upper Airway

Singeing of nasal and facial hair is a poor indicator for the need of airway control, which is almost never needed in the absence of a significant neck burn.

Burn injuries are associated with an underlying capillary leak, resulting in edema development causing subsequent swelling that is roughly proportional to the size of the cutaneous burn. Significant burns of the lower face, neck, and upper chest may be associated with sufficient pharyngeal and supraglottic swelling to occlude the upper airway, creating a high-mortality airway emergency. Isolated burns above the mandibular border rarely cause airway obstruction, while the unique anatomy of the supraglottic area makes it sensitive to edema development. This creates a one-way valve, initially allowing exhalation but not inhalation, especially under positive pressure.[5] Further swelling causes obstruction to both inhalation and exhalation.

Actual heat injury of the upper airway is relatively rare as the result of the thermal transfer capabilities of the upper airway. Singeing of nasal and facial hair is a poor indicator for the need of airway control, which is almost never needed in the absence of a significant neck burn. Progressive obliteration of the normal external anatomy of the neck (skin wrinkles, thyroid cartilage, and anterior border of the sternocleidomastoid muscle) are indirect signs indicating the need for airway control, while hoarseness is an indefinite indicator, dependent to some extent on the degree of preexamination screaming and yelling by the patient. Stridor is a very late sign of loss of airway integrity, signaling the need for immediate airway control. Neck and airway edema is very resuscitation and gravity dependent.

Elevation of the head of the bed to 45° and careful management of resuscitation volumes may abrogate the need for intubation or delay the need for emergent intubation. The smaller airway of children places them at increased risk for airway obstruction. Endotracheal intubation is performed in anticipation of continued swelling, which usually continues until 24 to 30 hours postinjury, with the procedure becoming progressively more difficult with increased swelling. The edema then gradually subsides over the next several days. When the patient is hypovolemic, infusion of even small volumes of resuscitation fluid may result in rapid catastrophic airway occlusion (Figure 15-1), mandating airway control before vigorous resuscitation.

A special case is the chronic obstructive pulmonary disease (COPD) patient who sustains a flash injury while smoking on home oxygen, the vast majority of whom do not require airway control. These patients should be treated with elevation of the head of the bed, oxygen at the same rate as they were receiving preburn, and transfer to a burn center.

Airway management in the acute burn situation is best approached as a "difficult airway" with an awake, sedated, and spontaneously breathing patient. Nasotracheal intubation is ideal in this situation. The technique requires significantly less sedation than does the

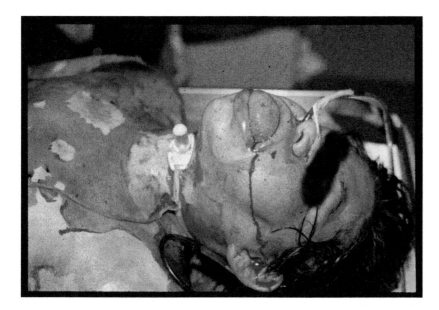

FIGURE 15-1

Catastrophic airway compromise, with failure of endotracheal intubation and subsequent insertion of cricothyroidotomy. Note the presence of flash pulmonary edema in the tube.
(Courtesy of Gary F. Purdue, MD)

orotracheal route, is very well tolerated, and may be performed with the patient in the head-up position. The nasotracheal route should be avoided in patients with a known history of sinusitis.[6]

Drug distribution and therapeutic effects in acute burn patients are often unpredictable due to third space distribution and variable pharmacokinetics. Our own protocol utilizes intravenous pharmacologic doses of morphine and diazepam (10 mg of each in the adult) given repeatedly until intubation can be accomplished. This may require more than 50 mg of each up to 90 mg. While midazolam has more rapid onset, its shorter duration makes repetitive stacking of doses more difficult. Although somewhat tedious, this technique is safe, because it avoids aspiration and the need for a surgical airway, and provides amnesia for the process.

PEARLS When the patient is hypovolemic, infusion of even small volumes of resuscitation fluid may result in rapid catastrophic airway occlusion. Therefore, airway control should be done before vigorous fluid resuscitation.

ON TARGET Avoid RSI. The apneic patient may have airway collapse and turn into a cannot-mask-ventilate/cannot-intubate patient if initial intubation is unsuccessful, causing the patient to need an emergent surgical airway.

We have used this technique in more than 1,000 consecutive patients with only two failures to intubate, both requiring a semi-urgent surgical airway. Fiberoptic intubation in this acute setting is made difficult by pharyngeal edema and friability, although the technique is very effective during later difficult elective airway intubations. Rapid sequence intubation is to be avoided because the apneic patient may have airway collapse and may not be able to be ventilated if initial intubation is unsuccessful, thus converting an urgent procedure into the need for an emergent surgical airway. All of our emergent surgical airways and most of the urgent ones are related to rapid sequence intubation, with subsequent inability to either intubate or ventilate the patient.

- Case 1: A 15-year-old male sustains a 10% total body surface area (TBSA) flash burn of his face and both arms while igniting trash with gasoline. His eyebrows and nasal hairs are singed, his lips are mildly edematous, and external neck anatomy (wrinkles, SCM, and thyroid cartilage) are visible. The patient is not having respiratory distress. Should this patient have his airway controlled? No. There is minimal if any risk of airway problems. Maintain minimal fluids during transport and keep the head of the bed elevated.

- Case 2: A 30-year-old female was using gasoline to clean tar tracked onto her kitchen floor, causing a 50% TBSA burn of her face, neck, chest, back arms, abdomen, and both lower legs. She is not discovered until two hours after injury. Physical examination is normal other than circumferential blistering of her neck. She is not in respiratory distress. Should this patient have her airway controlled? Yes. She is a setup for catastrophic upper airway obstruction. Endotracheally intubate using conscious sedation technique (morphine and valium) via either nasal or oral route. Do this prior to infusion of large amounts of resuscitation fluid because airway edema develops very rapidly under these circumstances. If facilities are not available for intubation, transport with the head of the bed elevated and KVO intravenous fluids. Intravenous access in some burn patients is not possible, necessitating the use of an intraosseous fluid line (Figure 15-2).

- Case 3: A 65-year-old male smoker sustains a presumed smoke inhalation injury and a 3% TBSA to both hands in a house fire. He is alert and oriented times three. His face has carbon staining, and there is carbon on his tongue and in his nares. He is not in respiratory distress. Should he be intubated and placed on mechanical ventilation? No. Treatment of smoke inhalation injury is expectant. Good **pulmonary toilet** and spot O_2 saturations are sufficient treatment, with intubation reserved for the same indications as any other surgical or medical patient (decreasing saturation, hypoventilation, tachypnea, work of breathing, and inability to protect the airway).

pulmonary toilet
Endotracheal suctioning of secretions.

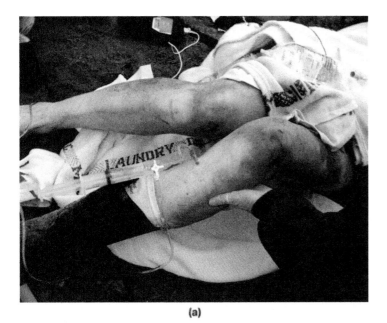

(a)

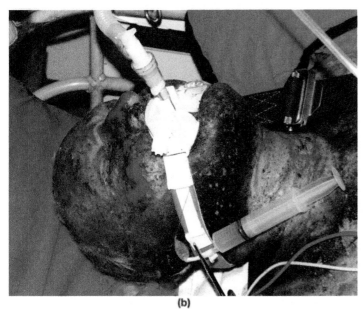

(b)

FIGURE 15-2

(a) Because of the extent of the burn injuries, no upper limb sites were available for venous cannulation, so an intraosseous needle was inserted into the upper tibia to allow administration of drugs prior to intubation.
(Courtesy of Dr. Andrew M. Mason)

(b) Casualty with 80% full-thickness burns, who had rapidly developing stridor due to burns to the upper airway. A supra-glottic device is not appropriate under these circumstances. A tracheal tube is in place en route to the hospital. The tube is stabilized and protected by means of a Thomas tube holder, which has an integral bite block.
(Courtesy of Dr. Andrew M. Mason)

Securing the endotracheal tube is paramount because inadvertent extubation of the acutely burned patient often results in death. The tube is secured in position with umbilical tape or a commercially available device (such as Endosecure®) because adhesive tape does not provide secure positioning due to adhesive lysis by burn fluid or topical antimicrobials (Figure 15-2). Fixation adjustments are made to compensate for early swelling of the face and tongue and its later resolution, thereby preventing either oral/facial necrosis or endotracheal tube misplacement. Appropriate sedation is maintained to ensure tube protection.

Lower Airway

microatelectasis
Microscopic collapse of alveoli.

Inhalation of the products of combustion creates a chemical pneumonitis, with distal airway swelling, closure, and **microatelectasis**, with a clinical course similar to **acute respiratory distress syndrome (ARDS)**. The products of combustion include hydrogen chloride,

acute respiratory distress syndrome (ARDS)
Severe respiratory distress due to inflammatory damage that causes increased permeability of the alveolar capillary membranes, which in turn causes fluid leakage into the alveoli.

hydrogen cyanide, chlorine, phosgene, formic acid, aldehydes, and the toxic oxides of nitrogen and sulfur. Two of these (phosgene and chlorine) are war gasses designed to produce pulmonary injury.

Burning synthetic materials are generally more toxic than natural ones. While the sine qua non of smoke inhalation is a history of being trapped in a closed, smoke-filled space, this injury is occasionally seen with brief open exposures to very toxic chemicals such as burning polyvinyl chloride (PVC) used in siding, pipes and electrical insulation, chemical fumes, and anhydrous ammonia (used as fertilizer and illicit manufacture of methamphetamines).

Carbon-stained oropharyngeal/nasal mucosa and carbonaceous sputum are poor indicators of a significant injury, as are singed nasal or facial hair. Initial chest x-ray and arterial blood gasses are usually within normal limits, even with severe, rapidly fatal injury. Early treatment is guided by the patient's clinical respiratory and neurologic status, not by the history of inhalation injury. Prophylactic intubation in the absence of face and neck burns is not indicated.

Pulmonary toilet is the cornerstone of care with endotracheal intubation and mechanical ventilation; it is utilized for the same indications as for any surgical or medical patient (inability to maintain the airway, inability to clear secretions and adequately oxygenate or ventilate the patient, tachypnea or increased work of breathing). Provision of adequate suctioning during early care and transport is paramount with inhalation patients because they are extremely prone to mucous/carbon plugging of the endotracheal tubes. Deteriorating respiratory status in the presence of newly developing bronchospasm manifested by wheezing and increased ventilatory pressures is the hallmark of a ball-valve obstruction of the tube, requiring replacement of the endotracheal tube or creation of a surgical airway, depending on the clinical situation.

PEARLS Deteriorating respiratory status in the presence of newly developing bronchospasm manifested by wheezing and increased ventilatory pressures is the hallmark of a ball-valve obstruction of the tube, requiring replacement of the ET tube or creation of a surgical airway.

inspissated secretions
Thickened secretions.

Diagnosis of inhalation injury is often a retrospective one based on the patient's clinical course, although fiberoptic bronchoscopy or xenon-133 scanning may assist in early evaluation. Treatment of smoke inhalation injury with high-frequency percussive ventilation (VDR) and clearance of **inspissated secretions** with nebulized heparin, acetylcystine, and albuteral may improve mortality.[7,8] Administration of steroids and prophylactic antibiotics are contraindicated.

Steam Inhalation

Burns below the pharynx are extremely rare, except where the mechanism is steam inhalation. This injury is usually of industrial origin involving heating systems or power generation. Steam carries approximately 2,000 times the amount of heat that air does and has the capacity to create burns to the level of the distal airways. The resulting scald-type injury is generally worse than originally expected (usually full thickness despite an initial superficial appearance) and is often associated with a large cutaneous burn. Treatment is endotracheal intubation and excellent pulmonary toilet of mucosal slough and hemorrhagic necrosis. The outcome is extremely poor.

PEARLS Steam carries approximately 2,000 times the amount of heat that air does.

Diagnosis and Treatment

The methods of diagnosis and treatment are individualized for the specific type of injury, as noted above, and are to a large extent influenced by burn size. Approximately 7% of burn patients (15% of electrical burns) sustain multiple trauma in addition to their burns and require appropriate modifications for those injuries (in-line stabilization, etc).

Special Considerations

Modifications of standard techniques are based on the pathophysiology associated with gradual edema formation and subsequent resolution and with later formation of scarring and contraction and poor pulmonary function.

Surgical Airway

Emergency creation of a surgical airway in the early postburn period is difficult at best because of swelling, with obliteration of both the midline and lateral landmarks; the presence of subcutaneous edema; and edema fluid in the surgical wound, making visualization difficult. Good lighting, functioning suction, and an adequate surgical incision are priorities. Choice of vertical or horizontal incisions depends on the comfort level of the provider, although we generally prefer a transverse incision. Blind techniques such as needle cricothyroidotomy have the risk of deep structure injury in the absence of visible or palpable landmarks resulting from thick burn eschar and swelling and should be considered only as a last resort.

If required in a patient with a large burn, early tracheostomy/cricothyroidotomy may necessitate insertion of an endotracheal tube through the stoma to prevent accidental decannulation of a standard-length tracheostomy tube as the result of continued postburn swelling. Cricothyroidotomy is contraindicated in children under age 10 years because inadvertent severing of the cricoid ring can cause tracheal collapse.

Summary

The burn patient has unique presentation and pathophysiology, which create needs for airway control and mechanical ventilation different from that of most trauma patients. The following points should be considered in prehospital management of the burn patient. Administer 100% oxygen by nonrebreathing mask. Elevate the head of the bed. Intubate only if the patient is in respiratory distress or when transport times will be long enough to risk airway loss by swelling. Avoid RSI if at all possible.

REVIEW QUESTIONS

1. What is the most common cause of death at the fire scene?

2. What is the field treatment for carbon monoxide poisoning?

3. What kinds of injury are most likely to lead to airway obstruction?

4. What prehospital measures may help in abrogating the necessity for intubation in the field?

5. What is the role of awake intubation in the burn patient?

6. Why should RSI be avoided in the burn patient?

7. What findings should guide treatment decisions of burn patients in the field?

8. What is the role of pulmonary toilet in intubated patients?

9. What complications can be encountered with surgical airway procedures?

The Pediatric Airway

Abid U. Ghafoor
Timothy W. Martin
James Michael Rich

Chapter Objectives

After reading this chapter, you should be able to:

- List at least five major differences between the normal pediatric and adult airways.

- Describe assessment of the pediatric airway.

- Describe at least 10 conditions that may be associated with difficult-airway management in children.

- Explain methods of providing supplemental oxygen to the child in whom oxygenation is impaired.

- Describe the various alternatives for nonintubation management of the pediatric airway.

- Describe the pharmacological agents and procedures involved in rapid sequence induction (RSI) of the child.

- Describe at least five alternative methods for intubation after classic RSI has failed.

- Discuss the role of the laryngeal mask airway (LMA) in pediatric airway management.

- Describe the options for emergency oxygenation and ventilation when attempts at intubation have failed.

- List at least five complications of intubation in the child.

CASE Study _____

Medic 3 is dispatched to the home of a 16-year-old female with severe abdominal pain. As they pull into the drive, the girl's mother runs out of the house and tells the crew that her daughter has just given birth to a baby on the bathroom floor. She adds that she had no idea that her daughter was pregnant. The paramedics immediately ask Medical Control to send a backup vehicle. Then they pick up their adult and pediatric grab bags and follow the woman into the house.

In the bathroom, the full-term infant is lying motionless in his mother's arms and has obvious central and peripheral cyanosis. His mother appears to be in a satisfactory condition, so the crew switch their attention to the baby. There is no sign of breathing, so the baby's mouth and nose are suctioned and the airway opened using the head-tilt/chin-lift maneuver. One of the paramedics spots a small hand towel, folds it, and places it beneath the infant's shoulders to maintain the airway in the correct position. The baby still makes no effort to breathe, so the crew make preparations for ventilation with a pediatric bag-valve-mask (BVM) fitted with an oxygen reservoir. One of the paramedics applies the mask to the infant's face and performs a jaw-thrust maneuver, while the other gently squeezes the bag at a rate of 60 per minute. There is good rise and fall of the chest.

After 30 seconds, the infant is still not breathing, so the correct size of oropharyngeal airway is selected and inserted while the pulse is being palpated. The brachial pulse rate is 50 per minute, so the crew start two-rescuer CPR. The paramedic performing chest compressions positions his hands to encircle the infant's chest and position his thumbs on the sternum, and gives compressions at a rate of 120 per minute. CPR is delivered with a ratio of 15 compressions to two ventilations. After 30 seconds, the pulse is rechecked and has risen to 60 per minute, so CPR is continued. After a further 30 seconds, the pulse has risen to 90 per minute, and the infant is beginning to make efforts to breathe, so chest compressions are stopped.

Monitoring electrodes are applied to the infant's chest, and the paramedics continue with mask ventilations until the monitored heart rate is seen to reach 120 per minute, by which time the central cyanosis has disappeared and the respiratory rate has increased to 30 per minute. Blow-by oxygen is then given as the umbilical cord is clamped and cut. The backup crew arrives, but Medic 3 can transport both mother and baby to the hospital without their assistance.

Introduction

The pediatric patient is *not* a little adult. This chapter focuses on emergency management of the pediatric airway and how it differs from the adult. It also illustrates how the pediatric patient may respond differently to medications in comparison to the adult patient. The chapter also discusses the important issue of oxygenation/ventilation versus tracheal intubation in pediatrics. American Heart Association Guidelines 2005 on confirmation of tracheal intubation, monitoring of lung ventilation, use of a cuffed tracheal tube, and the use of adjunctive ventilation devices in pediatrics are also reviewed.

KEY TERMS

arthrogryposis, pp. 273, 278

Beckwith-Wiedemann syndrome, pp. 273, 274

Bullard laryngoscope, p. 278

Carpenter syndrome, p. 273

commissure, p. 269

Crouzon syndrome, p. 273

Freeman-Sheldon syndrome, pp. 273, 274

glycopyrrolate, p. 281

Goldenhar syndrome, p. 278

hemangioma, pp. 273, 278

hypotonia, pp. 273, 278

Klipper-Feil syndrome, pp. 273, 278

lymphangioma, pp. 273, 277

micrognathia, pp. 273, 278

mucopolysaccharidosis (MPS), pp. 273, 277

neurofibroma, pp. 273, 277

Pierre-Robin syndrome, p. 273

Shikani seeing stylet, p. 278

Stickler's syndrome, p. 273

Treacher-Collins syndrome, pp. 273, 274

velocardiofacial syndrome, p. 273

Differences Between Pediatric and Adult Airway Anatomy and Respiratory Physiology

A clear understanding of pediatric airway anatomy is important in providing effective airway management in an emergency. The pediatric airway differs from that of the adult in its consistency, size, position, and shape. Understanding the differences between the normal pediatric and adult airways is the first step toward successfully managing the infant and pediatric airway

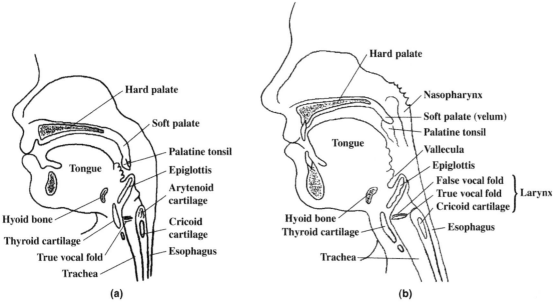

FIGURE 16-1

Sagittal section showing normal airway anatomy of (a) a child and (b) an adult. Note the position of the larynx, which is more anterior and cephalad in the neck of a child compared to the neck of an adult.
(Courtesy of Abid U. Ghafoor, MD)

ON TARGET

Young infants (less than approximately two to three months of age) are obligate nose breathers, and any obstruction in the nasal passages may severely impair air movement in and out of the lungs.

commissure
The place where two structures meet.

with skill and confidence. Anatomic differences (Figure 16-1) between the pediatric and the adult upper airways can affect both mask ventilation and endotracheal intubation.[1] These differences are listed in Table 16-1.

Young infants (less than approximately two to three months of age) are obligate nose breathers, and any obstruction in the nasal passages may severely impair air movement in and out of the lungs. The smaller diameter of the trachea in infants increases the significance of tracheal mucosal edema (Figure 16-2). One millimeter of edema of the tracheal mucosa may substantially reduce the airway cross-sectional area, causing stridor, an increase in the work of breathing, and even airway obstruction. Infants may also suffer from congenital vascular rings, slings, and other congenital cardiovascular anomalies, which may affect the airway and breathing. Because of the relatively high position of the pediatric larynx in the neck, laryngeal injuries are uncommon; the mandible generally provides protection against traumatic injuries.[4]

Table 16-1 Anatomic Differences Between the Adult and Pediatric Airways

- Children have a relatively larger tongue.
- Head is relatively larger in children, which is naturally flexed in supine position.
- Nasal passages are narrow in children compared to adults.
- Children have a larynx that is more anterior and cephalad in the neck at the C3–C4 level, as compared to C4–C5 in adults.
- Epiglottis is shorter and has a more acute angle over glottis.
- Vocal cords are slanted, and the anterior **commissure** is more inferior.
- Larynx is cone-shaped (Figure 16-2) and is narrowest at subglottic cricoid ring area in children younger than eight years, as opposed to the glottis in adults.[2]
- Airway is softer and more pliable.[3]
- Extension of head may result in tracheal extubation, while flexion may lead to mainstem intubation.

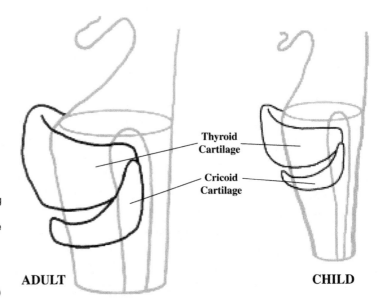

Certain points must be presented with regard to foreign-body airway obstruction in children. Prior to treating the patient, determine if the obstruction is partial or complete. Patients with a partial airway obstruction have a cough, hoarse voice or cry, stridor, or some other evidence that at least some air is passing through the airway. Avoid any maneuvers that may turn a partial obstruction into a complete one. The best thing to do in this situation is to place the patient in a comfortable position and transport as rapidly as possible. To treat a complete airway obstruction, Bledsoe et al. recommend the following age-specific maneuvers:[5] for children older than one year of age, perform a series of abdominal thrusts; for infants (younger than one year old), deliver a series of five back blows followed by five chest thrusts. Inspect the infant's mouth on completion of each series. Never check a pediatric patient's mouth with blind finger sweeps.

> **Note**
>
> According to AHA Guidelines 2005—Streamlining Actions for Relief of Foreign Body Airway Obstruction,[6] simplified terms like *mild airway obstruction* and *severe airway obstruction* are now used to distinguish choking victims who require intervention from those who do not. Rescuers should act if they observe signs and symptoms of severe airway obstruction: poor air exchange and increased breathing difficulty, a silent cough, cyanosis, or inability to speak or breathe. If, in response to the question, "Are you choking?" the victim nods yes, help is required. If the victim becomes unresponsive, all rescuers are instructed to activate the emergency response number at the appropriate time and provide CPR. Another change from previous guidelines: every time the rescuer opens the airway (with a head-tilt/chin-lift) to deliver rescue breaths, the rescuer should look in the mouth and remove an object if one is seen. The tongue-jaw lift is no longer taught, and blind finger sweeps should not be performed. The goal of these revisions is simplification. Experts could find no evidence that a complicated series of maneuvers is any more effective than simple CPR. Some studies showed that chest compressions performed during CPR increased intrathoracic pressure as high as or higher than abdominal thrusts. In addition, blind finger sweeps may result in injury to the victim's mouth and throat or to the rescuer's finger, and no evidence suggests that they are effective.

Children have:
- Increased rate of respiration.
- Increased chest wall compliance.
- Decreased lung elastic recoil.
- Decreased functional residual capacity (reduced oxygen reserve in lung).
- Increased metabolism and oxygen consumption.

Infants and children are more likely than adults to experience rapid arterial oxyhemoglobin desaturation due to several factors, which are listed in Table 16-2. Infants and children consume two to three times more oxygen per kilogram of body weight than do adults due to factors related to growth and higher basal metabolic rates.[7] In infants and small children, closing volume (defined as the lung volume at which terminal airways in the lung begin to close) equals or exceeds functional residual capacity (FRC) (the lung volume following a typical exhalation); this effect may be aggravated by the effects of sedatives and muscle relaxants. The net result of the infant's higher oxygen consumption and decreased oxygen reserve in the lungs is a tendency toward rapid oxyhemoglobin desaturation, which is often amplified in the presence of coexisting lung disease.

Recognizing the Difficult Pediatric Airway

The term *difficult airway* implies difficulty with mask ventilation, endotracheal intubation, or both. It is important to recognize the potential difficult airway before using sedative agents and neuromuscular relaxants. Failure to do so can result in life-threatening situations in which oxygenation, ventilation, and intubation are impossible. Both knowledge and considerable judgment are required. The guidelines for pediatric airway assessment are listed in Table 16-3.[8]

In children, it is unusual to encounter a difficult airway when the specific anatomic markers of the abnormal airway, facial and upper airway trauma, or inflammation are absent. When time permits, a history of previous difficult-airway management should be sought in children with conditions known to predispose to airway difficulty.

Examination of the oropharynx and detection of facial anomalies is the first step in assessing the pediatric airway. The patient's oral cavity is examined with the mouth open and tongue maximally protruded. The size of the tongue relative to the oral cavity and the degree of mouth opening is assessed. Mallampati et al. proposed a classification of the adult airway based on the degree of visualization of the soft palate, faucial pillars, and uvula.[9] The ability to visualize these structures may predict the adequacy of laryngeal visualization in adults.

Indications for tracheal intubation in children are the same as those for an adult:[15] ventilatory support with a BVM is inadequate; the patient is in cardiac or respiratory arrest; a route for drug administration or ready access to the airway for suctioning is needed; prolonged artificial ventilation is necessary.

PEARLS Failure to recognize the difficult airway before using sedatives and neuromuscular relaxants can result in a life-threatening situation in which oxygenation, ventilation, and intubation are impossible.

Because the full cooperation of the child is often difficult to achieve, it may not be possible to assign a Mallampati score. However, distinctive facial features such as a short neck or a small receding chin may predict the possibility of a difficult airway. Furthermore, it is unknown whether the Mallampati score is a reliable predictor of the degree of difficult endotracheal intubation in small children.[10]

Table 16-3 Airway Evaluation, Minimal Acceptable/Desirable Values/Endpoints, and Significance of the Airway Examination for Adults and Pediatric Patients

Airway Evaluation, Examination	Minimal Acceptable/ Desirable/Values/Endpoints	Significance of Airway Examination
Intercisor distance	Greater than 3 cm	A positive result (> 3 cm) means that the 2 cm deep phlange on a Macintosh and Miller blade can be easily inserted without hitting the teeth.
Oropharyngeal class	Less than or equal to Class II	A positive result (≤ Class II) means that the tongue is reasonably small in relation to the size of the oropharyngeal cavity and is relatively easy to retract out of the line of sight.
Mandibular space (MS) length (thyromental distance)	Greater than or equal to 1.5 cm in infants and ≥ 5 cm in adults	A positive result means that the larynx is reasonably posterior relative to the other upper airway structures, resulting in a favorable line of sight.
Mandibular space compliance	Qualitative palpation of normal resilience/softness	A laryngoscope retracts the tongue in the mandibular space. The compliance of the mandibular space determines its ability to accept the tongue and create a favorable line of sight.
Range of motion of head and neck	Neck flexed on chest 35° + head extended on neck 80° = sniffing position	The sniffing position aligns the oral, pharyngeal, and laryngeal axes to create a favorable line of sight.
Length of neck	Qualitative.	A short neck decreases the ability to align the upper airway axes.
Thickness of neck	Qualitative.	A thick neck decreases the ability to align the upper airway axes.
Length of incisors	Qualitative/relative	Long incisors unalign the oral axis from the pharyngeal axis (creates a sharper angle between the two axes).
Involuntary anterior over-riding of maxillary teeth on the mandibular teeth	No overriding of maxillary teeth on mandibular teeth	Same as long incisors.
Configuration of the palate	Should not appear very narrow or highly arched	A narrow palate decreases the oropharyngeal volume and the ability to continue to visualize the larynx when both the laryngoscope and endotracheal tube are in the mouth.

Reproduced, with permission, from Benumof JL. The Laryngeal Mask airway and the ASA Difficult airway algorithm. Anesthesiology News 1996; October: pp. 4–21.

Evaluation of neck mobility is important because neck extension is often required to create a straight line of vision through the mouth to the glottic structures. Successful laryngoscopy often can be performed without neck extension, as may be necessary in the patient with cervical-spine trauma; however, conditions involving limited neck extension are associated with an increased incidence of difficult intubation.

The ideal mandible length, measured from the thyroid cartilage to the chin, should be greater than 1.5 cm in infants.[11] Patients with shorter mandibles present greater difficulty during laryngoscopy because of difficulty lining up the oral, pharyngeal, and laryngotracheal axes. The fundamental problem in patients with small or receding mandibles is a relative lack of displacement space into which the soft tissues of the floor of the mouth may be moved during laryngoscopy.

Table 16-4 Some Conditions Associated with Possible Difficult-Airway Management

- Syndromes with micrognathia
  - **Pierre-Robin sequence**
  - **Stickler's syndrome**
  - **Velocardiofacial syndrome**
  - Fetal alcohol syndrome
  - Isolated micrognathia
  - **Carpenter syndrome**
  - **Crouzon syndrome**
  - **Freeman-Sheldon syndrome**
  - **Treacher-Collins syndrome**
- Syndromes with limited cervical-spine mobility
  - Klippel-Feil syndrome
  - Goldenhar syndrome
  - Arthrogryposis
- Arthritis of cervical spine and temporomandibular joint
- Cervical-spine trauma
- Conditions with increased tongue size
  - **Beckwith-Wiedemann syndrome**
  - **Mucopolysaccharidosis**
  - Congenital hypothyroidism
  - Hemangiomas of the tongue
  - **Lymphangiomas** and **neurofibromas** of the tongue
  - Down syndrome
- Life-threatening infections
  - Croup
  - Retropharyngeal abscess
  - Bacterial tracheitis

When determining an airway management strategy, it is important to take into account the degree of any airway abnormality, any previous history of difficult-airway management, and the ability of the patient to tolerate physiologically the proposed airway procedure. It is imperative to consider these factors carefully before attempting to control the airway in the spontaneously breathing child. There are many conditions and congenital anomalies in the pediatric population that are associated with difficult-airway management (Table 16-4).

In syndromes with **micrognathia** (small submandibular space), the relationship of the size of the tongue to the mandible has been postulated as the cause of airway management difficulties.[12] All of these conditions force the tongue to a relatively posterior position within the oropharynx and interfere with visualization of the vocal cords during direct laryngoscopy, sometimes making it impossible to intubate the trachea under direct vision.

Syndromes with limited cervical motion, such as **Klippel-Feil syndrome** (fusion of cervical vertebrae), **Goldenhar syndrome** (epibulbar dermoid appendages, preauricular skin tags, vertebral anomalies, hemifacial microsomia, micrognathia, cardiac and renal anomalies), **arthrogryposis**, and arthritis of the temporomandibular joint, have limitation of the mouth opening and cervical-spine mobility during direct laryngoscopy, making it difficult to intubate patients with these conditions using conventional techniques.

Life-threatening infectious diseases such as laryngotracheobronchitis (croup) and epiglottitis (Table 16-5), retropharyngeal abscess, and bacterial tracheitis may also present as a difficult airway because of local edema and infection in and around the airway, with the increased possibility of laryngospasm during direct laryngoscopy (Figure 16-3). In conditions that cause increased tongue size (macroglossia) (Table 16-4), the large size of the tongue and oropharyngeal soft tissue relative to the oral cavity may narrow the air passages and present as a difficult airway[13] during both mask ventilation and endotracheal intubation.

Children with Down syndrome (trisomy 21) can present airway management challenges because of the larger tongue, relative **hypotonia,** and potential cervical-spine instability. The large tongue can make mask ventilation difficult, necessitating the use of an oral or nasal airway.

Any extrinsic soft-tissue lesion that is sufficiently large or that develops surrounding inflammation may also affect the airway. These lesions include neoplasms of the soft tissue of the neck (teratomas, neuroblastomas, lymphomas, and rhabdomyosarcoma), cystic hygromas, **hemangiomas,** and thyroid tumors. Post-traumatic hematoma resulting from cervical-spine

Table 16-5	Symptoms of Croup and Epiglottitis in Pediatric Patients[5]	
Croup	**Epiglottitis**
• Slow onset	• Rapid onset
• Patient generally wants to sit up	• Patient prefers to sit up
• Barking cough	• No barking cough
• No drooling	• Drooling; painful to swallow
• Fever approximately 101°F to 102°F (38.3°C to 38.9°C)	• Fever approximately 102°F to 104°F (38.9°C to 40.0°C)

Used by permission of PCPP, Volume 5, p. 93, Table 2-12.

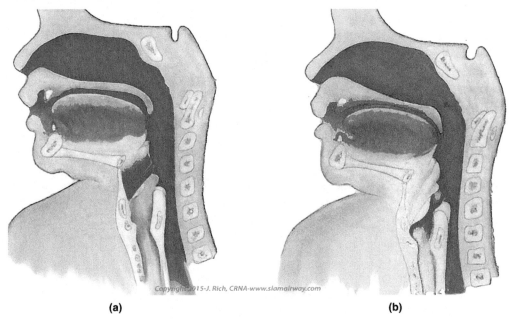

(a)   **(b)**

FIGURE 16-3

(a) Epiglottitis is characterized by inflammation of the epiglottis and supraglottic tissues. (b) Croup is characterized by subglottic edema.

injury and nontraumatic hematoma, as may occur with a bleeding disorder, can also compromise the airway.[14]

Emergency Pediatric Airway Management

Equipment

Proper equipment for pediatric airway management should be selected according to the age and weight of the patient (Table 16-6). New devices and medications have changed the emergency management of the pediatric airway in the past two decades. Most notable have been the rapid sequence induction and intubation (RSI) procedure, which employs cricoid pressure using Sellick's maneuver to help prevent aspiration as well as pharmacologic agents and other maneuvers to effect sedation and paralysis. RSI has dramatically improved the clinician's ability to secure the airway rapidly and support ventilation.[16] The success of airway management depends on the clinician's training, continual quality as-

Table 16-6 Equipment for Pediatric Airway Management[5,15]

Age/Weight	Oral Airway	Suction Catheter	Laryngoscope Blade	Tracheal Tube Size (age + 16 divided by 4)
Premature infant (1–2.5 kg)	Infant (00)	6–8	0 (straight)	2.5 to 3.0 (uncuffed)
Neonate (2.5–4.0 kg)	Infant (small) (0)	8	1 (straight)	3.0 to 3.5 (uncuffed)
6 months (7.0 kg)	Small (1)	8–10	1 (straight)	3.5 to 4.0 (uncuffed)
1–2 years (10–12 kg)	Small (2)	10	1 to 2 (straight)	4.0 to 4.5 (uncuffed)
2–5 years (16–18 kg)	Medium (3)	10–12	2 (straight or curved)	4.5 to 5.5 (uncuffed)
5–7 years (24–30 kg)	Medium large (4.5)	12	2 (straight) or 2 to 3 (curved)	5.5 to 6.5 (uncuffed)
7–15 years		12–14	2 (straight) or 3 (curved)	6.0 to 7.0 (cuffed)
16 years		14	2 to 3 (straight) or 3 (curved)	Greater than or equal to 7.0 (cuffed)

surance of proper techniques, and the frequency with which the clinician performs a particular intervention.[16,17] Medical personnel managing a difficult airway should devise a strategy according to personal preference, familiarity with the proposed procedure, and confidence level.

PEARLS Develop a personal strategy for difficult-airway management and practice until you are good at it.

The SLAM Universal Adult Airway Flowchart[18] (Chapter 1) was not designed for and is not intended for use in pediatric patients. The ASA difficult-airway algorithm has been in use for this purpose with some revision since 1991.[8,19,20] The ASA algorithm provides a guideline in the event one encounters a difficult airway in elective or emergent situations. Like most other algorithms, this serves as a helpful guideline and starting point; however, clinical expertise, judgment, and the experience of the practitioner managing the airway should guide the final approach.

As always, the management of the airway begins with evaluation of the airway. The evaluation of the airway should include assessment for the presence of all the conditions listed in Tables 16-3 and 16-4.[8] Indications for tracheal intubation in pediatrics are the same as those for an adult and should be understood and applied as needed.

For practical purposes, the emergency pediatric airway can be classified into three categories: the uncomplicated airway, the obviously difficult airway, and the difficult airway that is not anticipated.

PEARLS In young children and infants, particularly those with respiratory problems, change your RSI technique to provide gentle positive-pressure ventilation pending laryngoscopy and intubation to minimize desaturation.

Patients can generally be assumed to have a full stomach in situations where the need for emergent intubation arises. If the patient is assessed as having an uncomplicated airway, RSI should be performed (Table 16-7). RSI is an airway management technique that is designed

Table 16-7 Technique for RSI

1. Preoxygenate the patient with 100% oxygen using basic manual and adjunctive maneuvers and using a BVM, if indicated. Ensure that cricoid pressure is being applied during positive-pressure mask ventilation.

2. Prepare your equipment, your supplies, and the patient. In addition to the usual intubating equipment, be certain you have at least one, and preferably two, secure and working IV lines. Place the patient on a cardiac monitor and pulse oximeter. Draw the appropriate doses of medications into syringes and label them.

3. If the patient is alert, administer a sedative (induction) agent, such as midazolam (Versed), prior to administering any neuromuscular blocking agents.

4. Apply Sellick's maneuver. Do not release cricoid pressure until tracheal intubation is confirmed.

5. Per local protocols, consider premedicating the patient with a defasciculating dose of nondepolarizing neuromuscular blocking agent (e.g., rocuronium or vecuronium). This is especially important in children, where fasciculations from succinylcholine can cause musculoskeletal trauma. Also, if indicated in local protocols, consider premedicating with lidocaine and atropine.

6. Paralyze the patient, administering succinylcholine 1.5 mg/kg IV bolus and continue oxygenation. Alternatively, rocuronium can be used for muscle paralysis (1 mg/kg).

7. Once adequate relaxation is obtained (usually ≤ 1 minute), insert the laryngoscope and expose the glottic inlet (Figure 16-4). Insert the TT through the vocal cords. Positive-pressure ventilation is not required until the patient is intubated, unless the patient desaturates to ≤ 92% SpO_2. This helps prevent gastric insufflation of oxygen and decreases the risk of aspiration. If the patient desaturates during intubation attempts, stop trying to intubate, ventilate the patient with 100% oxygen, and reestablish the oxygen saturation as high as possible (preferably > 96% SpO_2). Only when the oxygen saturation has been reestablished should you proceed with further intubation attempts. Be sure to assess why the intubation was unsuccessful and make changes in any further attempts to improve the chances of successful intubation.

   Reasons for failed intubation include patient position, anatomical problems, equipment failure, wrong blade type (curved versus straight), wrong blade length, need for external laryngeal manipulation, and lack of operator skill. If intubation cannot be accomplished after several attempts or ≥ 10 minutes, do not continue to attempt intubation unless another practitioner with more skill becomes available to assist (see Chapter 1). Rather, proceed with BVM ventilation and, if available, use a laryngeal mask airway (see Chapter 8).

8. Connect the TT to an oxygen and ventilation source and confirm tracheal intubation using a combination of auscultation and an evidence-based method such as $ETCO_2$ or a self-inflating bulb (if appropriate). Auscultate. There should be no breath sounds over the abdomen and equal bilateral breath sounds should be heard over the chest and along the midaxillary lines.

9. Release the cricoid pressure.

10. Insert an oropharyngeal airway to prevent biting of the tracheal tube. Secure the tracheal tube by taping or through the use of a Thomas tube holder (see Chapter 4). Continuously monitor lung ventilation using pulse oximetry; EKG; and most important, continuous waveform capnography (see Chapter 5).

11. Follow protocols or medical direction concerning continued use of muscle relaxants and sedatives for postintubation management.

From Bledsoe, BE, RS Porter, RA Cherry. Paramedic Care: Principles & Practice, Volume 1, pp. 571–572 (Pearson/Prentice Hall).

to minimize the risk of aspiration of gastric contents as the patient is rendered unconscious and the trachea is intubated. In this procedure, the awake patient is first preoxygenated (or more accurately, denitrogenated) during spontaneous ventilation to fill the functional residual capacity (FRC) with oxygen. An induction agent and a muscle relaxant are then injected simultaneously into a rapidly running intravenous line. Cricoid pressure (Sellick's maneuver) is applied as the medications are administered and the patient begins to lose consciousness. The patient is allowed to breathe spontaneously until he or she becomes apneic, while positive-pressure ventilation is avoided. As soon as the patient becomes sedated and relaxed (ideally within 30 to 60 seconds), the clinician performs direct laryngoscopy and inserts the endotracheal tube into the trachea under direct visualization. Cricoid pressure is continued until correct placement of the endotracheal tube in the trachea is confirmed. The RSI technique provides optimal conditions for endotracheal intubation and minimizes the risk of gastric aspiration.

There are seven different varieties of MPS, with many different manifestations; however, the implications for airway management are short neck, macrocephaly (large head), spinal malformations, poor development of facial bones, cardiac valvular disease, and frequent respiratory infections.

lymphangioma

A tumor composed of lymphatic vessels.

neurofibroma

A tumor composed of the cells that form the myelin sheath of nerve fibers, the nerve fibers themselves, and connective tissue.

In younger children, especially in infants and those with severe lung pathology, rapid sequence induction should be modified because they are likely to experience oxyhemoglobin desaturation more quickly.[10] In this setting, a modified rapid sequence induction is selected. After preoxygenation, a sedative and paralytic medication is given intravenously as cricoid pressure is gently applied. The airway is gently ventilated with positive-pressure (which should not exceed 20 cm H_2O airway pressure) until laryngoscopy and endotracheal intubation are accomplished. Providing gentle positive-pressure ventilation prevents or minimizes the arterial oxygen desaturation that is often associated with brief periods of apnea in the sick infant. Insertion of an oral airway of the correct size (Chapter 3) often improves positive-pressure ventilation by decreasing the likelihood of gastric insufflation (Figure 16-5).

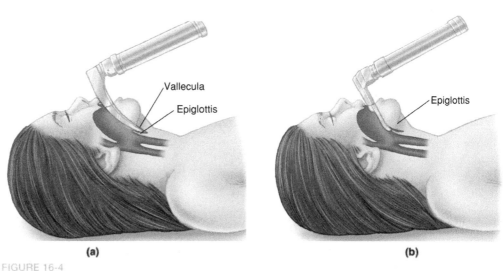

(a) (b)

FIGURE 16-4
Placement of the laryngoscope: (a) Macintosh (curved) blade and (b) Miller (straight) blade.

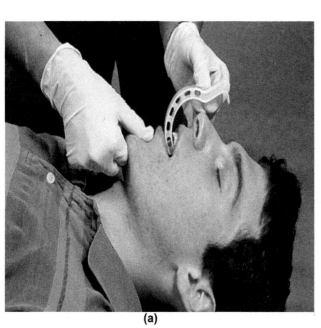

(a)

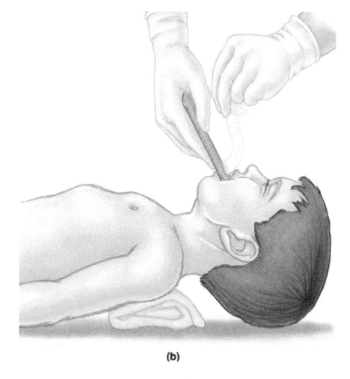

(b)

FIGURE 16-5
(a) In an adult, the oropharyngeal airway is inserted with the tip pointing to the roof of the mouth, then rotated into position. (b) In an infant or small child, the airway is inserted with the tip pointing toward the tongue and pharynx, in the same position it will be in after insertion.

The Pediatric Airway   277

Table 16-8	Alternative Approaches to Tracheal Intubation

• Awake flexible fiberoptic bronchoscopy
• Awake direct laryngoscopy
• Fiberoptic-assisted rigid devices
  • **Bullard laryngoscope**
  • **Shikani seeing stylet**
	• Blind nasotracheal intubation
	• Lightwand technique
	• Retrograde wire technique

It is imperative when working with children with a previous history or physical features suggestive of difficult intubation to avoid pitfalls that may lead to situations in which ventilation and intubation are difficult or impossible and thus avoid the resulting complications.

For patients in whom BVM ventilation is likely to be unsuccessful, it is important to avoid medications that abolish the respiratory drive and paralyze the respiratory muscles. In such instances, it is preferable to secure the airway while the patient is breathing spontaneously. Alternatives that serve to accomplish this goal are listed in Table 16-8. If the clinical situation permits these options should be attempted after judicious topical airway anesthesia.

The choice of technique depends on the preference and confidence level of the practitioner, age and degree of cooperation of the child, and the specific clinical circumstances. When BVM ventilation is likely to be easy but difficult endotracheal intubation is anticipated, techniques other than RSI should be used to secure the airway. In these situations, there is a real risk of aspiration during airway manipulation and ventilation; this risk should be weighed against the increased cooperation and lack of patient movement achieved by administration of sedatives and paralytic agents. In agitated and uncooperative patients, the risk benefit ratio may favor sedation and/or paralysis. The favorable conditions gained may more than offset the risk of aspiration. In addition to the techniques described previously, the spontaneously breathing patient can also be taken to the operating room and intubated while spontaneously inhaling volatile anesthetics.[10] However, this assumes that the patient can be ventilated adequately by other means in the prehospital setting.

If the initial intubation technique fails, then ventilation should be attempted by BVM ventilation. If the initial attempt to secure the airway was conventional direct laryngoscopy, as in RSI, then the practitioner should have some appreciation of the reasons that difficulties were encountered. And after optimizing the intubation conditions and equipment, the operator should repeat laryngoscopy.[21] The best attempt at laryngoscopy is defined as being

Note

According to AHA Guidelines 2005—Verify Correct Tube Placement with Clinical Exam and Device,[6] for infants and children with a perfusing rhythm, use a colorimetric detector or capnography to detect exhaled CO_2 to confirm endotracheal tube position in the prehospital and in-hospital settings (Class IIa) and during intrahospital and interhospital transport (Class IIb). The self-inflating bulb (esophageal detector device) may be considered to confirm endotracheal tube placement in children weighing more than 20 kg with a perfusing rhythm (Class IIb). Insufficient data exists to make a recommendation for or against its use in children during cardiac arrest (Class Indeterminate). The AHA's new emphasis is on the need to verify correct tube placement immediately after the tube is inserted, during transport, and especially when the patient is moved. The new wording also does not describe the use of devices as "secondary" confirmation but as "additional" confirmation with clinical assessment (i.e., part of the "primary" assessment).

Table 16-9 Indications for Use of Various Techniques for Ventilation and Intubation in Can-Mask-Ventilate/Cannot-Intubate Versus Cannot-Mask-Ventilate/Cannot-Intubate Situations

Technique	Indicated for Use in Can-Mask-Ventilate/Cannot Intubate?	Indicated for Use in Cannot-Mask-Ventilate/Cannot-Intubate?
Oral and nasopharyngeal airway[23]	Yes	Perhaps (based on the clinical situation)
LMA insertion[24,25]	Yes	Yes
Use of Combitube[26*]	Yes	Yes
Bullard laryngoscope	Yes	No
Lightwand	Yes	No
Use of transtracheal jet ventilation	Perhaps (based on the clinical situation)	Yes
Retrograde guide wire intubation technique	Yes	No
Creation of surgical airway	Yes	Yes

*Combitube 37 F SA can be used only in children taller than 4 feet independent of age. As an alternative, the Easytube 28 F can be used in children taller than 3 feet.

performed by a reasonably experienced laryngoscopist and using optimal position, optimal external laryngeal manipulation, and perhaps one change in laryngoscope blade length and/or type.[21,22]

If one cannot achieve intubation after the best possible attempt, then several alternative approaches that do not require conventional laryngoscopy may be considered (Table 16-9). One should avoid multiple attempts at conventional direct laryngoscopy; this may create trauma and make mask ventilation more difficult because of increased tissue edema and bleeding.[10]

In scenarios where BVM ventilation and endotracheal intubation are impossible and spontaneous ventilation is inadequate or absent, steps should be taken to bypass the airflow obstruction during ventilation in an effort to restore immediate gas exchange and avoid neurologic injury or loss of life. The acceptable alternatives for this cannot-ventilate/cannot-intubate situation are listed in Table 16-9.

Needle cricothyrotomy and transtracheal jet ventilation (TTJV) should be used only in patients who are too small for surgical cricothyrotomy and cannot be intubated or ventilated.[27] This technique is preferred over surgical cricothyrotomy because of the relatively high risk of injury to vital structures (such as the carotid arteries and jugular veins) that is associated with surgical cricothyrotomy in small children.[28] Commercial kits are available for needle cricothyrotomy that employ the Seldinger technique (the passage of a guide wire through a needle or catheter that has been placed in the cricothyroid membrane, followed by a dilator catheter and finally the cricothyrotomy tube). Such kits are available only for children above the age of 10 years.

Needle cricothyrotomy is a temporary measure that provides emergency oxygenation and some degree of gas exchange until a definitive airway can be obtained. It is prudent to pay close attention to the rise and fall of the chest wall and blood gas analysis to evaluate the arterial carbon dioxide (CO_2) tension because dangerously high levels of arterial carbon dioxide can develop using this technique.[10] Complications that can arise from misplacement of the needle and catheter include pneumothorax, subcutaneous emphysema (resulting in the loss of favorable conditions for subsequent attempts at correct catheter placement), mediastinal emphysema, esophageal injury, and bleeding.[29] In addition, venti-

ON TARGET Needle cricothyrotomy is a temporary measure that provides emergency oxygenation and some degree of gas exchange until a definitive airway can be obtained. It can be done quickly when a patient is in extreme danger of cardiac arrest due to hypoxia, and it will buy time while you are preparing to do a definitive airway technique.

lation with a self-filling resuscitation (e.g., AMBU bag) or anesthesia bag may be difficult because of the high resistance imposed by the relatively small catheter in the airway. Different methods have been suggested to identify correct needle placement in the trachea, including the aspiration of air from the trachea and the observation of bubbles as air is aspirated through saline.[23,30]

The so-called retrograde intubation technique first involves a needle cricothyrotomy and passage of a guide wire up and retrograde through the larynx into the oropharynx or nasopharynx. An endotracheal tube or tube exchange catheter is then passed over the guide wire through the vocal cords, using the wire as a guide. Following entrance of the endotracheal tube into the larynx, the guide wire is removed, allowing the endotracheal tube to enter the midtrachea. Complications of this technique include barotrauma, esophageal puncture, creation of a false passage, and bleeding.[31]

Surgical intervention for airway access may be the last resort but should be considered and implemented early once the cannot-ventilate/cannot-intubate scenario is encountered. Techniques of surgical intervention include incisional cricothyrotomy and emergency tracheostomy.

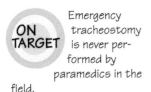

ON TARGET Emergency tracheostomy is never performed by paramedics in the field.

Emergency tracheostomy should be performed in an operating-room setting after consultation with appropriate surgical specialists such as those in otolaryngology or general surgery. The complication rate of emergency tracheostomy in the pediatric population is considerably high and may be as much as 44%.[32,33] This technique is not done in the prehospital setting.

In recent years, there has been a great controversy regarding the clinical outcome of patients who underwent prehospital endotracheal intubation performed by paramedics. Various studies have indicated a poor outcome and increased mortality associated with RSI performed by paramedics in a prehospital setting,[34-36] whereas other literature has suggested that the use of a proper drug-based RSI technique has been shown to improve the intubation success rates in a large urban prehospital setting.[37]

Current data suggest that prehospital RSI is potentially useful in only a select subset of prehospital patients, and the rate of successful intubations without complications depends on the practitioner's skill and experience level.[38] The factors that impede prehospital endotracheal intubation are not fully understood, and it is currently difficult to assess whether prehospital RSI would address these shortcomings.

Commonly Used Drugs in Children During RSI

Neuromuscular Blocking Agents

Succinylcholine is a depolarizing neuromuscular blocking agent (NMBA). It has been popular in both pediatric and adult populations for decades. Because of its various side effects (e.g., hyperkalemia, malignant hyperthermia trigger), however, several clinicians have encouraged avoiding its use in pediatric anesthesia practice.[39]

There have been several reports of cardiac arrest following administration of succinylcholine in patients with myopathies.[40-43] This led the U.S. Food and Drug Administration (FDA) in 1993 to accept the package insert text stating, "Except when used for emergency tracheal intubation or in instances where immediate securing of the airway is necessary, succinylcholine is contraindicated in children and adolescent patients." Subsequently, after claims from clinicians that this would increase rather than decrease the morbidity, the FDA considered another revision of the package insert in 1994. The label now states, "Since there may be no signs and symptoms to alert the practitioner to which patients are at risk, it is recommended that the use of succinylcholine in children should be reserved for emergency intubation or in instances where immediate securing of the airway is necessary, e.g. laryngospasm, difficult airway, full stomach, or for IM use when a suitable vein is inaccessible" (package insert for Anectine 1995). This revised language appears as a "boxed warning" rather than as a contraindication.

According to FDA recommendations, children and adolescent patients are more likely than adults to have undiagnosed myopathies; a nondepolarizing neuromuscular blocking drug should be used for routine elective surgery in these patients. Except when used for emergency tracheal intubation or in instances where immediate securing of the airway is necessary, succinylcholine is contraindicated in patients after the acute phase of injury following major burns, multiple trauma, extensive denervation of skeletal muscle, or upper motor neuron injury because succinylcholine administration to such individuals may result in severe hyperkalemia, which may result in cardiac arrest. The risk of hyperkalemia in these patients increases over time and usually peaks at 7 to 10 days after the injury. The risk depends on the extent and location of the injury. The precise time of onset and the duration of the risk period are not known.[44]

Rocuronium is a nondepolarizing neuromuscular blocker. It is the only nondepolarizing muscle relaxant (at a dose of more than 1.0 mg/kg) that has an onset of action similar to that of succinylcholine (60 to 90 seconds), making it suitable for RSI.[45,46]

 If succinylcholine is not available for paralysis, rocuronium is preferred over vecuronium because it has an onset of action similar to succinylcholine (60 to 90 seconds).

Anticholinergic Agents

glycopyrrolate
Also known as Robinul. An anticholinergic drug that may occasionally be used as an alternative to atropine and does not cross the blood–brain barrier.

Anticholinergic agents (atropine and **glycopyrrolate**) minimize the bradycardia and possibly even asystole that may result from vagal stimulation as a result of laryngoscopy, hypoxia, and succinylcholine administration. Anticholinergics are indicated for infants less than one year of age, in children 1 to 5 years of age receiving succinylcholine, and older children receiving a second dose of succinylcholine.[47] However, the routine use of atropine before a single dose of succinylcholine in older children should be reconsidered.[48]

Induction Agents

All children undergoing RSI should be appropriately sedated. Sedation blunts their awareness and decreases the sympathetic response associated with endotracheal intubation. Commonly used agents (Table 16-10) for sedation during RSI include benzodiazepines (e.g., midazolam or diazepam) barbiturates (e.g., thiopental), nonbarbiturate sedative hypnotics (e.g., etomidate and propofol), and the dissociative anesthetic ketamine.

Role of the Laryngeal Mask Airway (LMA)

The use of the LMA was first described in 1983, although it was introduced to the United States in 1992.[49] It has gained wide popularity around the world. The classic model of the LMA is reusable, and the insertion technique is generally readily mastered.[50,51] The LMA is a supraglottic device, and therefore it is ineffective in glottic and subglottic airway obstruction.[52] Also, it does not provide absolute protection against aspiration.[52] Laryngospasm and the inability to ventilate can still occur with the use of the LMA.[53]

The LMA-Classic™ is essentially a modified mask and, if properly inserted, it surrounds the larynx without entering the trachea or vocal cords. The inflatable mask of the LMA creates a seal over the laryngeal inlet the larynx (Chapter 8). It is supplied in eight sizes, as indicated in Table 16-11 (refer also to Chapter 8).

Table 16-10 Commonly Used Pharmacological Agents in RSI for Children

Drug	Dose	Route	Duration	Side Effects	Comments
Atropine	0.01 to 0.02 mg/kg, max 1 mg; IM dose 0.02 mg/kg	IV	More than 30 minutes	Paradoxical bradycardia can occur with dose if <0.01mg or pushed slowly.	Inhibits bradycardiac response to hypoxia, and vagal stimulation.
Midazolam	0.1 to 0.4 mg/kg	IV	30–60 minutes	Respiratory depression and hypotension.	No analgesic property. Potentiates respiratory depressive effect of narcotics and barbiturates.
Thiopental	2 to 4 mg/kg	IV	5 to 10 minutes	Hypotension and negative inotropic agent, hypotension with inadequate intravascular volume.	Ultra-short-acting, decreases cerebral metabolic rate (CMR) and intracranial pressure (ICP). Potentiates respiratory depressive effect of narcotics.
Etomidate	0.2 to 0.4 mg/kg	IV	10 to 15 minutes	Myotonic activity, adrenal suppression.	Decrease ICP and CMR, minimal cardiovascular and respiratory depression. No analgesic properties.
Ketamine (dissociative anesthetic)	0.5 to 1.0 mg/kg IV; 3 to 4 mg/kg IM	IV/IM	30 to 60 minutes	Increased ICP and blood pressure, increased secretions, hallucinations, and emergence reaction.	Bronchodilator; preserves the airway reflexes.
Propofol (general anesthetic)	2 to 3 mg/kg	IV	2 to 8 minutes	Hypotension, especially in patients with inadequate intravascular volume.	Highly lipid soluble with a short duration of action.
Succinylcholine (depolarizing neuromuscular blocker)	1 to 1.5 mg/kg in children; 2 mg/kg IV for infants; for IM use, double the IV dose	IV/IM	3 to 5 minutes	Fasciculations, increased ICP, increased intraocular and intragastric pressure, hyperkelemia.	Rapid onset and short duration of action should be avoided in hyperkelemia, patients with renal failure, and burns.
Rocuronium (nondepolarizing neuromuscular blocker)	0.6 to 1.2 mg/kg	IV	30 to 60 minutes	Minimal cardiovascular effect	In higher dose (>1.2 mg/kg) has a rapid onset of action equaling that of succinylcholine. May cause prolonged paralysis if given in cannot ventilate/cannot intubate scenario.

Table 16-11   Appropriate Sizes of LMA (Classic)

Size of LMA	Weight (kg)	Cuff Volume (mL)	I.D. of Endotracheal Tube (mm)
1	Less than 5	4	3.5
1.5	5 to 10	7	4.0
2	10 to 20	10	4.5
2.5	20 to 30	14	5.0
3	30 to 50	20	6.0
4	50 to 70	30	6.0
5	70 to 100	40	7.0
6	More than 100	50	7.0

Source: LMA North America.

The LMA has proven to be an extremely useful device in emergency situations.[8] Multiple case reports have demonstrated the value of the LMA for establishing and maintaining the airway when intubation and ventilation are extremely difficult.[54,55] In emergency situations, the LMA can be used as a temporizing airway while the definitive airway is established.

> **PEARLS**
> Every paramedic should be thoroughly familiar with multiple approaches to ventilation. It is not necessary that all available techniques be learned, but it is necessary to have backup plans for the difficult airway and the cannot mask-ventilate/cannot-intubate scenario. At a minimum, an LMA or similar device should be available in all pediatric sizes, remember that patients die from lack of ventilation, not lack of intubation.

Depending on the clinical scenario, the LMA Classic™ can be used for a variety of airway management indications, including use as a routine airway and as a rescue device in difficult-airway management. The LMA Classic™ makes an excellent airway for routine use during general anesthesia in patients who are appropriately selected.[56] Compared to the conventional face-mask ventilation, the LMA™ provides better ventilation during routine outpatient procedures requiring intubation,[57] neonatal resuscitation,[58] and use by inexperienced personnel.[59]

The LMA Classic™ has been successfully used as an conduit for the passage of an TT in a patient with a known difficult airway and who is easy to mask-ventilate but difficult to intubate using a conventional laryngoscope. A series of maneuvers have been described by Benumof[8] using LMA as a conduit for intubation. The LMA can also be used as a conduit for fiberoptic tracheal intubation in patients who require awake intubation for a variety of indications.[8] Compared to other awake intubation techniques, insertion of the LMA in awake patients is a relatively moderate stimulus, which results in minimal hemodynamic changes.[25]

The LMA Fastrach™ is an evolution of the LMA Classic™. It was specifically designed for the difficult and the emergency airway. It consists of an anatomically curved, stainless steel tube bonded to the LMA with a single moveable aperture bar. It can be used as an airway device on its own or as an intubating tool, with no interruption of patient oxygen. It is available only for children weighing more than 30 kg.

According to the AHA Guidelines 2005—Use of Advanced Airways[6]: Insufficient evidence exists for or against the routine use of an LMA during cardiac arrest (Class Indeterminate). When endotracheal intubation is not possible, the LMA is an acceptable adjunct for experienced providers (Class IIb), but it is associated with a higher incidence of complications in young children. Endotracheal intubation in infants and children requires special training because the pediatric airway anatomy differs from the adult airway anatomy. Success and a low complication rate are related to the length of training, supervised experience in the operating room and in the field, adequate ongoing experience, and the use of rapid sequence intubation (RSI). As experience with advanced airways has accumulated, endotracheal intubation by inexperienced providers appears to be associated with a high incidence of misplaced and displaced tubes. In addition, tubes may become displaced when the patient is moved. Providers should be experienced in BVM ventilation. If advanced airways are used, providers must evaluate placement and detect misplacement, and the health care system must monitor results.

Complications of Intubation

The complications resulting from endotracheal intubation in the pediatric population are well documented.[60,61] These complications bear significant morbidity and mortality risks. Some complications are listed in Table 16-12. Nasal mucosal injuries occur as a result of nasotracheal intubation. The tears are usually located on the nasal turbinates.[62] The use of an appropriately sized endotracheal tube is essential to prevent nasal mucosal injury. A topical nasal decongestant (such as phenylephrine nasal drops 0.125%, 1 to 2 drops per nostril in children six months to two years of age and 2 to 3 drops per nostril in children two to six years of age) should be applied before intubation. Sinusitis after prolonged nasal intubation is also well documented.[63] Appropriate antibiotic treatment is required to treat this condition. Dental trauma can occur during intubation and is usually caused by the laryngoscope blade. If the dental injury results in a loose or displaced tooth, it is imperative to recover the tooth so that aspiration of the tooth does not occur. Temporomandibular joint (TMJ) dislocation can occur if excessive force is applied on this joint during laryngoscopy. Patients with facial skeletal anomalies are particularly prone to this injury. The dislocation is identified at the time of the procedure when the jaw is locked in the open position and cannot be closed. Immediate reduction of the TMJ should be performed. The paramedic normally does not have training in this maneuver, and a TMJ dislocation can cause significant problems. The best option is to provide BVM ventilation and rapid transport to a hospital.

Table 16-12 Some Complications of Intubation

Acute	Mucosal tear False passage	1. Dental trauma 2. Temporomandibular joint dislocation 3. Mucosal injury	1. Mucosal injury 2. Arytenoid dislocation 3. Vocal-cord paralysis
Chronic	Sinusitis		1. Granulations/granulomas of larynx 2. Laryngotracheal stenosis

Complications such as TMJ dislocation or arytenoid cartilage dislocation must be dealt with in the hospital; if the paramedic suspects such a complication, rapid transport should be carried out.

Mucosal injuries in the laryngotracheal region occur commonly in patients with an anatomically difficult airway and when there has been an inappropriate choice of intubating equipment. These injuries can cause bleeding, which may further interfere with the process of securing the airway. Arytenoid cartilage dislocation, which can occur during intubation with suboptimal visualization of the larynx and in patients with pathology of the cricoarytenoid joint, as in rheumatoid arthritis, can lead to persistent hoarseness. Reduction of the dislocation should be attempted as soon as possible; delay may lead to abnormal adhesion and rigidity of the joint. This condition requires rapid transport to a hospital because paramedics are not normally trained in reduction of this dislocation. Vocal-cord paralysis is associated with long-term intubation. Pressure from the endotracheal tube cuff against the recurrent laryngeal nerve has been suggested as a cause of this complication.[60] After extubation, the patient may manifest a breathy voice and occasional aspiration because of inadequate glottic closure.

As mentioned earlier in this chapter, the narrowest part of the pediatric airway is located at the cricoid ring.[64] Therefore, it is desirable to intubate the trachea with an appropriate but not oversized endotracheal tube (TT) (Table 16-13).

It is recommended that the TT should allow a small air leak at a peak inflation pressure of 20 to 30 cm H_2O.[65] A variety of formulas and techniques have been used in an attempt to determine the appropriate TT size that minimizes both pressure-induced tracheal injury and aspiration potential or variable ventilation.[66] The air-leak test following tracheal intubation can be performed by measuring the minimum amount of air required to produce an audible rush of air around the TT while auscultating over the trachea and recording the airway pressure manometer reading.[67] In prehospital medicine, noise in the environment can make auscultation of air rushing around the TT tube difficult, if not impossible. Further, ambulances and paramedics do not normally have the necessary equipment to record airway pressure. Therefore, the methods described are unlikely to be successful in the ambulance and, additionally, the methods described are subjective and may not adequately differentiate between an appropriately sized and an oversized TT.[61] Furthermore, the air-leak test has a low sensitivity when used as a screening test to predict postextubation stridor in young children (younger than 7 years old), whereas in older children (7 years or older), the air-leak test may predict postextubation stridor.[68] In the

Table 16-13	Selecting an Appropriate Size Endotracheal Tube According to Age	
Age	Endotracheal Tube Size (mm I.D.)
Premature	2.5 to 3.0*
Term to 6 months	3.0*
6 to 12 months	3.5*
12 to 20 months	4.0*
2 years	4.5*
4 years	5.0*
6 years	5.5*
8 years	6.0*
10 years	6.5
12 years	7.5

*Uncuffed endotracheal tube

pediatric population, an inappropriately large endotracheal tube may contribute to the development of chronic laryngeal injuries.[60,61] Long-standing compression of the tracheal mucosa with an oversized tube can exceed the mucosal capillary perfusion pressure, leading to ischemic necrosis and ulceration of the tracheal wall, which in turn leads to granulation and stenosis.[69,70] The paramedic must pay particular attention to selection of the correct size ET tube.

> ### Note
>
> According to AHA Guidelines 2005—Use of Cuffed Endotracheal Tubes vs. Uncuffed Tubes[6]: In the in-hospital setting, a cuffed endotracheal tube is as safe as an uncuffed tube for infants (except the newborn) and children. In certain circumstances (e.g., poor lung compliance, high airway resistance, or a large glottic air leak) a cuffed tube may be preferable, provided that attention is paid to endotracheal tube size, position, and cuff inflation pressure (Class IIa). Keep cuff inflation pressure <20 cm H_2O. The formula used to estimate the internal diameter of a cuffed tube differs from that used for an uncuffed tube and is as follows: cuffed endotracheal tube size (mm I.D.) $=$ (age in years/4) $+$ 3.

Awareness of a potentially difficult airway and employment of appropriate techniques to maximize visualization and securing of the airway, including selection of an appropriately sized TT, can minimize the risk of these complications.

Summary

The overarching maxims that "Patients die from failure to ventilate/oxygenate rather than failure to intubate" and that "If your patient can't breathe, nothing else matters" are as important and as applicable in pediatric airway management as they are in adult airway management. The key to success and low complication rates is related to the length of training, supervised experience in operating rooms and in the field, adequate ongoing experience, and the appropriate use of RSI. Finally, it is important that one stay current with the latest AHA guidelines with regard to use of cuffed/uncuffed tracheal tubes, confirmation of tracheal intubation, monitoring of lung ventilation, and the proper application of adjunctive ventilation devices.

REVIEW QUESTIONS

1. Identify at least five differences between the pediatric airway and the adult airway.

2. Compare and contrast the difference between croup and epiglottitis.

3. What is the nondepolarizing paralytic agent that is recommended if succinylcholine is not available or contraindicated?

4. List at least five options for oxygenation and ventilation when attempts at intubation have failed.

5. List several complications of intubation in the pediatric patient.

CHAPTER 17

Sedation/Analgesia for Postintubation Management

Michael A. E. Ramsay
Michael A. Frakes
James Michael Rich

Chapter Objectives

After reading this chapter, you should be able to:

- Discuss the reasons for sedation in the intubated patient.

- Describe the risks and benefits of sedation.

- List agents for sedation commonly used in the prehospital setting.

- Discuss the significance of untreated pain.

- Discuss the side effects and contraindications of the use of analgesic agents.

- List the anxiolytic agents commonly used in prehospital care.

- Discuss the combined use of benzodiazepines and opioid analgesics.

- Discuss the side effects and contraindications for the use of benzodiazepines.

- Describe the methods used to assess and score a patient's level of sedation.

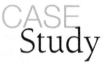

CASE Study _____

Medic 14 was dispatched to a nearby hospital's emergency department (ED) to transport an intubated patient to a larger tertiary care facility. The ED staff called for the flight crew, but the weather was below minimum so they were transferring by ground ambulance. The paramedics arrived and received the report from ED staff. The patient was a 27-year-old male who was found unconscious at work earlier in the day. He had no medical history and only took over-the-counter pain medicines for headaches. He was diagnosed with a subarachnoid bleed in his head. The ED physician elected to intubate the patient to secure the airway for transport.

The patient was evaluated by the paramedics. The airway was intact with an 8.0 tracheal tube secured at 22 cm. The patient was chemically paralyzed with vecuronium and was on a ventilator in an assist-control mode. His peripheral pulses were intact in all extremities. The patient had no motor response, would not open his eyes, and was intubated. The transport monitors were placed and revealed blood pressure of 117/80, sinus rhythm rate of 75, respiratory rate set at 14, with 100% oxygen saturations. Secondary assessment was unremarkable. They moved the patient to the stretcher and began ventilations with a bag-valve device. An end-tidal carbon dioxide ($ETCO_2$) monitor was attached, and the patient was secured into the ambulance for transport. The paramedic ventilated to keep the $ETCO_2$ between 35 and 40.

During transport, the patient's heart rate increased to 120 and his blood pressure increased to 180/110. The oxygen saturations and $ETCO_2$ remained unchanged. Reassessment was done with no change. Concerns about vital sign changes were discussed. The patient was given vecuronium prior to transport by the ED physician. They decided the patient lacked sedation but was paralyzed, so the assessment did not reveal expected signs. The paramedics administered morphine 4 mg and midazolam 4 mg. The patient's heart rate decreased and blood pressure improved. They continued to titrate small doses of morphine and midazolam throughout the remainder of the transport. The patient was delivered to the receiving hospital without further incident.

Introduction

Sedation—the effective management of pain, anxiety, and hypnosis—is essential for most intubated patients in the out-of-hospital environment. However, precise and safe control of sedation remains challenging. Poorly controlled sedation can lead to both undersedation and oversedation. Undersedation risks include patient or provider harm, adverse hemodynamic effects, and deleterious physiological consequences; oversedation may result in prolonged recovery times or unrecognized neurological changes. Optimal approaches require a multimodal regimen that combines analgesics, **anxiolytics**, and sedatives and considers the unwanted effects of each agent.

The routine use of sedation and analgesia scales provides objective assessment and close treatment control, thus reducing the need for muscle relaxants and their potential attendant complications. Sedation agents should be administered to a defined clinical end point, as opposed to a set dosage, allowing continual reassessment, care continuity, and cost effectiveness. Since the **Ramsay sedation scale (RSS)** was first used to describe the level of sedation in critical-care patients receiving sedation,[1] the management of critical-care patients has witnessed a number of advances, yet considerable room for improvement remains, and the effects of oversedation are still commonly seen.[2]

anxiolytic

A drug that relieves anxiety.

Ramsay sedation scale (RSS)

The Ramsay Sedation Scale (RSS) is a six-point assessment tool for recording the level of sedation in the unparalyzed patient.

KEY TERMS

Analgesia

Almost all critical-care patients, whether in or out of the hospital, suffer pain. It is possible that even extreme pain in intubated patients can go unrecognized for long periods of time due to communication barriers. Accordingly, the assessment and appropriate management of pain has to be a sedation priority.

PEARLS The sedated or unresponsive patient on mechanical ventilation may have an unmet analgesic need. Monitoring for signs of pain and the appropriate use of analgesics is essential for optimal patient care.

Untreated pain has significant physiological sequelae,[3] and effective pain management improves patient satisfaction, recovery times, and complication rates.[3] The importance of addressing pain in critical-care patients is emphasized by the Society of Critical Care Medicine (SCCM), whose practice guidelines recommend that adequate analgesia be a primary goal in the care of the critically ill.[4] Patients with pain in the out-of-hospital environment, however, receive analgesia as infrequently as 1.8% of the time, with the highest rates, up to 84.1% of patients, from specialty critical-care transport teams that include a nurse crew member.[5–13]

Intravenous opiates are the current mainstay of analgesic therapy. While these agents provide highly effective pain relief, their use is associated with a number of adverse effects, including respiratory depression, hypotension, gastric retention, ileus, pruritus, nausea, and vomiting.[14] In an effort to avoid these adverse effects and to address concerns over the potential for additive effects, adequate pain management is sometimes compromised.

ON TARGET Specialty critical-care transport teams that include a nurse have the best record in providing analgesia in the out-of-hospital environment.

Morphine sulfate is the most commonly used opioid, offering effective pain management at low cost. Sir William Osler once described it as "God's own medicine," and it is the standard against which other analgesics for acute pain are judged.[15] However, morphine has a narrow therapeutic window and has a relatively high frequency of the side effects associated with the opiate analgesics.

Fentanyl is often used as an alternative to morphine, particularly in hemodynamically unstable patients. A reduced histamine effect and greater lipid solubility give fentanyl a faster onset, fewer side effects, and more accurate titration of effects. The use and safety of fentanyl in transport is well documented as safe and effective.[6,11,13,16,17] Both of these opiates have active metabolites, so impaired drug clearance in critically ill patients may lead to accumulation and prolonged effects.

Extremely high fentanyl doses may cause chest wall and glottic rigidity. This adverse effect, although commonly discussed, does not occur until single doses in excess of 8.8 mcg/kg have been administered, well beyond typical analgesia and sedation doses of between 2 and 7 mcg/kg. Although less well-described, muscle rigidity significant enough to prevent ventilation may also occur with IV morphine and meperidine. Regardless of the agent, rigidity may be reversed with either naloxone or neuromuscular blockade.[18] Alfentanil has an even more rapid onset and elimination than does fentanyl, but it is used almost exclusively in the operating room.

PEARLS The long term use of morphine analgesia in the multiorgan failure patient may result in unintentional accumulation because of the build up of active metabolites. More precise pain mangement may be obtained by the administration of fentanyl, alfentanil, or remifentanil.

The synthetic opiate meperidine is metabolized to normeperidine, a metabolite with a number of central nervous system effects that include tremors, disorientation, hallucinations, multifocal myoclonus, and seizures. Meperidine offers no real clinical advantages over morphine, and there is essentially no indication for the use of meperidine in acute-care analgesia.[19,20]

To provide an appropriate level of analgesia, it is essential that regular assessments be conducted. A number of behavioral observation systems have been developed, and the verbal rating, visual analog, or numerical rating scales assess patient reports of pain. Picture scales have the benefit of being successfully used in children and illiterate, nonverbal patients, or those who have difficulty understanding other scales.[21] Although these approaches to pain assessment are highly subjective, physiological indicators such as tachycardia and increased blood pressure are not reliable as indications of pain intensity.[22–24] While physiological signs are useful indications that a patient is suffering pain, particularly if they are nonverbal or semiconscious, they are not considered suitable parameters for establishing the absence of pain.

There is some preliminary data that the processed spectral array analysis of brain cortical activity with monitors such as the **bispectral index (BIS) monitor** may be an indicator

bispectral index (BIS) monitor
A monitoring system that measures the effects of anesthetics and sedatives on the brain. Using a sensor placed on the patient's forehead, the device translates the patient's electroencephalogram (EEG) into a number from 0 to 100, indicating the patient's level of consciousness.

of unmet analgesic needs of the patient. The patient state index has been demonstrated to correlate well with the need for morphine in the semiconscious intensive care unit (ICU) patient.[25] These monitors are now used extensively in the operating suite and ICU, but they are not currently available in the field. Perhaps in the future, these devices will become routinely used in prehospital medicine.

Anxiolysis and Hypnosis

Opiates have no real amnesic properties, although some debate on this topic continues. It is intuitive that patients experiencing the unpleasant nature of a critical illness, the critical-care environment, and associated pain are best managed by aiming to ensure they have no recollection of the experience. However, this view is not universally held, with the suggestion that patients with no recall of their critical-care period may have unrealistic expectations of their recovery.[26] Regardless of this debate, the needs for anxiolysis and hypnosis are also important components in providing sedation.

GABA agonist
An amino acid derivative, g-aminobutyrate (GABA) is a well-known inhibitor of presynaptic transmission in the central nervous system. Benzodiazepines exert their soothing effects by potentiating the responses of GABA-A receptors to GABA binding.

The classic anxiolytic agents are the benzodiazepines. These indirect **GABA agonists** produce amnesia and reduce anxiety. Of the many available agents, midazolam has a faster onset, shorter duration, and narrower dosing range than lorazepam or diazepam.[27,28] Midazolam is a negative inotrope, but traditional sedative doses cause little hemodynamic change.[18,27] Diazepam requires titration through a wide dosage range to achieve satisfactory effects, and it is rarely used. Lorazepam produces no active metabolites and may provide the most manageable and cost-effective option for sedation lasting longer than a few intermittent doses.[19]

The combination of benzodiazepines and opiate analgesics provides extremely effective sedation with anxiolysis and analgesia at reduced doses of both agents individually. The synergistic effect greatly increases the likelihood of hypoventilation or apnea, an important consideration in the management of patients without a backup mechanical ventilatory rate.[29]

Hypnosis can also be achieved with propofol. This lipid-soluble agent is widely used in the operating room and with increased frequency in other critical-care settings. It combines rapid onset with rapid awakening because unconsciousness and excellent amnesia occur within 30 seconds of a usual dose and awakening occurs within 10 minutes.[29] Propofol, however, is a significant cardiovascular depressant, more so than the barbiturates, and is somewhat expensive. It requires both a bolus and continuous infusion to maintain hypnosis, and there is a risk of patient allergy.

Sedation Assessment and Scoring

In the past, heavily sedated patients were not uncommon in the majority of critical-care areas, but it is now generally considered that an ideal level of sedation maintains the patient in a cooperative, orientated, and tranquil state when roused, but asleep when not disturbed.[30,31] For most patients, a certain degree of awareness is important to allow them to communicate their needs to the care team. An alert and aware patient is also better able to participate in his or her own care and to gain a sense of control. This situation is also less worrisome for relatives than seeing the patient unconscious for prolonged periods.

Despite recognition of the general goals of patient sedation, achieving an appropriate level of sedation presents a number of clinical and practical problems and there is little standardization of sedative approaches.[32] As with any drug regimen, regular assessment of effect, patient status, and emergent adverse effects is essential. Sedative and analgesic agents should be no exception, but patient assessment is by no means routine practice. A survey of Danish intensive care units has demonstrated that only 16% of the units used a sedation scoring system.[33] This likely reflects the approach in the majority of intensive care units, and it is unclear whether any out-of-hospital providers are using a sedation scoring system.

Table 17-1 Ramsay Sedation Scale

Score	Definition
1	Patient anxious, agitated, or restless
2	Patient cooperative, oriented, and tranquil
3	Patient responds to commands
4	Asleep, but with brisk response to light glabellar tap or loud auditory stimuli
5	Asleep, sluggish response to light glabellar tap or loud auditory stimuli
6	Asleep, no response

Ramsay et al. BMJ. 1974;2:656-659.

Since the RSS was first presented in 1974,[1] it has become a universally recognized standard test of arousability of the sedated patient, providing a numerical ranking of a patient's level of consciousness (Table 17-1). However the RSS level 1 does not differentiate among anxiety, delirium, and agitation, and level 6 does not discriminate between light general anesthesia and deep coma. Furthermore, the scale is not appropriate for the paralyzed patient. Despite these criticisms, it has proven to be a practical and robust tool that has stood the test of time, and it is the only instrument that has received any degree of general acceptance and utilization.[34]

In recognition of the limitations of the RSS, a number of new assessment instruments have been developed in recent years. The most frequently used and best validated are the sedation-agitation or Riker scale; the motor assessment scale; the COMFORT scale; and the latest to join the total of over 30 scales, the Richmond agitation sedation score.[35-40] The use of the bispectral index (BIS) monitor and the patient state index (PSI) monitor are gaining popularity.[41,42]

Summary

Safe postintubation management of the patient hinges on administration of an effective and appropriate level of sedation and analgesia. A good level of each improves patient and practitioner safety and reduces anxiety for both. Vital signs are maintained with better stability when medications are titrated to effect rather than given according to strict dosage regimens or protocols. Frequent assessment of the level of sedation and analgesia is paramount to the success of both airway management and the clinical outcome of the patient.

The best method of controlling sedation is to use medications and assessment techniques with which the practitioner is trained and effective. The adept use of one or two medications is frequently preferable to the juggling of a myriad of medications (e.g., polypharmacy) in which the practitioner is apt to find him- or herself treating the combined effects of medications rather than the patient. The combined wisdom found in the sayings "Practice makes perfect" and "Keep it simple" readily apply to this critical aspect of postintubation management.

Prehospital care would benefit from implementation of methods and programs aimed at the standardization of approaches for the administration and monitoring of sedation and analgesia. Sedation scales such as the RSS have proven beneficial and have received generalized acceptance in the care of critically ill hospitalized patients, and there is no reason to believe that such scales would not assist equally well in the care and monitoring of sedated prehospital patients. BIS and PSI monitors may well prove beneficial for future prehospital care, but further research in this regard is needed. Such research could facilitate standardization of sedative approaches, which could assist in providing solutions to the clinical and practical problems that currently exist in the administration of sedation/analgesia for postintubation management in the prehospital environment.

REVIEW QUESTIONS

1. Can an intubated patient who is not reactive to a painful or noxious stimulus still feel pain?

2. Which intravenous analgesics are currently recommended for out-of-hospital use?

3. List the adverse side-effects associated with the use of fentanyl and ways to prevent them.

4. What drugs are used most often for their anxiolytic and hynotic properties?

5. Why is it important to titrate narcotic analgesics and sedatives rather than administer them as a large bolus or according to a set protocol?

Legal Implications of Emergency Airway Management

William E. Gandy

Chapter Objectives

After reading this chapter, you should be able to:

- Identify the legal basis for a medical malpractice suit.
- Discuss standard of care in airway management.
- Discuss reasons why malpractice cases are filed.
- List the elements that must be proved in a negligence case.
- Describe the documents that make up the pleadings in a lawsuit.
- Describe actions that take place after a suit is filed.
- Describe how a lawsuit may be resolved or concluded.
- Describe post-trial remedies.
- List the essential elements of risk management.
- Demonstrate legally sufficient documentation in an airway case.
- Discuss the peer-review process.
- Formulate a risk-management plan.

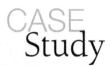

CASE Study _____

Medic 3 and Engine 14 respond to an injured person at a local construction site. When they arrive, the crew members are directed to the back of the building, where a 28-year-old man has fallen 40 feet from scaffolding. They find the man lying on the ground in a combative state and being held down by colleagues. A rapid primary survey reveals that the patient has an open airway, is breathing spontaneously, and has a palpable radial pulse. There is spontaneous eye opening and the patient is localizing pain, but his best verbal response consists of inappropriate words.

With the patient's head and neck held in neutral alignment, the paramedics begin treatment by assisting spontaneous ventilation using a bag-valve-mask (BVM) device. An IV cannula is inserted and, because it is proving difficult to control the patient, a decision is made to perform rapid sequence intubation (RSI). A paramedic administers etomidate 20 mg and vecuronium 10 mg and, once the drugs have taken effect, direct laryngoscopy is attempted.

During the procedure, the patient begins to regurgitate gastric contents. The crew members discover that the suction machine has been left in the ambulance, so the patient is quickly turned onto his side. A second attempt at laryngoscopy is made with the patient in this position and, despite a poor view of the larynx, an endotracheal tube (TT) is inserted. The TT cuff is inflated, and the patient is returned to his back. Ventilations are administered by means of the BVM device, and the patient is moved to the ambulance.

As they begin transport to the hospital, various monitors are applied. They reveal that the patient is bradycardic with a heart rate of 30 beats per minute, his blood pressure is 60/32 mm Hg, and pulse oximetry shows an SpO_2 reading of 58%. They administer atropine 1 mg and a 1-liter bolus of normal saline. At the same time, the patient is hyperventilated in an attempt to improve oxygenation. There is no response to these measures, and the patient's cardiac rhythm soon changes into asystole. Chest compressions are started, and the advanced cardiac life support (ACLS) asystole protocol is followed.

On arrival at the emergency department, the physician listens for breath sounds, finds none, and discovers that the TT has been placed in the esophagus. The tube is removed, and bag-valve-mask ventilation is commenced. After intubation by the physician, the patient has bilateral breath sounds with good rise and fall of the chest and no epigastric sounds. A gastric tube is inserted, and a large amount of air is evacuated from the patient's stomach. The patient fails to respond to treatment, so resuscitation attempts are eventually abandoned and the patient is certified dead.

Crew members had placed the ET tube blindly, failed to properly verify tube placement, and failed to correctly interpret clear signs that something was drastically wrong with the patient. Unfortunately, they chose to treat his symptoms rather than to seek and correct the underlying causes of his deterioration. Several months after this incident, the patient's survivors filed a suit against the emergency medical service (EMS) and each individual member of the crew, alleging gross negligence for failure to properly intubate the patient, failure to recognize that the patient was not properly intubated, failure to provide necessary ventilation to the patient, and for directly causing the patient's death.

After the suit was filed and depositions were taken by both sides, the EMS insurer decided to settle the case. Based on the patient's age, earning power, loss of future earnings, and the loss of his services to the family, settlement was for $1,479,000. Because the patient's survivors have also filed complaints against the EMS service and the paramedics involved, the paramedic who took care of the patient had his certificate suspended for one year by the regulatory authority and chose to leave the EMS profession. The EMS service was fined $15,000, placed on probation by the regulatory authority, and required to conduct remedial classes in airway management for all personnel.

ON TARGET *Failure to ventilate has no legal defense.*

Introduction

Mismanagement of a patient's airway brings serious legal risks. Failure to maintain continuous ventilation has no legal defense because the consequences are so grave.[1] Failures to ventilate are fairly easy to detect and prove. Either one did or did not maintain adequate ventilation. Failure to ventilate results in death or irreversible brain injury in many cases. This chapter will explore the legal implications of airway management.

KEY TERMS

gross negligence, p. 295

malfeasance, p. 295

misfeasance, p. 295

negligence, p. 295

nonfeasance, p. 295

proximate cause, p. 297

standard of care, p. 296

tortfeasor, p. 297

Legal Basis for a Malpractice Case

Medical malpractice cases are usually brought under concepts of the law of torts. A tort is a civil wrong, as opposed to a criminal wrong, although the same act may give rise to both civil and criminal sanctions, as when an assault and battery has occurred. However, malpractice cases may also be brought under contractual concepts such as breach of contract and breach of warranty. Some cases involve failure of medical devices and may result in suits against both the manufacturers and users of the devices.

Negligence implies that something that ought to have been done was not done, something was done that should not have been done, or something that should have been done was done carelessly. **Gross negligence**, sometimes referred to as *negligence with malice*, infers a greater degree of negligence, generally including actions that are reckless in nature.

 The law of torts addresses both negligence and intentional civil wrongs.

negligence
Failure to act as a reasonable and prudent person would have acted under the same or similar circumstances.

gross negligence
Negligence committed with an element of reckless or wanton disregard for the person affected.

Intentional wrongs occur when intentional harm is inflicted. Intentional wrongs may, and often do, result in the filing of criminal charges as well as civil suits.

Why Malpractice Cases Are Filed

Malpractice cases are filed for many reasons, but most involve disappointment with the outcome of the care given. Expectations of care arise from many sources, not the least of which is common human experience. Expectations may also be influenced by cases portrayed on television and in movies, information readily available to lay persons on the Internet, advertising by lawyers, and discussions with medically trained friends and acquaintances.[2]

Expectations may or may not be reasonable. The lay public's expectations may be quite different from the realities of medical practice and realistic outcome possibilities. Patients and their significant others may have a personality conflict with a caregiver that skews their perceptions of the care given. Some practitioners have poor communication skills, appear to be arrogant and uncaring, and may infuriate their patients by their personal actions. All these factors play into the decision by a patient or his or her representatives to seek legal advice and to start a lawsuit.

People are less apt to sue those they genuinely like and respect than those whom they perceive to have offended them in some way. One study that explored reasons for filing complaints against medical providers found that 53% of potential plaintiffs had what they viewed as an unsatisfactory relationship with their provider before the alleged injury happened.[2]

nonfeasance
Failure to do what was required.

misfeasance
Doing a lawfully required act in an improper manner.

malfeasance
Doing a wrongful act, sometimes intentionally.

Understanding the Lawsuit

Understanding the workings of a lawsuit can help prevent claims from being filed and win those that are. All states have statutes of limitations, which provide time limits on filing claims. These limits vary from state to state. Care should be taken to determine whether or not a claim is barred by the statute of limitations.

Most suits against medical practitioners are brought as medical malpractice suits. Negligence occurs when a caregiver fails to "do the right thing" for the patient. Negligence can consist of **nonfeasance**, or failure to do what was required; **misfeasance**, or doing something that was lawful and required but in an improper manner; and **malfeasance**, doing a wrongful or improper act.[3]

People are less apt to sue those they genuinely like and respect than those whom they perceive to have offended them in some way.

Negligence and malpractice suits require the plaintiff to prove at least four standard elements by a preponderance of evidence. The "preponderance" standard in civil cases is different from the "beyond a reasonable doubt" standard in criminal cases. A preponderance of the evidence is only a slight tipping of the scales, whereas beyond a reasonable doubt is the ultimate tipping of the scales. Thus, proof that something is 50.01% more likely than not is a preponderance of the evidence.

The four standard elements that a plaintiff must prove in a negligence case are:

- The defendant had a duty to treat the patient.
- The defendant breached that duty.
- The breach of duty caused injury to the patient (proximate cause).[4]
- There were damages to the patient that can be proven.

Duty to Treat

What constitutes a duty to treat? There was no general duty to treat at common law, and there is no duty to treat unless duty arises in some way. Many cases discuss duty to treat a patient, but they can be reduced to these considerations: the caregiver's employment or status as a volunteer EMS provider requires him to treat, he contracts independently to treat, he accepts the patient for treatment, or he begins treatment unilaterally.

Providing the standard of care in a gracious and friendly way is the best defense against a lawsuit.

Breach of Duty

standard of care

Care that is recognized as acceptable and appropriate by reasonably prudent health care providers.

What constitutes breach of duty? Breach of duty is breach of the **standard of care**. Although there are varying definitions of standard of care in literature and case law, all of them basically say the same thing: standard of care is doing what is reasonable under the circumstances.

A typical definition can be found in Florida law, which defines standard of care as that level of care, skill, and treatment, which, in light of all relevant surrounding circumstances, is recognized as acceptable and appropriate by reasonably prudent similar health care providers.[5] Florida has extended the provisions of its Good Samaritan law, which normally applies only to out-of-hospital care, to treatment in a hospital's emergency department, barring recovery unless treatment demonstrates a reckless disregard for the consequences to the life or health of the patient.[6] This elevates the standard, which will trigger vulnerability to a suit in an emergency department to what is sometimes referred to as gross negligence. This differs from state to state and is not universally true.

All practitioners must be thoroughly familiar with the prevailing standard of care for airway maintenance and evolving changes in concepts. For example, American Heart Association (AHA) ACLS guidelines now suggest that airway adjuncts such as the esophageal tracheal Combitube and the laryngeal mask airway should be present and available for airway care, cervical immobilization devices may minimize the possibility of endotracheal tube displacement, and secondary methods of tube placement confirmation are now required. The Combitube and LMA are presently the only supraglottic devices given the IIa (recommended) rating by the AHA. Secondary methods include self-inflating bulb syringe and similar devices, end-tidal carbon dioxide ($ETCO_2$) detection devices, and waveform capnography.[7] Constant attention to the process of care and continuing education to stay abreast of changes in standards are essential.

Standard of care and *guidelines* are sometimes confused. Standard of care implies a more rigid standard, one universally accepted, deviation from which will result in legal blame, while guidelines may be more suggestive and flexible. However, lines between standard of care and guidelines become blurred, and an expert witness may include guidelines in descriptions of standard of care, and it may be difficult for experts, attorneys, judges, and juries to differentiate between them. The finder of fact (judge or jury) may not perceive the fine distinctions between the two and come to the conclusion that a guideline is in fact a recognized standard of care. Semantic differences may make the point at which a guideline becomes accepted practice difficult to spot.

The standard of care is ultimately decided by the trier of fact, either the judge in a case without a jury, or the jury in a jury case. Even though the world's most eminent medical experts may testify as to the standard of care, it is usually the jury, composed of lay persons, that decides what is the applicable standard of care.

Nationally accepted guidelines such as AHA's ACLS guidelines are difficult to overcome when presented as standard of care.[7] Further, publications such as the American Association of Nurse Anesthetists published "Scope and Standards for Nurse Anesthesia Practice" and the American Society of Anesthesiologists Standards for Basic Intra-Operative Monitoring may have particularly great weight for nurse anesthetists and anesthesiologists.[7–10]

Prehospital emergency medical service providers may find that the same standards and guidelines are applied to their practices. There is no logical reason why they should not be because prehospital providers now have access to a majority of the same airway equipment and supplies that are available inside the hospital.

Causation

The alleged breach of duty must be the cause of the patient's injury. While there may be intervening and superseding injuries, the defendant's alleged negligence must be the direct or **proximate cause** of the injury complained of. Further, the injury must have been foreseeable by the defendant in order for liability to be established.[11] Foreseeability means that a reasonable person would have known or should have known that the injury was a likely result of the conduct involved.

proximate cause
An event that sets off a continuous and unbroken chain of events that results, in law, in injury.

Damages

There must be damages that can be proved to have arisen from the defendant's alleged negligence. Damages fall into three basic categories: economic damages, noneconomic damages, and punitive damages. Economic damages are the tangible costs of medical care, noneconomic damages are for pain and suffering and other intangible factors, while punitive or exemplary damages are meant to punish the negligent party.

Recent legislation in many states has set limits to the noneconomic damages in certain cases. The most common limit on noneconomic damages is $250,000 against one person. Some statutes impose a $250,000 limit on all damages, no matter how many separate **tortfeasors** are involved, and there are also varying formulas for noneconomic damages that can be recovered against hospitals. Most of the statutes do not limit the damages that can be recovered against EMS providers.

tortfeasor
One who commits an act of negligence that is actionable under the law of torts.

The Lawsuit

A lawsuit has many aspects. Understanding them can make dealing with the legal system less stressful. Nomenclature may vary from state to state, but the concepts are generally the same. Table 18-1 illustrates the differing kinds of documents that are filed during a typical case.

Table 18-1   Anatomy of a Lawsuit

Term	Definition
Pleading	Document filed in court to begin a lawsuit, answer a lawsuit, or assert charges against a codefendant or third party.
Motion	A motion asks the court to do something within a lawsuit, such as delay a hearing, dismiss the case, or force a party to do or not do something.
Complaint or petition	Initial pleading filed to begin a lawsuit.
Res ipsa loquitur	Literally "the thing speaks for itself," a special kind of pleading used when an act of negligence is readily inferred from the facts of the case, and the defendant was able to control the facts. Has the effect of shifting the burden to the defendant to prove that negligence was not present. Typical use: when a surgical instrument is left inside the patient or when an endotracheal tube is found to be in the esophagus.
Prayer for relief	Closing portion of a complaint or petition where the plaintiff asks the court to grant him or her judgment and damages.
Answer	The pleading filed by a defendant in response to a plaintiff's complaint or petition for relief.
Counterclaim	A pleading in which a defendant files a claim against the plaintiff.
Reply to counterclaim	The plaintiff's answer to a counterclaim.
Cross claim	A claim by one defendant against another defendant.
Third-party complaint	A defendant's claim against a third party alleging that the third party, not the defendant, is actually responsible for the plaintiff's damages.
Summons or citation	A document issued by the clerk of the court where the case is filed that commands the defendant to answer the plaintiff's complaint or petition. Normally served by a sheriff, constable, or private-process server.

ON TARGET Anyone who receives a summons or citation in a lawsuit should immediately seek legal counsel and prepare to defend the case.

The defendant usually has around 20 days from the date the citation or summons is served on her in which to file an answer to the plaintiff's claims with the clerk of the court. Failure to defend by filing an answer allows the plaintiff to take a default judgment. Default judgments can sometimes be set aside for good reason shown, but not always. One who ignores a court summons or citation does so at his or her peril.

Actions Within a Lawsuit

After a case is filed, many actions take place. Other than trial, the most important is the development of the facts of the case. This is done through a process called discovery, perhaps the most important part of a lawsuit. During this process, the true facts of the case may be developed. Table 18-2 illustrates actions that may take place after a lawsuit is filed.

Table 18-3 illustrates items that a party may be required to produce for inspection by the other side. Production of documents and release of a patient's protected health information are governed by both federal and state laws. The Health Insurance Portability and Accountability Act of 1996, commonly known as HIPAA, provides extensive protections for a patient's health information. HIPAA is a long and complex set of laws and regulations, beyond the scope of this chapter, and all providers should be familiar with its basic provisions.[12] There are numerous nuances and exceptions to its provisions, both contained within the law and regulations, and in other federal and state laws. In a lawsuit brought by a patient, however, the general rule is that all records and other items relative to that patient's care must be produced. HIPAA specifically requires that medical records be produced in response to a valid subpoena.

Table 18-2 Actions Within a Lawsuit

Term	Definition
Discovery	Process by which parties to a lawsuit develop the facts of the case, gain access to documents, and place parties under oath and take their depositions before trial.
Written interrogatories	Written questions an adverse party sends to another party that he or she must answer under oath; for example, "Did you attend the plaintiff on July 2, 2001?"
Request for admissions	A powerful tool used by attorneys to force opposing parties either to admit or deny pertinent facts of a case. Failure to respond properly can result in sanctions against the party.
Request for production of documents	A request that an adverse party produce certain documents for inspection by the requesting party and his or her attorneys.
Subpoena duces tecum	A document commanding a person to appear at a deposition or in trial and bring with him or her documents and items listed in the subpoena.
Notice of intent to take deposition	A notice sent by mail or served by a process server notifying a witness or party that his or her deposition will be taken on a certain day and at a specified time and place and commanding his or her presence.

Resolution of the Lawsuit

Lawsuits may be resolved in many ways, including settlement either before or during trial, through mediation or arbitration, or by court award or jury verdict. Table 18-4 illustrates the most common ways in which a lawsuit is resolved.

Table 18-3 Items Typically Included in *Subpoena Duces Tecum*

- All patient care forms, records, and information relative to the plaintiff, including but not limited to, results of diagnostic tests and studies done on the plaintiff, such as ECG and capnography strips, lab reports, and radiographic studies.
- Patient care policies, protocols, treatment standards, recommendations, and procedures.
- Quality assurance and quality improvement documents.
- Tapes or transcripts of radio and telephone communications between caller, call-taker, dispatcher/controller, and field units, and ambulance to hospital communications.
- Billing information, including Medicare/Medicaid/insurance filings and correspondence.
- Log of disclosures of information and other requests received pursuant to the Health Insurance Portability and Accountability Act of 1996 (HIPAA).
- Correspondence with the patient and other health care providers relative to the incident.
- Incident reports relevant to the patient's care.
- Notes and diaries maintained by the defendant regarding the patient's care.
- Photographs relevant to the case, including pictures of patient's injuries, vehicle wreckage, and so forth.
- Peer-review materials relative to the case. Note, however, that these may not be subject to discovery, but the privilege against discovery may be waived by producing the documents. Care should be taken to clearly identify peer-review materials and keep them separate from patient records.
- Notes taken by the witness in preparation for deposition.
- List of materials looked at in preparation for deposition, including medical reference books, journal articles, films, recordings, photographs, computer data, and Internet sites.
- Records and data maintained on any computer known to the deponent to exist or which could reasonably be discovered to exist, whether or not under the control of the deponent.
- Any records, materials, data, or information relative to the case, not otherwise covered in the request.

Table 18-4	Methods of Lawsuit Resolution
Resolution out of Court	
Settlement before trial	Great majority are settled before trial.
Mediation	Mediator acts as a go-between, assisting the parties in assessing their strengths and weaknesses and assisting them in arriving at a settlement.
Arbitration	An arbitrator or arbitrators act as the finder of fact and render a decision in the matter. The arbitrator's decision may be binding or nonbinding according to the agreement to arbitrate.
Resolution by a Court	
Dismissal	Judge dismisses the case for whatever reason.
Summary judgment	Judge grants summary judgment to a party based on affidavits and depositions, finding that there is not sufficient disputed evidence to be placed before the jury.
Court award or jury verdict	After the evidence is presented, the judge or the jury renders a verdict finding in favor of one party or another.

Standard of Care

Standard of care is nothing more than what should have been done, how it should have been done, and when. When it is applied to airway management, it includes not only the proper methods, devices, and techniques to be employed in airway management, but also the total scope of management, from initial patient contact to documentation. Knowledge, skills, planning, practice, assembly of the proper equipment, supplies and drugs, patient monitoring, and overall performance are all part of the standard of care.[10,13]

Standard of care is generally proved by opinion testimony from experts for each side. Experts may be asked the basis for their opinions, and they generally cite textbooks and other written materials generally recognized as being authoritative; policies, protocols, and procedures; peer-reviewed research findings that have been published in recognized medical journals; and practice guidelines promulgated by medical societies such as the American Heart Association, American Society of Anesthesiologists, American Association of Nurse Anesthetists, and the American College of Emergency Physicians; and personal professional experience. Hospital and EMS protocols and practice standards are admissible and have the practical effect of setting the standard of care. Deviation from one's own protocols is difficult to defend.

Thus, a recommendation by a national organization to employ at least one secondary tube placement confirmation device may arguably become standard of care.[7] Deviation from a practice guideline may be explainable and found not to violate standard of care, but experts may disagree and present conflicting evidence. Some courts recognize a "respected minority" view. The jury will make the ultimate decision.

PEARLS Deviation from the emergency medical service's own protocols sets up a presumption of violation of standard of care that must be overcome by testimony showing that the deviation was reasonable. Protocols are the best evidence of an emergency medical service's standard of care.

An expert should expect to be cross-examined on the bases for his opinions and asked to justify them, especially if they differ substantially from nationally recognized standards or guidelines. At one time, standard of care was said to be the prevailing standard in the geographical region where the physician or other provider practices, suggesting that rural practitioners ought not be held to the same standards as urban practitioners; however, such a locality rule is rather meaningless because airway management practices are much the same the world over.[13]

While said to be the ultimate search for truth, a trial is in fact a duel by experts and attorneys to influence the trier of fact, whether that be judge or jury. The judge or jury weigh the evidence presented and decide what it believes to be the proper standard of care. While the jury's finding may be at odds with the opinions of one or more parties or experts, if there was credible and properly admissible evidence to support the jury's verdict, it generally will not be overturned.

Damages

Many states have now placed limits on the amount that can be awarded for noneconomic damages. Typically, noneconomic damages such as for pain and suffering, emotional stress, or loss of the companionship of one's mate or family member can be capped at $250,000. Noneconomic damages are intangible damages.

The plaintiff's lawyers typically try to link testimony about inability to perform normal functions—sleep and eating disturbances, sexual dysfunction, and other corporal manifestations of intangible damages—to testimony about pain and suffering, mental anguish, and depression to demonstrate measurable and recordable events. Videos of the injured party may be shown, and computer-generated reenactments may be used by either side. For example, a video of a plaintiff who claims substantial disability playing basketball will have considerable impact on a jury. On the other hand, "a day in the life" videos are often presented, depicting in gruesome detail the injured party's life and disabilities after the injury.

Economic damages generally include hospital bills, doctor bills, ambulance bills, future medical bills, and other tangible damages. They are not capped. Notwithstanding the caps on damages, a patient who suffers hypoxic brain damage and who is in a persistent vegetative state will be entitled to damages for future care, and these damages can be astronomical. Economists usually testify as to these damages, and they take into consideration factors such as inflation, increased medical costs, and loss of income.

Post-Trial Remedies

Either side may appeal a court's or jury's findings and award, but unless the judge made a significant mistake in allowing evidence to be heard or examined by the jury, he or she erred in ruling on an issue of law or in granting a motion, or there was insufficient evidence to support the jury's findings, appeals courts generally do not overturn judgments and verdicts.

Risk Management

Each practitioner should practice risk management on his or her own. Risk management consists of protection of the individual and institution from loss. Key factors in risk management are:

- Identification of risks.
- Planning to minimize risks.
- Knowledge of standard of care and adherence to it.
- Adequate practice, planning, and assembling of helpers and equipment.
- Competence in all medical techniques employed.
- Proper monitoring of the patient at all times.
- Recognition of changes in the patient's condition that signal an adverse event.
- Proper documentation of the case.

Both the American Society of Anesthesiologists and the American Association of Nurse Anesthetists have conducted closed case studies over the last two decades in which insurance carriers made available extensive case materials to reviewing panels for analysis of the factors leading to the filing of lawsuits.[1,14–16] As a result of the first of these studies, three situations—inadequate ventilation, esophageal intubation, and difficult endotracheal intubation—were identified as the principal causes of lawsuits against anesthesiologists and anesthetists. Other adverse outcomes resulted from airway obstruction, bronchospasm, aspiration, premature tracheal extubation, unintentional tracheal extubation, inadequate oxygenation, endobronchial intubation, esophageal or pharyngeal perforations or lacerations, injury to other airway structures, and temporomandibular injuries.[16]

Risk Identification

Since those studies were undertaken, airway management practices have changed significantly, particularly with the advent of pulse oximetry, end-tidal carbon dioxide monitoring, and waveform capnography. The percentage of claims based on esophageal intubations and inadequate ventilation declined, while claims based on difficult airway problems proportionally increased, with emphasis being placed on injuries resulting from inadequate patient monitoring. Awards have diminished given the reduction in catastrophic outcomes.[1]

Evidence that an injury was preventable is admissible; therefore, it is essential that patients be monitored using the methods now available at all levels of practice. Monitoring must be coupled with critical thinking and analysis so that changes in the patient's condition are neither ignored nor rationalized.[10,15]

While significant closed claims studies involving prehospital airway management have not been done, the principles learned from the anesthesia studies logically apply to the prehospital setting. Airway management in the prehospital setting is more difficult than in the controlled hospital environment. Noise levels in ambulances may effectively prevent auscultation of breath sounds; poor lighting, patient movement, presence of clothing, dressings, bandages, stretcher straps, and other equipment may make observation of chest excursion unreliable, and limited numbers of crew members available to attend the patient during transport make the use of careful evaluation of tube placement with the esophageal detector device, pulse oximetry, capnometry, and capnography and proper documentation even more critical.

Risk-management plans should develop a system of information retrieval following critical incidents to follow all contributing factors. Extenuating circumstances may exist, and it is essential that those be documented.

Risk management involves continuing education, training, and practice in best practices and procedures, monitoring, and interpretation of findings. Preoxygenation prior to tube placement may delay onset of cyanosis. Practitioners must learn not to ignore or rationalize hemodynamic changes (changes in heart rate, hypotension, cardiac dysrhythmias) and to seek the causes of such changes rather than attempting simply to treat the emergent condition.[14]

In one study, auscultation of the airway resulted in the mistaken conclusion that the ET tube was in the trachea in 48% of cases involving esophageal intubation.[14] Practitioners may be tempted to explain distant breath sounds by factors such as obesity, background noise, and lack of signs of abdominal distention. Having an attitude that capnometry, waveform capnography, and oximetry are subject to interpretation, and a mind-set toward everything being okay can lead to a spiral of unrecoverable events.

Peer Review

Peer review is a process by which an incident may be reviewed and evaluated by one's peers to determine ways in which to improve patient care. Peer review has been established by statute both at the federal[17] and state levels[18] and has been the subject of extensive discussion and review by the courts. A review of existing peer-review statutes and court rulings far exceeds the scope of this chapter.

The peer-review process is supposed to be confidential and not subject to discovery in a legal proceeding. However, peer-review protections range from near absolute[17,18] to a system of balancing interests, in which a court looks at the materials involved in the peer-review process and determines which information can be disclosed.[19] A recent federal case held that peer-review organizations (PROs) conducted under the Health Care Quality Improvement Act of 1986, as administered by the Department of Health and Human Services Centers for Medicare and Medicaid Services (CMS), have a duty to notify patients when the investigations have been completed. The court further held that a PRO operating under CMS must disclose findings of physician misconduct to patients who seek such information.[20]

All PROs are not conducted under the federal law, however. Individual organizations such as hospitals, medical societies, and other organizations may use the peer-review process to improve health care. State laws may govern their proceedings. The Minnesota Court of Appeals ruled in 1999 that the peer-review statute protects an organization from disclosing peer-review information.[20] A similar result occurred in Texas.[21]

The Health Insurance Portability and Accountability Law of 1996 (HIPAA) contains a complex scheme of rules regarding release of protected health information (PHI). HIPAA gives the patient powerful tools to determine the uses of his or her PHI.[12] To date, there are no court interpretations of HIPAA regarding peer-review materials.

Each provider should become familiar with the provisions of the peer-review laws that govern him or her. Nuances abound. Some states may not protect nurses and prehospital providers in the same way that physicians are protected. Protections may inadvertently be lost unless the peer-review process is conducted in the proper procedural way. Committees should avoid mixing evaluation of medical care activities with non-peer-review functions, opening a meeting to public participation and input, and inadvertently releasing portions of a peer-review file.[22]

Recent legislation has been introduced into Congress that would affect peer-review matters, but no final legislation has been passed at this writing.

Documenting the Airway Case

Documentation is the foundation of defense because it is one of the strongest methods by which the facts are established and verified. Good documentation often dissuades lawyers from filing a case, while bad documentation can have the opposite effect. Because few cases are filed until months or years after the incident, and most depositions and trials occur even later, the defendant and his or her witnesses may not remember the facts or details of the case. Documentation at the time of the incident can counter these natural memory lapses.

 Always document that the patient received adequate ventilations at all times.

Documentation should be clear and comprehensive, and should tell a story that the court and jury can understand because they will usually see it during their deliberations. Misspellings and errors in grammar and punctuation can send a negative message about the writer to the jury. Check boxes do not tell a complete story unless they are accompanied by a narrative statement.

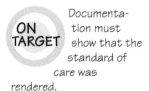 Documentation must show that the standard of care was rendered.

All documentation should reflect that the patient was either breathing adequately by her- or himself or was being adequately ventilated at all times by the defendant or his or her associates. It is not negligence to place an endotracheal tube into a patient's esophagus if the mistake is discovered and corrected before injury occurs. It is negligence, and probably gross negligence, to misplace an endotracheal tube and fail to discover it before the patient has suffered hypoxic injury.

Further, it is not wrong not to intubate a patient if his or her airway can be protected and he or she can be ventilated adequately by other means. Adequate ventilation and protection of the airway, not intubation, is the standard of care.

Good care and good documentation are your best defenses against a lawsuit. Good documentation requires a narrative report that tells a clear story of the patient's condition and treatment for the jury. Check-box documentation is useful as a reminder, but it is no substitute for a clear and complete narrative report.

Good documentation includes the following facts: a summary of the patient's ventilatory status prior to intervention, the need for assisted ventilation, all steps taken to ventilate the patient, and the outcome of the steps taken in terms of patient condition. Documentation of endotracheal tube placement should be done not only immediately after placement but serially after each time the patient is moved, another procedure is done, or at least every three to four minutes. Use of other airway adjuncts such as tube introducers, Combitube, LMA, or other adjunctive devices should be documented similarly.

Documentation of endotracheal tube placement should include at least the following:

- Summary of the need for intubation and the time of the start of the procedure.
- Preoxygenation of the patient and by what means.
- Type and size of laryngoscope blade or other device used.
- Statement of visualization of the cords or other structures (eg. Cormack & Lehane laryngeal grade).
- Statement of visualization of the tube passing through the vocal cords, if applicable.
- Statement of the usage of a tube introducer, if applicable.
- Statement of inflation of the cuff.
- Tube depth to the teeth or gums, in centimeters.
- How the tube was secured.
- Statement of observation of chest rise and fall with ventilation.
- Statement of auscultation of equal breath sounds at the apices and along the midaxillary lines.
- Statement of auscultation over the epigastrium with absence of breath sounds.
- Verification by at least one AHA recommended secondary device, such as end-tidal carbon dioxide detector, esophageal detector device, or preferably waveform capnography.
- Patient condition after intubation in terms of skin color, pulse oxymetry, heart rate, ECG, and improvement in level of consciousness, if present.

Once this documentation is written and the time is noted, further serial placement checks can be documented with just the times (e.g., further tube placement verifications done as above, beginning with checking cuff inflation, at 1021, 1025, 1029, 1033, and 1035 hours, and found to be correctly placed each time). Further supporting documentation is provided by the SpO_2 log, ECG strips, capnography graphs, and patient vital signs recorded.

Summary

Careful attention to standard of care, planning, practice, technique, and documentation can discourage lawsuits and help you win if you should be unfortunate enough to be sued. Remember that airway mistakes can result in devastating legal and medical consequences. Consider the following: adequate assessment of the airway prior to attempting intubation, adequate preparation, recognition of risk factors, adequate technique, adequate use of adjuncts for airway management, continuous ventilation, adequate patient monitoring, greater opportunity for dislodgment, and difficulty in assessing clinical signs. Documentation should demonstrate standard of care. Airway maintenance is an ongoing process and requires ongoing checks and serial documentation.

REVIEW QUESTIONS

1. What situation has no legal defense in airway management?

2. How can one minimize the likelihood of a lawsuit filed against him or her?

3. What action should be taken when you are served with a citation or summons showing that a lawsuit has been filed against you?

4. At a minimum, what should be documented with regard to airway management?

5. Who ultimately determines the "standard of care" in a lawsuit?

Nosocomial Risks of Airway Management

W. Patrick Monaghan

Chapter Objectives

After reading this chapter, you should be able to:

- State the specific risks of nosocomial infections to both patients and health care providers.

- Discuss the rate of nosocomial infections that may occur and what steps health care providers can do to protect themselves and their patients.

- Discuss commonly contaminated items and medical incidents leading to nosocomial infections in both patients and health care providers.

- Discuss the need for proper and standardized cleaning and sterilization of equipment.

- List steps to take in preventing nosocomial infections.

CASE Study _____

Medic 1 responds to a medical emergency at a nursing home following a report that a resident has collapsed. Within four minutes of the call, they arrive on scene. They are directed to a room where they find two staff members performing CPR on a 68-year-old man who is lying on the floor. They are told that the man is a heavy smoker and has a history of coronary artery disease and emphysema. He had called staff to report an attack of severe central chest pain, and he collapsed as two care assistants entered his room to investigate. The staff at the home are all BLS-trained, so one assistant started CPR while the other called 911.

The paramedics instruct the staff to continue CPR while they attach adhesive defibrillation/monitoring pads to the man's chest. Once the pads are applied, they ask the staff to suspend resuscitation to permit analysis of the cardiac rhythm. Coarse ventricular fibrillation is seen on the monitor. A single biphasic shock of 150 joules is delivered from the defibrillator, and chest compressions are resumed immediately at a rate of 100 per minute. An oropharyngeal airway is inserted, and CPR is continued for an additional two minutes, with two bag-valve-mask (BVM) ventilations given after every 30 chest compressions.

At the end of two minutes, CPR is suspended a second time, and the heart rhythm is analyzed again. Normal sinus rhythm is seen on the monitor, but there is no palpable carotid pulse and no spontaneous respirations, so CPR is resumed. An IV cannula is inserted, and preparations are made for intubation. The intubating paramedic opens his airway bag and removes an 8.0 mm endotracheal tube (ETT). This is a tube that he keeps out of its packaging ready for use with a stylet already inserted. Direct laryngoscopy is performed with a #3 Miller blade. There is a clear view of the larynx, and chest compressions are briefly suspended as the ETT is passed between the vocal cords. The tube cuff is inflated, correct placement of the ETT is confirmed, and CPR is immediately resumed.

With the patient safely intubated, uninterrupted chest compressions are given, and the patient is simultaneously bagged at a rate of 10 ventilations per minute. As the ambulance pulls into the hospital, the patient begins to show signs of life, so the chest compressions are discontinued. He is making some attempts to breathe, so his respirations are assisted by manual bagging. He is admitted to the intensive care unit and soon regains consciousness. Two days later, the patient becomes febrile, and his chest x-ray reveals a right-side infection. Sputum cultures show a heavy growth of gram negative rods and, despite antibiotic treatment, his condition deteriorates and he dies the following day from septicemia secondary to a fulminating chest infection.

Introduction

Intubation and airway management procedures pose significant nosocomial risks to both patients and health care providers.[1] According to Occupational Safety and Health Administration (OSHA) regulations, all health care providers are required to wear gloves whenever a risk of exposure to blood or infectious microorganisms exist.[2] Quite often, the proper wearing of gloves and protective clothing is not done. It was reported by Bready in 1988 that 1.5 to 2.5 million patients had acquired **nosocomial infections** and at least 15,000 had died as a direct result.[3] A recent report by the Centers for Disease Control (CDC) estimates that 2 to 3 million cases of nosocomial infections occur annually in patients hospitalized in the United States.[4] About 90,000 of these patients actually die each year as a result of these acquired infections. It is obvious that these rates of nosocomial infection will continue to soar, especially with the increased occurrence of antibiotic-resistant strains of microorganism.

nosocomial infection

An infection acquired in a hospital.

 The use of protective gloves and frequent hand washing are the fundamental practices that can limit the spread of infection. Gloves should be changed frequently during a paramedic call to avoid contaminating objects in the ambulance and the emergency department.

methicillin-resistant S. aureus (MRSA)

A type of bacteria that is resistant to certain antibiotics, such as methicillin and other more common antibiotics, such as oxacillin, penicillin, and amoxicillin.

It is well documented that each year an estimated 100,000 individuals are hospitalized with **methicillin-resistant S. aureus (MRSA)** infections.[5] In many of those MRSA cases, vancomycin is the antibiotic of choice for treatment, but several of these cases have also become vancomycin-resistant. This increasing trend in the occurrence of resistant bacteria and too few new antibiotics in the research and development pipeline all indicate frequent hospital-acquired infections with increasing morbidity and mortality. All personnel in the medical environment, including all cleaning personnel and administrative and clinical groups, obviously need to take a proactive role in reducing these infections and fatalities. The specific role that airway management techniques play and the degree to which these procedures may result in nosocomial infections are difficult to fully define.[6,7] All aspects of airway management need to be assessed completely to more fully understand what part these procedures may contribute to these incredibly high rates of morbidity and mortality. These assessment categories of airway management include equipment, personnel, and the environment.

KEY TERMS

Equipment

The Centers for Disease Control estimates that 2 to 3 million cases of nosocomial infections occur annually in patients hospitalized in the United States, and about 90,000 of the patients die each year from those infections.

Almost all advanced airway management procedures begin with the use of laryngoscopes. It is well documented that many of these instruments are contaminated due to the fact that they receive inadequate terminal sterilization.

Several significant studies conducted throughout the previous 15 years have documented the occurrence of improperly cleaned equipment used for airway management.[7-17] Most notably have been the studies that consistently exhibit the frequency with which laryngoscope blades and handles are contaminated. Almost all airway management procedures begin with the use of laryngoscopes. Presently, there is well-documented evidence that many of these laryngoscopes and bronchoscopes are frequently contaminated with occult blood prior to use.

In 1989, Kanefield, et al.[7] reported an elegant study that investigated whether visible or occult blood was present on airway management equipment that was in routine use in their anesthetic practice. They examined the equipment used in 100 general anesthetic cases that involved intubation. After completion of the cases, the equipment was collected and placed in a vat of water, and after a few minutes the water was tested for occult blood. Visible gross blood or positive occult blood occurred in 86 of their cases. Morell et al. sampled 38 laryngoscope blades and handles from two different hospitals. Using a guiac-based assay, they found 10.5% of the blades and 50% of the handles were contaminated with occult blood.[12]

Phillips reported in 1997 a study on the incidence of visible and occult human blood that occurred on laryngoscope blades and handles that were all labeled as "ready for patient use."[16] All of these instruments were located in various operating-room suites. A modified three-stage phenolphthalein blood forensic test was used. Of the total 65 blades and handles tested, 20% of the blades and 40% of the handles tested positive for occult blood. Afternoon samples were consistently higher in testing positive, indicating that it was likely that cross-contamination throughout the day may have been occurring.

As a direct result of many of these studies, Tobin, et al. (1995) developed and made commercially available a simple laryngoscope handle protection device in an attempt to lessen the frequency of using contaminated laryngoscope blades and handles.[17] These devices consisted of small disposable plastic bags that were placed over the laryngoscope blades and handles. Several manufacturers have also advocated the use of disposable plastic laryngoscope blades. Another alternative was the development of a disposable latex or polyethylenelike sleeve that fits over the laryngoscope and contains a one-way valve, which allowed air to be evacuated to achieve a closer fit. An example of one such sleeve is the Pogo. The Pogo developed by Pogo, Inc. of Rochester, MN, was felt by many users to be somewhat cumbersome to adapt and has not apparently achieved widespread use.

One alternative to using potentially contaminated reusable equipment is to use disposable laryngoscope blades and fiberoptic devices. One example of sterile stainless steel disposable fiberoptic laryngoscope blades are the Greenline/d disposable laryngoscope blades (SunMed USA, Largo, FL [www.airwaystore.com]). An example of clean disposable ABS plastic laryngoscope spatel blade that is non-sterile, yet clean is the Heine XP® (Heine Medical, http://www.heinemedical.com). Several commercial manufacturers have marketed suitable disposable equipment. Many manufacturers now market disposable supraglottic airways. A single-use bougie introducer (eg., endotracheal tube introducer by SunMed USA, Largo, FL [www.airwaystore.com] and also by Smiths Medical, Keene, NH [www.smiths-medical.com]) is also available, as are single-use airway exchange catheters. (Cook Critical Care, Bloomington, IN [www.cookmedical.com]).

Nikkola in 1999 sampled 211 pieces of ready-to-use airway management equipment in seven different sites within a large military hospital.[13] Three percent of the items inspected contained visible blood, and 17% were found to be positive for occult blood. This data further support the lack of compliance with adequate cleaning and decontamination procedures. The improperly cleaned airway management equipment is often used to perform lifesaving procedures and may needlessly expose both patients and health care workers to life-threatening diseases carried on these fomites.

Perry in 1997 (later published in 2001) sampled 210 items of anesthesia equipment and monitoring devices such as pulse oximeter probes and blood pressure cuffs commonly used in the operating room at two different hospitals. Thirty-three percent of the items tested were found to be positive for occult blood.[15]

In 2003, Nolen examined laryngoscope blades and handles at both a community and major teaching facility hospital.[14] Thirty percent of the 120 samples were tested using the forensic phenolphthalein blood test and found to be positive for occult blood. Statistically significant, more morning blades and handles tested positive. The community hospital in this sample also had a higher rate of positively tested equipment.

Endoscopes have also been a source of documented hospital-acquired infections. In 1997, two separate studies reported that multiple patients contracted mycobacterium tuberculosis (TB) from inadequately disinfected bronchoscopes.[9,11] Both of these studies demonstrated the growth of bacteria or the presence of blood on the surfaces of medical equipment after they were supposedly decontaminated.

In addition to several bacterial and parasitic diseases that can be spread by blood, both human immunodeficiency virus (HIV) and hepatitis are common viral diseases that have been proven to be blood-borne. Hepatitis B has been shown to survive from between seven to ten days on dry surfaces.[10] The HIV organism was originally reported to be detectable on surfaces for up to 15 days;[8] however, current advisories from the CDC report no recorded instances of HIV transmission from surfaces.[18]

The common thread exhibited by these frequency and epidemiological studies show several significant findings.[8-11,13-17] Approximately 30% of the reusable medical equipment that is ready for patient use may have remnants of human blood on their surfaces. Some of these studies have documented the occurrence of visible organic matter on the equipment. The finding of occult blood on this equipment serves as an indicator that these items were not properly cleaned. The fact that many of these studies were done in different medical facilities in various geographical locations over a long period of time, yet portray similar findings, speak for the veracity of this data. Because of the complexity, very few microbiological and viral studies are performed on medical equipment. Blood contamination frequency studies can therefore be more easily performed and indicate the improper cleaning of these devices. It is obvious that these high rates of blood contamination on various pieces of commonly used medical equipment most certainly contribute to the estimated 2 to 3 million cases of nosocomial infections that occur each year.

The performance of venipunctures, collection of blood for arterial blood gases, and the insertion of catheters pose relatively common risks, most notably the potential spread of infectious agents or injury involved in the handling of sharp instruments. According to the National Institute for Occupational Safety and Health (NIOSH), 600,000 to 800,000 needle-stick accidents are reported each year.[19] Judicious care in performing all invasive procedures must be rigidly adhered to in order to minimize the spread of infectious organisms. All sharp instruments used in the collection of blood specimens must be appropriately handled. Of paramount importance is the proper handling and disposal of all sharp instruments according to local facility policies to minimize exposing these hazardous materials to others.

A great deal of recent interest has been directed toward the potential role that **prions** may play in disease transmission.[20,21] Human prion diseases include Creutzfeldt-Jakob disease (CJD), which has several variants. These mutations of the prion protein gene include the close relative of bovine spongiform encephalopathy (BSE). The human variant form of this disease may not become symptomatic until 5 to 20 years after initial infection. Medical equipment contaminated with infective material may transmit these diseases to other patients.[22]

Laryngeal mask airways and other sterilized reusable rubber anesthesia products have been shown to contain protein contaminants.[23] An erythrosin B dye used in a test that stains for protein has found that 90% of the airway masks were positive for protein remnants. The current cleaning methods appear to be inadequate in removing all proteinaceous material.

prion

A proteinaceous infectious particle; an infectious particle made entirely of protein.

Personnel

The maintenance of proper personal hygiene of all health care providers is of paramount importance in preventing the spread of infections throughout the health care environments. The wearing of clean protective garments and shoes clearly plays a vital role in protecting the health care provider from becoming contaminated with harmful substances (Table 19-1).

Table 19-1 Frequently Contaminated Personal Items

Frequently contaminated personal items on or near the health care provider that contribute to the spread of nosocomial infections include:

- Hands.
- Pens.
- Stethoscopes.
- Computer keyboards.
- Clothing.
- Shoes.
- Cell phones.
- Neckties.

Adequate and frequent hand washing is reputed to be the most critical and fundamental practice one can perform to limit the spread of infections. The routine use of sterile gloves in the performance of all procedures in which contact with any patient occurs also needs to be done.

Many individuals who were trained prior to the 1990s may have performed routine procedures like venipuncture without being gloved. Because of the potential for blood-borne infections, it is imperative that gloves be worn. These practices help protect both the health care providers and the patients. The provision of waterless cleansers and decontamination solutions need to be readily available to airway management personnel, anesthesia providers, and operating-room personnel when sinks and soaps are not easily accessible. Protective gloves are now being developed that are better than the latex, vinyl, nitrile, and powder-free variety currently available. Bernard Technologies has developed a new antimicrobial glove designed to reduce the cross-contamination that frequently occurs in hospitals.[24] These gloves actually emit a gaseous form of chlorine dioxide, which can effectively kill bacteria, spores, viruses, fungi, and parasites. They are being used in the Asian and European markets and should be available in other markets soon.

Protective clothing—including operating-room scrubs and outer laboratory coats—are worn to protect both the patients and providers. Frequently, individuals in hospitals are observed wearing blood-stained and soiled garments and shoes. Most of us have observed individuals with these contaminated clothing in the food-service and vending areas, getting their food and eating their lunch. It is highly unlikely that they change their clothing each time prior to performing subsequent patient cases. The actual role that these garments have in the spread of nosocomial infections is difficult to ascertain but relatively easy to envision.

Physical items carried and used by the health care provider are frequently found to be contaminated. Recently, reported that frequently contaminated items included the cell phones carried and used by various health care providers.[25] Writing implements like pens were also reported to be contaminated with bacteria and blood residue. Stethoscopes are frequently found to be contaminated. Computer keyboards are a common site of contamination, and some facilities have advocated the use of latex protective coverings for these keyboards. These coverings of the computer board, of course, need to be changed and routinely cleaned by housekeeping personnel.

Most recently reported at the American Society for Microbiology meeting (Lori Rackl, *Chicago Sun-Times*) was a study that identified neckties worn by health care providers as harboring disease-causing bacteria.[26] Fifty percent of the clinicians sampled had ties that carried common bacteria capable of causing pneumonia and urinary tract and blood infections. Ten security guards who wore neckties also had their ties cultured. The clinicians were eight times more likely to be wearing neckties that were contaminated with pathogenic bacteria. The average office environment may harbor large amounts of bacteria; common items include the desktop, doorknobs, microwave handles, keyboards, and telephone receivers.[27,28]

Environment (Aerosols, Ambient Microorganisms, Sound, Stress, Decreased Immune System)

The physical environment where one works can adversely affect individuals because of exposure to gases, aerosols, ambient microorganisms, and highly variable sound levels. All of these factors are known to increase stress and have an adverse effect on various physiological processes such as the immune system.

Aerosols in the operating room environment are a common event and can be hazardous to individuals. Although most hospitals provide air filtration, some nonhospital work environments may require more efforts to minimize exposure to dust, vapor, fumes, and other materials. It is prudent that these common contaminants be minimized and kept away from both the patient and the health care provider's breathing zone. Some commercial filtering units such as the Winged Sentry[*] (Sentry Air Systems, Inc., Houston, TX) are available which exhibit efficiencies up to 99.97 percent and at removing particles as small as 0.3 microns in providing clean air. Continued efforts at improving the clinical environment are needed. Improved methods at decreasing the adverse effects of environmental factors on all health care personnel necessitate upgrading.

Summary

A more comprehensive understanding of the inherent risks associated with all airway management procedures will greatly assist in reducing the number and frequency of nosocomial infections. This will most likely occur when every health care provider has increased his or her body of knowledge and awareness of these exceedingly high rates of morbidity and mortality. Such knowledge serves as a challenge to everyone to practice clean and safe procedures to reduce the spread of all infections.

The recently documented high rates of hospital-acquired infections and the subsequent morbidity and mortality is a cause for concern for all personnel involved in providing health care. Everyone, from the first responders to nurses, doctors, rehabilitationists, and the patient's family, must be aware of the risks in the spread of infectious agents. Awareness can help decrease the spread of these agents to both patients and health care providers. Specific actions that have proven useful in reducing the frequency of these nosocomial infections include vigilance, monitoring, performance of proper procedures, incidence reporting, case management, and the conduction of sampling and frequency studies.

Clearly the best defense against nosocomial infections of any sort relies on frequent hand washing and changing gloves between each patient contact. In prehospital care, disposable devices and equipment should be the rule rather than the exception because of the challenge imposed by transporting, handling, and processing contaminated equipment and products.

REVIEW QUESTIONS

1. What measures should be assessed to understand how to limit nosocomial infections?

2. What item of equipment used in airway management is frequently contaminated prior to being used for patient care?

3. What measures should be taken to ensure that laryngoscope blades and handles are not contaminated and ready for patient use?

4. Approximately how many needle-stick incidents occur annually in the U.S.?

5. Name several personal items that have been shown to be frequently contaminated.

Answers to
Review Questions

Chapter 1

1. The patient should be oxygenated by spontaneously breathing 100% oxygen by nonrebreathing mask, be manually ventilated using positive-pressure mask ventilation with the BVM, or a supraglottic airway device, as needed.

2. Generally limit intubation attempts to less than 10 minutes or no more than three attempts by an experienced laryngoscopist because attempting further laryngoscopies beyond this will probably not be successful using the same failed methods and will likely cause trauma and swelling which can lead to a cannot-mask-ventilate/cannot-intubate situation, a much more serious critical airway event.

3. Three simple methods to rescue failed intubation (among others) are external laryngeal manipulation, head-elevated laryngoscopy position, and bougie-assisted intubation.

4. Auscultation of the lungs and epigastrium, compliance of the ventilation bag, and tube condensation are unreliable and nonfailsafe signs of correct tube placement and should not be used without first using evidence-based devices such as waveform or colormetric capnography or an esophageal detector device or relying on a second laryngoscopy to ensure that the tracheal tube lies appropriately within the glottis as is evidenced by the visible presence of laryngeal anatomy.

5. The Combitube or LMA Classic or LMA Unique should be used for rescue ventilation in the presence of a critical airway event such as inability to intubate or mask ventilate the patient, three or more failed intubation attempts or attempting intubation for longer than 10 minutes, or sustained hypoxemia that does not respond to positive-pressure mask ventilation with 100% oxygen despite the use of oropharyngeal and/or nasopharyngeal airways.

6. Mason's PU-92 concept works as follows. If the patient is either 1) responsive only to pain (AVPU = P), or 2) unresponsive to any stimuli (AVPU = U) and the $SpO_2 \leq 92\%$ despite maximal attempts at ventilation with 100% oxygen, the patient is deemed to have a "crash" airway and needs to receive immediate lung ventilation with 100% oxygen. Pulse oximeters generally have a tolerance of $\pm 2\%$. Since the threshold for hypoxemia is an SaO_2 of 90%, the threshold when using a pulse oximeter is an SpO_2 of 92%.

7. The SLAM Universal Adult Airway Flowchart depends heavily on assessment of SpO_2. If SpO_2 measurement is not possible, rescuers should proceed using their best clinical judgment concerning oxygenation. However, hypoxemia is difficult to diagnose clinically, and doubly so in the prehospital setting, so every effort should be made to obtain a pulse oximeter reading. No algorithm can be created to fit all situations; thus, the SUAAF must be interpreted, modified, and applied according to individual patient assessment and good clinical judgment. Additionally the algorithm has not been designed for use in children.

Chapter 2

1. Two methods of manipulating the thyroid cartilage are external laryngeal manipulation (ELM) and backward, upward, rightward pressure (BURP).

2. The cricoid cartilage lies at the most inferior aspect of the larynx.

3. The cricoid cartilage is the narrowest part of the pediatric larynx. The glottis is the narrowest part of the adult larynx.

4. The bougie can be slipped posterior to the epiglottis when the vocal cords cannot be seen. As it is moved through the cords and into the trachea, vibrations can be felt as the tip travels over the tracheal rings (tracheal clicking). The tracheal tube can then be railroaded over the bougie into the airway.

5. A Cormack and Lehane Grade 4 view shows only soft tissue, with no identifiable laryngeal anatomy. This indicates a difficult intubation, generally requiring advanced techniques other than direct laryngoscopy.

Chapter 3

1. The functions of the respiratory system are to: a) move air to and from the gas-exchange surfaces of the lungs, b) help control the pH (acidity/alkalinity) of the body fluids, c) permit vocal communication, and d) provide specific defenses against the invasion of pathogens and other foreign material.

2. The intercostal muscles are innervated via the ventral rami of the thoracic nerves (intercostal nerves).

3. The diaphragm is innervated by cervical nerve roots three, four, and five. Neural transmission via cranial nerves C_3, C_4, and C_5 is necessary for diaphragmatic contractions to occur.

4. The result of a C7-level transection is immediate and complete paralysis of the intercostal muscles, but diaphragmatic contractions are not affected.

5. When the arms are in a fixed position and the patient is sitting up and leaning forward, the pectoral muscles that attach between the chest wall and upper arms can assist in raising the chest wall.

6. An increase in hydrogen ion concentration results in a rightward shift of the oxygen dissociation curve whereas a decrease in hydrogen ion concentration has the opposite effect. The affinity that hemoglobin has for oxygen alters according to the chemical environment, an increased affinity resulting in a shift of the oxygen dissociation curve to the left and a decreased affinity shifting it to the right. Factors that decrease the oxygen affinity and allow greater quantities of oxygen to dissociate from the hemoglobin molecule include an increase in both temperature and the acidity of the blood. Factors such as an increase in hydrogen (H^+) increase the acidity of the blood and cause a shift of the oxygen dissociation curve to the right. A decrease in affinity of hemoglobin for oxygen allows greater quantities of oxygen to dissociate from the hemoglobin, thereby making more oxygen available for exchange with cells.

7. Partial pressure of oxygen in the alveoli at sea level is 102 mm Hg (760 mm Hg $\times$ 13.4%). For carbon dioxide, it is 40 mm Hg (760 mm Hg $\times$ 5.2%). Venous blood perfusing through the alveolar capillaries has about 40 mm Hg of O_2, so that oxygen at a high partial pressure of 102 mm Hg diffuses into the blood. Remember that a gas moves from a high concentration to a lower concentration.

8. The four general methods of ventilating the high-risk patient are: a) spontaneous ventilation by the patient (with or without supplemental oxygen and an NPA or OPA), b) mask ventilation (assisted or controlled), c) placement of an endotracheal tube or supraglottic airway device, or 4) creation of a surgical airway.

9. The standard of care for airway management is lung ventilation, not intubation.

Chapter 4

1. General indications for tracheal intubation are: a) the need to protect the airway from aspiration and obstruction from blood in the airway, gastric contents, secretions, or foreign bodies; b) apnea, soft-tissue obstruction, hypercarbia; c) impending airway obstruction: facial fractures, nasopharyngeal hematoma, and inhalation injury; d) excessive work of breathing; e) shock (SBP < 80 mm Hg); f) persistent hypoxia (SpO$_2$ $\leq$ 92%); g) definitive maintenance of airway patency; h) head injury and a Glasgow Coma Scale score of $\leq$9; i) AVPU score of P or U; j) mechanical ventilation; k) respiratory failure; l) airway management during emergency surgery and requirement for general anesthesia; m) cardiopulmonary arrest secondary to illness or injury; n) application of advanced cardiac life support and drug administration; o) maintenance of oxygenation or positive end-expiratory pressure; p) hypoxemia after application of optimal attempts to ventilate the patient using 100%; q) maintenance of pulmonary toilet oxygen and positive-pressure ventilation.

2. Three critical airway events include: a) failed intubation, b) inadequate ventilation, and c) any cannot-mask-ventilate/cannot-intubate situation.

3. If not contraindicated, the airway should be aligned by placing the patient's head in the sniffing position prior to intubation in order to better align the pharyngeal axis, laryngeal axis, and oral axis; whereas the recumbent position, with the head lying flat on the same surface as the shoulders, results in misalignment of the airway.

4. Stop an intubation attempt and reoxygenate when the patient's oxygen saturation falls below 93%.

5. Laryngoscopic pitfalls include: a) inserting the blade too deeply, b) using a blade that is too short or too long, c) not controlling the tongue, and d) placing your eye too close to the laryngoscope.

6. Bougie-assisted intubation can facilitate overcoming a difficult intubation (Cormack and Lehane Grade 3). As the bougie is inserted posterior to the epiglottis and enters the glottis, the tip will bump against the tracheal

rings, causing vibrations to be felt (tracheal clicking) by the hand holding the bougie. The bougie is advanced until the 25 cm mark is at the level of the corner of the lip. The tracheal tube is then advanced over the bougie and into the trachea. Doing this allows the trachea to be intubated atraumatically using direct laryngoscopy, even though the optimal laryngeal view does not expose the glottis inlet.

7. When caring for a large or morbidly obese patient, elevate the patient's shoulders and upper back by placing them upon pillows, folded blankets, or a specially designed "head-elevated laryngoscopy" pillow. Enough elevation is attained when an imaginary horizontal line runs from the inner ear canal to the xiphoid process.

Chapter 5

1. An SaO_2 of 90% correlates to a PaO_2 of 60 mm Hg, which is the laboratory threshold for hypoxia.

2. End-tidal changes in hypoventilating patients precede pulse oximetry changes and can provide sufficient advance warning to prevent patient deterioration.

3. Arterial carbon dioxide levels are affected by both metabolic and ventilatory changes, and ventilation is a primary method of managing acid-base balance.

4. To rule out the presence of an esophageal intubation and the cola complication, 6 to 12 ventilations may be required to wash out the carbon dioxide that may be residing in the stomach prior to reliance on a colorimetric device. Colorimetric caponmetry is more sensitive to carbon dioxide than capnographic waveform capnometry. Because capnographic waveform capnometry is not as sensitive to carbon dioxide it can be relied upon after only 5 ventilations. It should be understood also that the shape of the capnographic waveform seen during the cola complication is quite different than the shape of the normal capnogram.

5. Situations in which capnometry devices may give false readings (tube in the trachea but no detection of carbon dioxide) include nonperfusing rhythms, shock, low cardiac output states, and rapid ventilatory rates.

6. Increased PIP may indicate endotracheal tube occlusion, pneumothorax, increasing bronchospasm, or pulmonary edema, and high peak pressures are clearly associated with lung tissue injury.

Chapter 6

1. In low flow states where perfusion of the liver and splanchnic system is limited, drug clearance is decreased. Conditions such as hypovolemia, cardiogenic shock or dysfunction, and endogenous or exogenous adrenergic stimulation all decrease the splanchnic and hepatic blood flow and have profound effects on the pharmacokinetics of anesthetics and sedatives with high and intermediate liver extraction ratio.

2. Succinylcholine.

3. Rocuronium and vecuronium.

4. Succinylcholine has a faster onset time than rocuronium which has a faster onset time than vecuronium.

5. The most commonly used drugs in emergency airway management are the sedative hypnotics etomidate, midazolam, and ketamine, and muscle relaxants such as succinylcholine, rocuronium, and vecuronium.

Chapter 7

1. The six principles of RSI are that: a) the trachea needs to be intubated, b) the patient is at risk of aspiration, c) intubation is predicted to be successful, d) cricoid pressure is not contraindicated, e) the operator is skilled at airway management, and f) contingency plans are available for failed intubation.

2. Drugs used in RSI include induction agents (thiopental, etomidate, ketamine), neuromuscular blocking agents (succinylcholine, rocuronium), and adjunctive agents (fentanyl, lidocaine, midazolam).

3. Equipment necessary for RSI includes a working laryngoscope with good batteries and light; oropharyngeal and nasopharyngeal airways; tracheal tubes in varying sizes; both straight and curved blades; malleable stylet; end-tidal CO_2 detector; esophageal detector device; capnography, if available; RSI drugs, drawn up and labeled; stethoscope; cardiac monitor connected and functioning; pulse oximeter; and a means of securing the tube properly (tincture of benzoin or mastisol if using tape or a tracheal tube holder); esophageal tracheal Combitube or laryngeal mask airway; and a cricothyrotomy kit.

4. Special equipment available for facilitating difficult intubation includes a bougie introducer, HELP pillow, alternative blades of various lengths and shapes, LMA Fastrach, and a cricothyrotomy kit.

Chapter 8

1. Two devices given Class IIa (recommended) status by the American Heart Association are the LMA Classic and the esophageal tracheal Combitube.

2. Elective use of the LMA is contraindicated where there is a significant risk of aspiration (e.g., full stomach, morbid obesity, etc.) and where high inflation pressures are necessary (e.g., low compliance of lungs/chest wall or high airway resistance); however, the presence of any of these conditions do not preclude emergency use of the LMA for rescue ventilation.

3. The practitioner should go directly to transtracheal jet ventilation (TTJV) cricothyrotomy when a cannot-mask-ventilate/cannot-intubate situation cannot be overcome using a Combitube or LMA (or BVM ventilation). The cricothyrotomy equipment should always be readily available when deploying an LMA or Combitube, in the unlikely event that rescue ventilation is not successful.

4. Overinflation of the cuff simply distorts periglottic tissues and aggravates leakage of air around the mask during positive-pressure ventilation. When sizing has been performed correctly, the cuff volume producing the best seal is often half the recommended maximum cuff volume. Consequently, if a leak is detected, it is often worth removing some air from the cuff, especially when it has been inflated initially to the maximum recommended volume. The manufacturer recommends that the cuff should be inflated with just enough air to obtain an intracuff pressure of 60 cm H_2O.

5. The Combitube should not be used in patients less than four feet tall, those with known esophageal pathology such as esophageal ulcers or esophageal varices, those who have ingested caustic substances, those with a gag reflex or a clenched jaw, and patients with obstructions at or below the level of the glottic openings.

6. The LMA is the only Class IIa ventilation device that is available in pediatric sizes.

Chapter 9

1. Three specific reasons for problems with tracheal intubation are poor access, poor view of the glottis, and the inability to advance the tracheal tube.

2. The goal of laryngoscopy is to visualize the vocal cords, whereas the goal of tracheal intubation is to introduce the tracheal tube between the vocal cords.

3. The advantages of blind nasotracheal intubation are that patients need not be paralyzed to perform the procedure, and patients may be supine, sitting, or in the prone position.

4. Available devices for use with the difficult airway include but not limited to: a) bougie-assisted intubation; b) external laryngeal manipulation; c) head-elevated laryngoscopy position; d) fiberscopic and video-assisted devices; e) McCoy or levering-laryngoscope, f) blind nasotracheal intubation, g) airway exchange catheters; g) retrograde intubation; and h) the LMA Fastrach.

Chapter 10

1. Reasons for failed FOB intubation include excessive secretions or blood, inadequate topicalization, oversedation, and laryngospasm.

2. The nasal approach is the preferred route for awake fiberoptic intubation.

3. Prolonged mechanical ventilation via a nasotracheal tube may be associated with infectious sinusitis and pneumonia.

4. The steps to be taken when exchanging a tracheal tube for the Combitube while using an FOB include: a) deflate the distal oropharyngeal balloon, b) advance the FOB loaded with a standard tracheal tube past the distal balloon and then reinflate the distal balloon of the Combitube, c) pass the FOB through the glottis, d) keep the distal balloon of the Combitube inflated until tracheal intubation is confirmed, and e) when tracheal intubation is confirmed, deflate all Combitube cuffs and remove the Combitube.

5. The LMA Fastrach may be especially suitable in the prehospital setting because positioning is easy, tidal volumes are adequate, and tracheal intubation is possible through the device.

6. Particular indications for the use of an FOB include: a) airway management in cervical-spine injury, b) the exchange of temporary for definitive airways (e.g., exchange of Combitube or laryngeal mask airway for a standard tracheal tube), c) the placement of double-lumen tubes, and d) the confirmation of correct placement of a tracheal tube.

Chapter 11

1. The laryngoscope is not required or used in lighted stylet intubation.
2. Lighted stylets may be used in infants and children.
3. You must be able to visualize the anterior neck.
4. The practitioner can be positioned behind the patient, in front, or on either side when performing a lighted stylet intubation.
5. No, lighted stylet intubation cannot be used in bright sunlight. Ambient light in the field may make it somewhat more difficult to appreciate the transillumination, and particularly the difference in brightness of the light when the patient has a thin neck and the esophagus can transilluminate through the neck. Using a blanket or shade over the head and neck may be very helpful or, if possible, move the patient into the ambulance.

Chapter 12

1. The cricothyroid membrane or ligament is located between the inferior border of the thyroid cartilage and the superior border of the cricoid cartilage (Figure 12-1). It is derived from the fibroelastic membrane of the larynx, being its inferior portion, and connects the thyroid, cricoid, and posterior cartilages of the larynx. It is approximately 10 mm in vertical dimension and 22 mm in horizontal dimension. Performance of cricothyrotomy examination includes palpation and identification of the cricoid cartilage over its entire anterior surface. From below, placing the little finger in the suprasternal notch, then laying the hand on the anterior neck can help in estimating the position of the cricoid cartilage. The position of the cricothyroid membrane should generally coincide with one's index finger. This is a useful maneuver if the anterior anatomy of the neck is poorly defined (e.g., as in extreme obesity). Identification of the cricothyroid membrane can be performed from above, by first locating the hyoid bone, the laryngeal prominence at the notch of the thyroid cartilage (i.e., Adam's apple) and then sliding the palpating finger downwards until a depression is encountered on the thyroid cartilage. In general, the laryngeal prominence is generally easier to palpate in males than in females. Palpation of the laryngeal prominence in females is generally more challenging, which can make placement of cricothyrotomy more difficult. Frequent elective practice in the palpation of the cricothyroid membrane and the surrounding anatomy should improve the skill required in locating the cricoid cartilage when an emergency situation occurs. Superficial to the membrane lies the skin, the anterior cervical fascia, and generally a small quantity of subcutaneous tissue.
2. The most disastrous immediate complication is death from failure to establish an airway. Other immediate complications include: bleeding, pneumothorax, pneumomediastinum, subcutaneous emphysema, difficult cannulation, incorrect tube placement, damage to recurrent laryngeal artery, damage to thyroid gland, esophageal perforation, damage to cricoid cartilage, and aspiration. Intermediate complications include: subglottic stenosis, trachea-esophageal fistula, vocal cord dysfunction, stomal granulations, accidental decannulation, tracheal edema, acute respiratory failure secondary to decannulation, and infection. Delayed or long-term complications include: tracheal granulation, persistent wound, lower airway injury, vocal cord dysfunction, trachea-esophageal malacia, dysphonia, hemorrhage from trachea-innominate fistula, and infection.
3. The common methods of percutaneous needle cricothyrotomy include: a) transtracheal (i.e. translaryngeal) jet ventilation; b) percutaneous dilational cricothyrotomy (Seldinger technique); and c) non-Seldinger percutaneous cricothyrotomy.
4. The four steps of the rapid 4-step technique include: a) palpation of the cricothyroid membrane; b) stab incision through both the skin and the cricothyroid membrane; c) traction; and d) tracheal tube insertion.
5. The percutaneous dilational cricothyroidotomy or the vertical, or longitudinal, incision may be considered more appropriate in the prehospital environment and in a world of deadly communicable blood-borne pathogens.

Chapter 13

1. The goal of airway intervention is to relieve or prevent airway obstruction and to secure the unprotected airway from aspiration.

2. The most common facial fractures involve the mandible and midface maxilla, or Le Fort's fracture.

3. Réné Le Fort, a French physician, described three different types of facial fractures: Le Fort I, a transverse fracture of the body of the maxilla just under the nasal septum features motion of the maxilla independent of the remainder of the face. Le Fort II, a fracture of the central maxilla and palate, wherein the nose and its structures are displaced so that the whole facial skeleton separates from the skull. Le Fort's II fracture can extend through the orbital rim, medial orbital wall, ethmoid sinuses, nose, and cribriform plate. Le Fort's III fracture involves a transverse fracture above the malar, or zygomatic bone extending through the orbits, resulting in complete separation of the maxilla from the craniofacial skeleton. Le Fort IV, not one of Le Fort's original classifications, involves the frontal bone as well as the facial skeleton. Le Fort's IV is similar to Le Fort's III but also involves separation of the frontal bone from the facial skeleton. These serious injuries usually require aggressive airway management.

4. Cervical-spine injury coexists in up to 4% of the patients suffering facial trauma.

5. The major concern with blunt trauma to the neck is swelling and hematoma, which can occlude the airway and make intubation difficult as well as fractures to the cartilaginous parts of the airway.

6. Rapid sequence orotracheal intubation, the laryngeal mask airway, and the esophageal obturator are contraindicated in patients suspected of having laryngotracheal discontinuation.

Chapter 14

1. Approximately 55% of spinal injuries are to the cervical spine.

2. Injury at C3–C5 can disrupt the innervation of the diaphragm, resulting in loss of respiration.

3. Indicators for field immobilization of the c-spine are spine pain or palpation tenderness, any neurologic abnormality or symptoms, altered level of consciousness, or suspected intoxication.

4. **Never:** Axial traction is contraindicated in field management of trauma patients.

5. MIAS of the c-spine resulted in a 22% incidence of Grade 3 views in which the vocal cords were not seen, although the epiglottis was visualized. MIAS reduced the optimal view of the larynx in 45% of patients.

6. Techniques and devices that can be used to achieve airway control and ventilation in the spine-injured patient are the use of: a) bougie-assisted intubation, b) the BURP technique or use of ELM (external layngeal manipulation), c) the McCoy levering laryngoscope blade, d) fiberoptic laryngoscopy, e) the Combitube, f) the LMA, g) the intubating LMA, and h) other supraglottic devices.

Chapter 15

1. Hypoxia is the most common cause of death at the fire scene and is most often associated with burns sustained in a closed-space environment.

2. Treatment for carbon monoxide poisoning in the field is high-flow oxygen by nonrebreathing mask, followed by endotracheal intubation as indicated by the patient's clinical status.

3. Significant burns of the lower face, neck, and upper chest are associated with sufficient pharyngeal and supraglottic swelling to occlude the upper airway, creating a high-mortality airway emergency. Burns above the mandibular border rarely cause airway obstruction.

4. Elevation of the head of the stretcher 45° and judicious management of fluid resuscitation volumes may abrogate or delay the need for emergent intubation.

5. Airway management in the acute burn patient is best approached as a difficult airway with an awake, sedated, and spontaneously breathing patient. Nasotracheal intubation is ideal in this situation.

6. RSI can result in airway collapse as the muscles relax, and if the first intubation attempt is unsuccessful, a cannot-ventilate-by-any-means/cannot-intubate situation may arise.

7. Early treatment is guided by the patient's clinical respiratory and neurologic status, not by the history of inhalation injury. Singed nasal and facial hair, carbon-stained oropharyngeal and nasal mucosa, and carbonaceous sputum are poor indicators of a significant airway injury.

8. Pulmonary toilet, involving adequate suctioning during early care and transport, is essential given the fact that inhalation-burn patients are extremely prone to mucous/carbon plugging of tracheal tubes. If the tracheal tube becomes obstructed, it must be exchanged or a surgical airway must be performed. Tube exchange may be difficult due to swelling.

9. Swelling, causing difficulty in identifying landmarks; the presence of subcutaneous edema; and edema fluid in the surgical wound can make it extremely difficult to successfully complete surgical airway procedures. The initial surgical airway should be a tracheal tube because subsequent swelling of the anterior neck can completely envelop and obstruct a shorter tracheostomy tube. Cricothyroidotomy is contraindicated in children under age 10 because of anatomy causing tracheal collapse.

Chapter 16

1. Differences between the pediatric and adult airway include: a) children have a relatively larger tongue; b) the head is relatively larger in children, which is naturally flexed in the supine position; c) nasal passages are narrow in children compared to adults; d) children have a larynx that is more anterior and cephalad in the neck at the C3–C4 level, compared to C4–C5 in adults; e) the epiglottis is shorter and has a more acute angle over the glottis; f) the vocal cords are slanted and the anterior commissure is more inferior; g) the larynx is cone-shaped and is narrowest at the subglottic cricoid ring area in children younger than eight years, as opposed to the glottis in adults.

2. Epiglottitis is characterized by inflammation of the epiglottis and supraglottic tissues. Croup is characterized by subglottic edema. Croup is slow and epiglottitis is rapid in onset. In both croup and epiglottitis, the patient will want to sit up. Croup produces a barking type cough but epiglottitis does not. In croup there is no drooling and in epiglottitis there is excessive drooling in addition to very painful swallowing. Fevers with croup will range between 101°F to 102°F (38.3°C to 38.9°C) and fevers with epiglottitis will range between 102°F and 104°F (38.9°C to 40°C).

3. Rocuronium is the most suitable nondepolarizing muscle relaxant for RSI because it has a similar time of onset to that of succinylcholine (60 to 90 seconds).

4. Options for oxygenation and ventilation when attempts at intubation have failed include: a) BVM ventilation with oropharyngeal or nasopharyngeal airway, b) laryngeal mask airway, c) needle cricothyroidotomy, d) surgical cricothyroidotomy, e) retrograde wire-guided intubation, and f) fiberoptic intubation.

5. Complications of intubation in the pediatric patient include: a) dental injury, b) TMJ dislocation, c) mucosal injuries in the laryngotracheal region, d) ischemic ulceration and necrosis of the tracheal wall, e) bleeding into the airway, f) arytenoid cartilage dislocation, g) vocal cord paralysis, and h) aspiration.

Chapter 17

1. Yes, intubated paralyzed patients who are undersedated or have been given inadequate analgesia can feel pain, but because they are intubated they cannot vocalize this and if they are deeply paralyzed, they cannot grimace or move when they feel pain. Therefore it is important that patients who are deeply paralyzed be given judicious amounts of analgesia and sedation to help prevent this from occurring. It is important to note that if the patient is too unstable hemodynamically to receive analgesics or sedation, because of the adverse effects these drugs may have on their already unstable condition, they should at least receive an amnestic agent such as scopolamine 0.4 mg to diminish the likelihood of recall.

2. The intravenous opioids morphine and fentanyl are both recommended and used frequently.

3. The most common adverse side effect of any narcotic to include fentanyl is respiratory depression or respiratory arrest which can be prevented by limiting the dosage of the medication and monitoring respiration. Fentanyl administration should be titrated to between 25 and 50 microgram increments to prevent chest wall and glottic rigidity which have been seen with rapidly administered high dosages (e.g., more than 8.8 mcg/kg [which are unlikely to be required in the prehospital environment]). Chest wall rigidity can be reversed with the use of naloxone or the use of skeletal muscle relaxants. Itching (pruritus) is a common side effect of fentanyl which is caused by histamine release. This is usually tolerated by the patient but if it is not, a small amount of naloxone or diphenhydramine can be used to treat it.

4. Benzodiazepines are the classic anxiolytic and hypnotic drugs.

5. Fewer side effects are seen when drugs are titrated to effect. Additionally, vital signs are maintained with better stability when medications are titrated to effect rather than given according to strict dosage regimens.

Chapter 18

1. Failure to ventilate the patient has no legal defense.

2. Patients will generally sue those who they perceived to have been offended by in some way. Maintaining good rapport with a patient can help a practitioner minimize the likelihood of a lawsuit being filed, even if he or she makes a mistake. However, an airway disaster will almost always subject one to a lawsuit regardless.

3. When notified that a suit has been filed, one should immediately inform their employer and find out what legal options exist.

4. All patient care documentation should paint a picture for the judge and jury showing that the standard of care was met. This should be evident from the documentation without much requirement for interpretation.

5. The trier of fact, whether that is the judge or the jury, makes the final determination concerning what the standard of care is and whether or not it was met.

Chapter 19

1. All aspects of airway management, including equipment, personnel, and the environment, should be assessed to understand the role these procedures may play in morbidity and mortality from nosocomial infections.

2. The laryngoscope handle and blade are frequently contaminated prior to patient use even though they have received terminal sterilization.

3. Alternatives to ensuring that laryngoscope blades and handles are not contaminated prior to use is to: a) use disposable blades and handles; b) use sterile or clinically clean covers or sleeves over the handles and blades; c) ensure that blades and handles are decontaminated according to strict CDC guidelines after use and that they are placed in sterile packaging and that they are not removed from this packaging until just prior to use.

4. Approximately 600,000 to 800,000 needle-stick incidents happen each year in the United States.

5. Frequent contamination has been shown to exist on hands, pens, stethoscopes, computer keyboards, clothing, shoes, cell phones, pagers and neckties. Therefore, frequent handwashing or changing of gloves is mandatory between patient encounters and after coming into contact with blood and body fluids. If personal items are touched during patient care, hands must be washed and gloved prior to resuming patient care.

References

Chapter 1

1. Rich J. Street Level Airway Management (SLAM): If your patient can't breathe—nothing else matters. Anesthesia Today 2005; 16: 13–22.

2. Rich J: The SLAM (Street Level Airway Management) Concept, 2000. http://www.airwayeducation.com/concept.asp

3. Knacke A. Fallbeispiel: Atemwegsmanagement bei eingeklemmtem Polytrauma-Patienten [Case report: Prehospital airway management of a trapped person with polytrauma]. Rettungsdienst 2001; 24: 994–996.

4. Mason AM. Use of the intubating laryngeal mask airway in pre-hospital care: a case report. Resuscitation 2001; 51: 91–95.

5. Peterson G, Posner K, Domino K, Lee L, Caplan R, Cheney F. Management of the difficult airway in closed malpractice claims, 2003. Anesthesiology, University of Washington, Seattle, WA. http://depts.washington.edu/asaccp/ASA/ASAAbstracts/2003_99_A1252.pdf

6. Katz S, Falk J. Misplaced endotracheal tubes by paramedics in an urban emergency medical services system. Ann Emerg Med 2001; 37: 32–37.

7. Li J, Murphy-Lavoie H, Bugas C, Martinez J, Preston C. Complications of emergency intubation with and without paralysis. Am J Emerg Med 1999; 17: 141–143.

8. Schwartz DE, Matthay MA, Cohen NH. Death and other complications of emergency airway management in critically ill adults. A prospective investigation of 297 tracheal intubations. Anesthesiology 1995; 82: 367–376.

9. Caplan RA, Posner KL, Ward RJ, Cheney FW. Adverse respiratory events in anesthesia: A closed claims analysis. Anesthesiology 1990; 72: 828–833.

10. Caplan RA, Posner KL. Medical-Legal Considerations: The ASA Closed Claims Project, in *Airway Management: Principles and Practice*. Edited by Benumof JL. St. Louis, Mosby, 1996, pp. 944–955.

11. Crosby ET, Cooper RM, Douglas MJ, Doyle DJ, Hung OR, Labrecque P, Muir H, Murphy MF, Preston RP, Rose DK, Roy L. The unanticipated difficult airway with recommendations for management. Can J Anaesth 1998; 45: 757–776.

12. Domino K, Posner K, Caplan R, Cheney F. Airway injury during anesthesia: A closed claims analysis. Anesthesiology 1999; 91: 1703–1711.

13. Practice guidelines for management of the difficult airway: An updated report by the American Society of Anesthesiologists Task Force on Management of the Difficult Airway. Anesthesiology 2003; 98: 1269–1277.

14. Baskett P, Bossaert L, Carli P, Chamberlain D, Dick W, Nolan J, Parr M, Scheidegger D, Zideman D. Guidelines for the advanced management of the airway and ventilation during resuscitation: A statement by the Airway and Ventilation Management Working Group of the European Resuscitation Council. Resuscitation 1996; 31: 201–230.

15. Benumof JL. The American Society of Anesthesiologists' Management of the Difficult Airway Algorithm and Explanation-Analysis of the Algorithm, in *Airway Management: Principles and Practice*. Edited by Benumof JL. St. Louis, Mosby, 1996, pp. 143–158.

16. Henderson J, Popat M, Latto I, Pearce A. Difficult Airway Society guidelines for management of the unanticipated difficult intubation. Anaesthesia 2004; 59: 675–694.

17. Mason A, Rich J, Ramsay M. Mason's PU-92 concept: Rapid recognition and treatment of the crash airway. TraumaCare 2003; 13: 46.

18. Rich J, Mason A, Ramsay M, Osborn I, Miro R, Beeson J, Hancock R. SLAM Emergency Airway Flowchart: Universal Considerations for the Emergency Airway (Educational/Scientific Exhibit), 57th Post

Graduate Assembly of Anesthesiologists, New York State Society of Anesthesiologists. New York, NY, 2003.

19. Walls R. The emergency airway algorithms, in *Manual of Emergency Airway Management*. Edited by Walls R. Philadelphia, Lippincott Williams & Wilkins, 2000, pp. 16–26.

20. Brain A. The laryngeal mask airway—a possible new solution to airway problems in the emergency situation. Arch Emerg Med 1984: 229–232.

21. Frass M, Frenzer R, Zdrahal F, Hoflehner G, Porges P, Lackner F. The esophageal tracheal combitube: Preliminary results with a new airway for CPR. Annals of Emergency Medicine 1987; 16: 768–772.

22. Rich J, Mason A, Bey T, Krafft P, Frass M: The critical airway, rescue ventilation and the Combitube: Part 1 (available at http://www.airwayeducation.com/PDFs/AANA_ARTICLE_2–04.pdf). AANA J 2004; 72: 17–27.

23. Rich J, Mason A, Bey T, Krafft P, Frass M. The critical airway, rescue ventilation and the Combitube: Part 2 (available at http://www.airwayeducation.com/PDFs/AANA_ARTICLE_4–04.pdf). AANA J 2004; 72: 115–124.

24. Nunn J. The oesophageal detector device (letter). Anaesthesia 1988; 43: 804.

25. Rich J, Mason A, Ramsay M. AANA Journal Course: Update for Nurse Anesthetists. The SLAM Emergency Airway Flowchart: A new guide for advanced airway practitioners (available at http://www.airwayeducation.com/PDFs/flowchart_AANA_journal_course.pdf). AANA J 2004; 72: 431–439.

26. Sum-Ping ST, Mehta MP, Anderton JM: A Comparative Study of Methods of Detection of Esophageal Intubation. Anesth Analg 1989; 69: 627–632.

27. Thomas S, Wedel S, Wayne M. *Oxygenation, Ventilation, and Monitoring, Prehospital Trauma Care*. Edited by Soreide E, Grande C. New York, Marcel Dekker, 2001, pp. 255–272.

28. Wee M. The oesophageal detector device: Assessment of a method to distinguish oesophageal from tracheal intubation. Anaesthesia 1988; 43: 27–29.

29. Benumof J. The ASA Difficult Airway Algorithm: New thoughts and considerations, Handbook of Difficult Airway Management. Edited by Hagberg C. Philadelphia, Churchill Livingstone, 2000, pp. 31–48.

30. Stoneham M. Pulse oximetry, in *Complications in Anesthesia*. Edited by Atlee J. Philadelphia, W.B. Saunders, 1999, pp 591–594.

31. Mason A. The Laryngeal Mask Airway (LMA) & Intubating Laryngeal Mask Airway (ILMA), in *Prehospital Trauma Care, Royal College of Anaesthetists—May 13, 2002*. London, UK, 2002.

32. Rich J. Use of an elevation pillow to produce the head-elevated laryngoscopy position for airway management in morbidly obese and large-framed patients (letter). Anesth Analg 2004; 98: 264–265.

33. Larson S, Jordan L. Preventable adverse patient outcomes: A closed claims analysis of respiratory incidents. AANA J 2001; 69: 386–392.

34. Petty WC, Kremer M, Biddle C. A synthesis of the Australian Patient Safety Foundation Anesthesia Incident Monitoring Study, the American Society of Anesthesiologists Closed Claims Project, and the American Association of Nurse Anesthetists Closed Claims Study. Aana J 2002; 70: 193–202.

35. Dunham CM, Barraco RD, Clark DE, Daley BJ, Davis FEI, Gibbs MA, Knuth T, Letarte PB, Luchette FA, Omert L, Weireter LJ, Wiles CEI. Guidelines for Emergency Tracheal Intubation Immediately after Traumatic Injury. J Trauma 2003; 55: 162–179.

36. Rich J. Airway time travel: Avoiding the pitfalls of the past. The International Symposium on Crisis Management and the Sixth Symposium of Saudi Anesthetic Association in Anesthesiology and Intensive Care. Dhahran, Saudi Arabia, 2002, pp. 72–75.

37. Rich J, Mason A, Ramsay M, Beeson J, Hancock R. The Universal Emergency Airway Flowchart: Preventing accidents associated with emergency airway management (abstract A 33). AANA J 2003; 71: 462.

38. Rich J. The Universal Emergency Airway Flowchart: Avoiding accidents associated with emergency airway management (oral presentation), American Association of Nurse Anesthetists Annual Meeting. Boston, MA, 2003.

39. Rich J. The Universal Emergency Airway Flowchart: Preventing accidents associated with emergency airway management (poster presentation), American Association of Nurse Anesthetists Annual Meeting. Boston, MA, 2003.

40. Rich J, Ramsay M, Frass M, Osborn I, Beeson J, Hancock R. The SLAM Emergency Airway Flowchart: Universal considerations for the emergency airway (scientific exhibit), International Anesthesia Research Society 77th Congress. New Orleans, LA, 2003.

41. Rich J. SLAM Emergency Airway Flowchart: Universal considerations for the emergency airway. TraumaCare 2003; 13: 46–47.

42. Baylor News. Baylor University Medical Center Proceedings 2004; 17: 209.

43. Mason A. Method of securing the laryngeal mask airway in pre-hospital care. Prehospital Immediate Care 1999; 3: 167–169.

44. Melker RJ, Orlando G. Florete J. Cricothyrotomy: Review and Debate, in *Anesthesiology Clinics of North America*. Edited by Benumof JL. Philadelphia, W. B. Saunders, 1995, pp. 565–584.

45. Melker RJ, Florete OG. Percutaneous dilational cricothyrotomy and tracheostomy, in *Airway Management: Principles and Practice*. Edited by Benumof JL. St. Louis, Mosby, 1996, pp. 484–512.

46. Baskett P. The use of the laryngeal mask airway by nurses during cardiopulmonary resuscitation. Multicentre trial. Anaesthesia 1994; 49: 3–7.

47. Ochs M, Davis D, Joyt D, Bailey D, Marshall L, Rosen P. Paramedic-performed rapid sequence intubation of patients with severe head injuries. Ann Emerg Med 2002; 40: 159–167.

48. Smith C. Rapid sequence induction in adults: Indications and concerns. Clinical Pulmonary Medicine 2001; 8: 147–165.

49. Rabitsch W, Schellongowski P, Staudinger T, Hofbauer R, Dufek V, Eder B, Raab H, Thell R, Schuster E, Frass M. Comparison of a conventional tracheal airway with the Combitube in an urban emergency medical services system run by physicians. Resuscitation 2003; 57: 27–32.

50. Smith C: Cervical Spine Injury and Tracheal Intubation: A Never Ending Conflict (available at http://www.airwayeducation.com/PDFs/SpringSummer_2000.pdf). TraumaCare 2000; 10(1): 20–26.

51. Rich J. Recognition and management of the difficult airway with special emphasis on the intubating LMA-Fastrach/whistle technique: A brief review with case reports. BUMC Proceedings 2005; 18: 220–227.

52. Mallampati S. Clinical assessment of the airway. Anesthesiol Clin North Am 1995; 13: 301–308.

53. Mallampati SR. Recognition of the difficult airway, in *Airway Management: Principles and Practice*. Edited by Benumof JL. St. Louis, Mosby, 1996, pp. 126–142.

54. Mallampati SR, Gatt SP, Gugino LD, Desai SP, Waraksa B, Freiberger D, Liu PL. A clinical sign to predict difficult tracheal intubation: A prospective study. Can Anaesth Soc J 1985; 32: 429–434.

55. Wilson W. Difficult intubation, in *Complications in Anesthesia*. Edited by Atlee J. Philadelphia, W.B. Saunders, 1999, pp. 138–147.

56. Beck G. Blind nasal intubation. Emerg Med Serv. 2002; 31(1): 79.

57. Levitan RM. Patient safety in emergency airway management and rapid sequence intubation: Metaphorical lessons from skydiving. Ann Emerg Med 2003; 42: 81–87.

58. Parmet J, Colonna-Romano P, Horrow J, Miller F, Gonzales J, Rosenberg H. The laryngeal mask airway reliably provides rescue ventilation in cases of unanticipated difficult tracheal intubation along with difficult mask ventilation. Anesth Analg 1998; 87: 661–665.

59. Barnes T, MacDonald D, Nolan J, Otto C, Pepe P, Sayre M, Shuster M, Zaritsky A. Airway devices. Ann Emerg Med 2001; 37: S145–S151.

60. American Heart Association guidelines for cardiopulmonary resuscitation and emergency cardiovascular care. Circulation 2005; 112: IV-1–IV-211.

61. Ornato J, Callaham M. International Guidelines 2000: The story and the science. Ann Emerg Med 2001; 37(4 suppl): S3–S4.

62. McKay C, Burke D, Burke J, Porter K, Bowden D, Gorman D. Association between the assessment of conscious level using the AVPU system and the Glasgow coma scale. Pre-hospital Immediate Care 2000; 4: 17–19.

63. Levitan R. Rescuing intubation. Simple techniques to improve airway visualization. JEMS 2001; 26: 36–42, 44–46, 48–49.

64. Levitan R, Mechem C, Ochroch E, Shofer F, Hollander J. Head-elevated laryngoscopy position: Improving laryngeal exposure during laryngoscopy by increasing head elevation. Ann Emerg Med 2003; 41: 322–330.

65. Miller GT. LMA Fastrach. EMS discovers the intubating laryngeal mask airway. J Emerg Med Serv JEMS 2002; 27: 68–74.

66. Pinchalk M, Roth R, Paris P, Hostler D. Comparison of times to intubate a simulated trauma patient in two positions. Prehosp Emerg Care 2003; 7: 252–257.

67. Schmitt J, Mang H. Head and neck elevation beyond the sniffing position improves laryngeal view in cases of difficult direct laryngoscopy. J Clin Anesth 2002; 14: 335–338.

68. Heidegger T, Gerig H, Keller C. Comparison of algorithms for management of the difficult airway. Anaesthetist 2003; 52: 375–376.

69. Stone B, Chantler P, Baskett P. The incidence of regurgitation during cardiopulmonary resuscitation: A comparison between the bag valve mask and laryngeal mask airway. Resuscitation 1998; 38: 3–6.

70. de Latorre F, Nolan J, Robertson C, Chamberlain D, Baskett P. European Resuscitation Council Guidelines 2000 for Adult Advanced Life Support. A statement from the Advanced Life Support Working Group(1) and approved by the Executive Committee of the European Resuscitation Council. Resuscitation 2001; 48: 211–221.

71. Benumof JL. Management of the difficult adult airway. With special emphasis on awake tracheal intubation. Anesthesiology 1991; 75: 1087–1110.

72. Sanchez A, Morrison D. Preparation of the patient for awake intubation, in *Handbook of Difficult Airway Management*. Edited by Hagberg C. Philadelphia, Churchill Livingstone, 2000, pp. 49–82.

73. Ferson DZ, Rosenblatt WH, Johansen MJ, Osborn I, Ovassapian A. Use of the intubating LMA-Fastrach in 254 patients with difficult-to-manage airways. Anesthesiology 2001; 95: 1175–1181.

74. Minkowitz H. Airway gadgets, in *Handbook of Difficult Airway Management*. Edited by Hagberg C. Philadelphia, Churchill Livingstone, 2000, pp. 149–170.

75. Ovassapian A, Wheeler M. Flexible fiberoptic tracheal intubation, in *Handbook of Difficult Airway Management*. Edited by Hagberg C. Philadelphia, Churchill Livingstone, 2000, pp. 83–114.

76. Cooper R, Pacey J, Bishop M, McCluskey S. Early clinical experience with a new videolaryngoscope (GlideScope) in 728 patients. Can J Anaesth 2005; 52: 191–198.

77. Agro F, Cataldo R, Carassiti M, Costa F. The Seeing Stylet: tracheal intubation. Resuscitation 2000; 44: 177–180.

78. Benumof JL. Conventional (laryngoscopic), orotracheal, and nasotracheal intubation (single-lumen tube), in *Airway Management: Principles and Practice*. Edited by Benumof JL. St. Louis, Mosby, 1996, pp. 261–276.

79. Knill RL. Difficult laryngoscopy made easy with a "BURP." Can J Anaesth 1993; 40: 279–282.

80. Latto I. Management of difficult intubation, in *Difficulties in Tracheal Intubation*. Edited by Latto I, Vaughan R. London, W.B. Saunders Company Ltd, 1997, pp. 107–160.

81. Ochs M, Vilke GM, Chan TC, Moats T, Buchanan J. Successful prehospital airway management by EMT-Ds using the Combitube. Prehosp Emerg Care 2000; 4: 333–337.

82. Salem MR, Baraka A. Confirmation of tracheal intubation, in *Airway Management: Principles and Practice*. Edited by Benumof JL. St. Louis, Mosby, 1996, pp. 531–560.

83. Anderson K, Hald A. Assessing the position of the tracheal tube: The reliability of different methods. Anaesthesia 1989; 44: 984–985.

84. Anderson K, Schultz-Lebahn T. Oesophageal intubation can be undetected by auscultation of the chest. Acta Anaesthesiologica Scandinavica 1994; 38: 580–582.

85. Baraka A, Khoury PJ, Siddik SS, Salem MR, Joseph NJ. Efficacy of the self-inflating bulb in differentiating esophageal from tracheal intubation in the parturient undergoing cesarean section. Anesth Analg 1997; 84: 533–537.

86. Zaleski L, Abello D, Gold MI. The Esophageal Detector Device: Does it work? Anesthesiology 1993; 79: 244–247.

87. Baraka A, Choueiry P, Salem M. The esophageal detector device in the morbidly obese (letter). Anesthesia and Analgesia 1993; 77: 400.

88. Baraka A. The oesophageal detector device (letter). Anaesthesia 1991; 45: 697.

89. Asai T, Appadurai I. LMA for failed intubation. Can J Anaesth 1993; 40: 802; author reply, 803.

90. Asai T, Latto P. Role of the laryngeal mask in patients with difficult tracheal intubation and difficult ventilation, in *Difficulties in Tracheal Intubation,* Second Edition. Edited by Latto IP, Vaughn RS. London, W.B. Saunders Ltd., 1997, pp. 177–196.

91. Frass M, Frenzer R, Zahler J, Ilias W, Leithner C. Ventilation via the esophageal tracheal combitube in a case of difficult intubation. Journal of Cardiothorasic Anesthesia 1987; 1: 565–568.

92. Frass M, Frenzer R, Rauscha F, Schuster E, Glogar D. Ventilation with the esophageal tracheal Combitube in cardiopulmonary resuscitation: Promptness and effectiveness. Chest 1988; 93: 781–784.

93. Moller J, Johannessen N, Berg H, Espersen K, Larsen L. Hypoxaemia during anaesthesia—an observer study. Br J Anaesth 1991; 66: 437–444.

Chapter 2

1. Langdon, JD. Surface anatomy of the head and neck. In Gray's Anatomy: The anatomical basis of clinical practice. 39 edition. Edited by Standring S and Berkovitz KB. Elsevier Churchill Livingstone, New York, 2005 p. 444.

2. Benumof J. The ASA Difficult Airway Algorithm: New thoughts and considerations, in *Handbook of Difficult Airway Management.* Edited by Hagberg C. Philadelphia, Churchill Livingstone, 2000, pp. 31–48.

3. Knill R. Difficult laryngoscopy made easy with a "BURP." Can J Anaesth 1993; 40: 279–282.

4. Sellick BA. Cricoid pressure to control regurgitation of stomach contents during induction of anaesthesia. Lancet 1961; 2: 404–406.

5. Butler J. Cricoid pressure in emergency rapid sequence induction. Emerg Med J 2005; 22: 815–816.

6. Levitan R, Ochroch EA. Airway management and direct laryngoscopy. A review and update. Crit Care Clin 2000; 16: 373–388.

7. Cormack RS, Lehane J. Difficult tracheal intubation in obstetrics. Anaesthesia 1984; 39: 1105–1111.

8. Benumof JL. Definition and incidence of the difficult airway, in *Airway Management: Principles and Practice.* Edited by Benumof JL. St. Louis, Mosby, 1996, pp. 121–125.

9. Henderson J, Popat M, Latto I, Pearce A. Difficult Airway Society guidelines for management of the unanticipated difficult intubation. Anaesthesia 2004; 59: 675–694.

10. Rich J. Recognition and management of the difficult airway with special emphasis on the intubating LMA-Fastrach/whistle technique: A brief review with case reports. BUMC Proceedings 2005; 18: 220–227.

11. Mallampati S. Clinical assessment of the airway. Anesthesiol Clin North Am 1995; 13: 301–308.

12. Rich J, Mason A, Ramsay M. The SLAM Emergency Airway Flowchart: A new guide for advanced airway practitioners (available at http://www.airwayeducation.com/PDFs/flowchart_AANA_journal_course.pdf). AANA J 2004; 72: 431–439.

13. Rich J. If your patient can't breathe—nothing else matters! Alternative techniques to manage the difficult airway, American Association of Nurse Anesthetist's 72nd Annual Meeting. Washington, DC, AANA, 2005, pp. 40–42.

14. Crosby ET, Cooper RM, Douglas MJ, Doyle DJ, Hung OR, Labrecque P, Muir H, Murphy MF, Preston RP, Rose DK, Roy L. The unanticipated difficult airway with recommendations for management. Can J Anaesth 1998; 45: 757–776.

15. Wilson W. Difficult intubation, in *Complications in Anesthesia.* Edited by Atlee J. Philadelphia, W.B. Saunders, 1999, pp. 138–147.

16. Karkouti K, Rose DK, Ferris LE, Wigglesworth DF, Meisami-Fard T, Lee H. Inter-observer reliability of ten tests used for predicting difficult tracheal intubation. Can J Anaesth 1996; 43: 554–559.

17. Mallampati SR, Gatt SP, Gugino LD, Desai SP, Waraksa B, Freiberger D, Liu PL. A clinical sign to predict difficult tracheal intubation: A prospective study. Can Anaesth Soc J 1985; 32: 429–434.

18. Benumof JL, Scheller MS. The importance of transtracheal jet ventilation in the management of the difficult airway. Anesthesiology 1989; 71: 769–778.

19. Mallampati SR. Recognition of the difficult airway, in *Airway Management: Principles and Practice*. Edited by Benumof JL. St. Louis, Mosby, 1996, pp. 126–142.

20. Rich J. Street Level Airway Management (SLAM): If your patient can't breathe—nothing else matters (available at http://www.airwayeducation.com/PDFs/Anesthesia_Today_16_2005.pdf). Anesthesia Today 2005; 16: 13–22.

21. Benumof JL. Conventional (laryngoscopic), orotracheal, and nasotracheal intubation (single-lumen tube), in *Airway Management: Principles and Practice*. Edited by Benumof JL. St. Louis, Mosby, 1996, pp. 261–276.

22. Latto I. Management of difficult intubation, in *Difficulties in Tracheal Intubation*. Edited by Latto I, Vaughan R. London. W.B. Saunders Company Ltd, 1997, pp. 107–160.

23. Levitan R, Mechem C, Ochroch E, Shofer F, Hollander J. Head-elevated laryngoscopy position: Improving laryngeal exposure during laryngoscopy by increasing head elevation. Ann Emerg Med 2003; 41: 322–330.

24. Minkowitz H. Airway gadgets, in *Handbook of Difficult Intubation*. Edited by Hagberg C. Philadelphia, Churchill Livingstone, 2000, pp. 149–170.

25. Rich J. Use of an elevation pillow to produce the head-elevated laryngoscopy position for airway management in morbidly obese and large-framed patients (letter). Anesth Analg 2004; 98: 264–265.

26. Smith C: Cervical spine injury and tracheal intubation: A never ending conflict (available at http://www.airwayeducation.com/PDFs/SpringSummer_2000.pdf). TraumaCare 2000; 10(1): 20–26.

27. Benumof JL. Management of the difficult adult airway. With special emphasis on awake tracheal intubation. Anesthesiology 1991; 75: 1087–1110.

28. Sanchez A, Morrison D. Preparation of the patient for awake intubation, in *Handbook of Difficult Airway Management*. Edited by Hagberg C. Philadelphia, Churchill Livingstone, 2000, pp. 49–82.

29. Beck G. Blind nasal intubation. Emerg Med Serv 2002; 31: 79.

30. Ferson DZ, Rosenblatt WH, Johansen MJ, Osborn I, Ovassapian A. Use of the intubating LMA-Fastrach in 254 patients with difficult-to-manage airways. Anesthesiology 2001; 95: 1175–1181.

31. Sanchez A, Pallares V. Retrograde intubation technique, in *Airway Management: Principles and Practice*. Edited by Benumof JL. St. Louis, Mosby, 1996, pp. 320–341.

32. Minkowitz H. Airway gadgets, in *Handbook of Difficult Airway Management*. Edited by Hagberg C. Philadelphia, Churchill Livingstone, 2000, pp. 149–169.

33. Ovassapian A, Wheeler M. Flexible fiberoptic tracheal intubation, in *Handbook of Difficult Airway Management*. Edited by Hagberg C. Philadelphia, Churchill Livingstone, 2000, pp. 83–114.

34. Cooper R, Pacey J, Bishop M, McCluskey S. Early clinical experience with a new videolaryngoscope (GlideScope) in 728 patients. Can J Anaesth 2005; 52: 191–198.

35. Agro F, Cataldo R, Carassiti M, Costa F. The seeing stylet: A new device for tracheal intubation. Resuscitation 2000; 44: 177–180.

Chapter 3

1. Benumof JL. Conventional (laryngoscopic), orotracheal, and nasotracheal intubation (single-lumen tube), in *Airway Management: Principles and Practice*. Edited by Benumof JL. St. Louis, Mosby, 1996, pp. 261–276.

2. Levitan R, Ochroch EA. Airway management and direct laryngoscopy. A review and update. Crit Care Clin 2000; 16: 373–388.

3. Knacke A. Fallbeispiel: Atemwegsmanagement bei eingeklemmtem Polytrauma-Patienten [Case report: Prehospital airway management of a trapped person with polytrauma]. Rettungsdienst 2001; 24: 994–996.

4. Smith C, Grande C, Wayne M, Gonzalez D, Murphy M, Barton C, Lacombe D, Kloeck W, Sorede E, Lipp M, Parr M, Nolan J. Rapid sequence intubation (RSI) in trauma (poster), Trauma Care '97; The 10th Annual Trauma Anesthesia and Critical Care Society Symposium, May 1997. Baltimore, MD, USA, 1997.

5. Rich J. Street Level Airway Management (SLAM): If your patient can't breathe—nothing else matters. Anesthesia Today 2005; 16: 13–22.

6. Rich V, Mason A, Ramsay M. AANA Journal Course: Update for nurse anesthetists–part 5–The SLAM Emergency Airway Flowchart. A new guide for advanced airway practitioners. AANA J., Vol 72, Number 6, December 2004, pp. 431–439.

7. Bledsoe B, Porter R, Cherry R. Airway management and ventilation, in *Paramedic Care, Principles & Practice,* Vol. 1. Upper Saddle River, NJ, Pearson Prentice Hall, 2006, pp. 504–611.

8. Stewart C. Oxygenation and ventilation aids, in *Advanced Airway Management.* Upper Saddle River, NJ, Prentice Hall, 2002, pp. 59–75.

9. Bledsoe B, Porter R, Cherry R. Pulmonology, in *Paramedic Care: Principles & Practice—Medical Emergencies,* Second Edition, Vol. 3. Upper Saddle River, NJ, Prentice Hall, 2006, pp. 2–63.

10. Roberts K, Whalley H, Bleetman A. The nasopharyngeal airway: Dispelling myths and establishing the facts. Emerg Med J 2005; 22: 394–396.

11. Bledsoe B, Porter R, Cherry R. Thoracic Trauma, in *Paramedic Care: Principles and Practice—Trauma Emergencies,* Vol. 4. Upper Saddle River, NJ, Prentice Hall, 2006, pp. 378–425.

12. ILCOR/ERC. Guidelines 2000 for Cardiopulmonary Resuscitation and Emergency Cardiovascular Care—An International Consensus on Science. Part 6: Advanced Cardiovascular Life Support. Section 3: Adjuncts for Oxygenation, Ventilation, and Airway Control. Resuscitation 2000; 46: 115–125.

13. Langeron O, Masso E, Huraux C, Guggiari M, Bianchi A, Coriat P, Riou B. Prediction of difficult mask ventilation. Anesthesiology 2000; 92: 1229–1236.

14. Latto I. Management of difficult intubation, in *Difficulties in Tracheal Intubation.* Edited by Latto I, Vaughan R. London, W.B. Saunders Company Ltd, 1997, pp. 107–160.

15. Sellick BA. Cricoid pressure to control regurgitation of stomach contents during induction of anaesthesia. Lancet 1961; 2: 404–406.

16. Caplan RA, Posner KL. Medical-legal considerations: The ASA Closed Claims Project, in *Airway Management: Principles and Practice.* Edited by Benumof JL. St. Louis, Mosby, 1996, pp. 944–955.

17. Caplan RA, Posner KL, Ward RJ, Cheney FW. Adverse respiratory events in anesthesia: A closed claims analysis. Anesthesiology 1990; 72: 828–833.

18. Rich J, Mason A, Bey T, Krafft P, Frass M. The critical airway, rescue ventilation and the Combitube: Part 1 (available at http://www.airwayeducation.com/PDFs/AANA_ARTICLE_2-04.pdf). AANA J 2004; 72: 17–27.

19. Levitan R. Rescuing intubation. Simple techniques to improve airway visualization. JEMS 2001; 26: 36–42, 44–46, 48–49.

20. Levitan RM. Patient safety in emergency airway management and rapid sequence intubation: Metaphorical lessons from skydiving. Ann Emerg Med 2003; 42: 81–87.

21. American Heart Association guidelines for cardiopulmonary resuscitation and emergency cardiovascular care. Circulation 2005; 112: IV-1–IV-211.

22. Ornato J, Callaham M. International Guidelines 2000: The story and the science. Ann Emerg Med 2001; 37(4 suppl): S3–S4.

23. Rich J. Recognition and management of the difficult airway with special emphasis on the intubating LMA-Fastrach/whistle technique: A brief review with case reports. BUMC Proceedings 2005; 18: 220–227.

24. Practice guidelines for management of the difficult airway: An updated report by the American Society of Anesthesiologists Task Force on Management of the Difficult Airway. Anesthesiology 2003; 98: 1269–1277.

25. Genzwurker H, Isovic H, Finteis T, Hinkelbein J, Denz C, Groschel J, Ellinger K. Equipment of physician-staffed ambulance systems in the state of Baden-Wuerttemberg. Anaesthesist 2002; 51: 367–373.

26. Ridgway S, Hodrovic I, Woollard M, Latto I. Prehospital airway management in ambulance services in the United Kingdom. Anaesthesia 2004; 59: 1091–1094.

27. Barnes T, MacDonald D, Nolan J, Otto C, Pepe P, Sayre M, Shuster M, Zaritsky A. Airway devices. Ann Emerg Med 2001; 37: S145–S151.

28. Stone B, Chantler P, Baskett P. The incidence of regurgitation during cardiopulmonary resuscitation: A comparison between the bag valve mask and laryngeal mask airway. Resuscitation 1998; 38: 3–6.

29. Benumof J. The ASA Difficult Airway Algorithm: New thoughts and considerations, in *Handbook of Difficult Airway Management*. Edited by Hagberg C. Philadelphia, Churchill Livingstone, 2000, pp. 31–48.

30. Brain A. The laryngeal mask airway—a possible new solution to airway problems in the emergency situation. Arch Emerg Med 1984: 229–232.

31. Haskell G. Prehospital Airway Devices, E-Medicine, 2005.

32. Barbieri S, Michieletto E, Giulio MD, Feltracco P, Gorlato P, Salvaterra F, Scalone A, Spagna A. Prehospital airway management with the laryngeal mask airway in polytraumatized patients. Prehosp Emerg Care 2001; 5: 300–303.

33. Hagberg C, Samsoe-Jensen F, Genzwuerker H, Krivosic-Horber R, Schmitz B, Hinkelbein J, Contzen M, Menu H, Bourzoufi K. International, multi-center study of the ambu laryngeal mask in nonparalyzed, anesthetized patients. Anesth Analg, 2005 Dec; 101(6):1867–6.

34. Agro F, Cataldo R, Alfano A, Galli B. A new prototype for airway management in an emergency: the laryngeal tube. Resuscitation 1999; 41: 284–286.

35. Asai T, Moriyama S, Nishita Y, Kawachi S. Use of the laryngeal tube during cardiopulmonary resuscitation by paramedical staff. Anaesthesia 2003; 58: 393–394.

36. Genzwuerker HV, Dhonau S, Ellinger K. Use of the laryngeal tube for out-of-hospital resuscitation. Resuscitation 2002; 52: 221–224.

37. Genzwuerker HV, Hilker T, Hohner E, Kuhnert-Frey B. The laryngeal tube: A new adjunct for airway management. Prehosp Emerg Care 2000; 4: 168–172.

38. Dorges V, Ocker H, Wenzel V, Schmucker P. The laryngeal tube: A new simple airway device. Anesth Analg 2000; 90: 1220–1223.

39. Frass M, Frenzer R, Zdrahal F, Hoflehner G, Porges P, Lackner F. The esophageal tracheal Combitube: Preliminary results with a new airway for CPR. Annals of Emergency Medicine 1987; 16: 768–772.

40. Rich J, Mason A, Bey T, Krafft P, Frass M. The critical airway, rescue ventilation and the Combitube: Part 2 (available at http://www.airwayeducation.com/PDFs/AANA_ARTICLE_4–04.pdf). AANA J 2004; 72: 115–124.

41. Thierbach A, Piepho T, Mayrbauer M. A new device for emergency airway management: The Easytube. Resuscitation 2004; 60: 347.

42. Akca O, Wadhwa A, Sengupta P, Durrani J, Hanni K, Wenke M, Yucel Y, Lenhardt R, Doufas A, Sessler D. The new perilaryngeal airway (CobraPLA) is as efficient as the laryngeal mask airway (LMA) but provides better airway sealing pressures. Anesth Analg 2004; 99: 272–278.

Chapter 4

1. Benumof JL. Indications for tracheal intubation, in *Airway Management: Principles and Practice*. Edited by Benumof JL. St. Louis, Mosby, 1996, pp. 255–260.

2. Levitan R, Ochroch EA. Airway management and direct laryngoscopy. A review and update. Crit Care Clin 2000; 16: 373–388.

3. Rich J, Mason A, Ramsay M. AANA Journal Course: Update for Nurse Anesthetists. The SLAM Emergency Airway Flowchart: A new guide for advanced airway practitioners (available at http://www.airwayeducation.com/PDFs/flowchart_AANA_journal_course.pdf). AANA J 2004; 72: 431–439.

4. Smith C, Grande C, Wayne M, Gonzalez D, Murphy M, Barton C, Lacombe D, Kloeck W, Sorede E, Lipp M, Parr M, Nolan J. Rapid sequence intubation (RSI) in trauma (poster), Trauma Care '97; The 10th Annual Trauma Anesthesia and Critical Care Society Symposium, May 1997. Baltimore, MD, USA, 1997.

5. Biegner A. Management of the difficult airway in a combat environment, American Association of Nurse Anesthetist's 72nd Annual Meeting, Washington, DC, AANA, 2005, pp. 74–75.

6. Mason A, Rich J, Ramsay M. Mason's PU-92 concept: Rapid recognition and treatment of the crash airway. TraumaCare 2003; 13: 46.

7. Benumof J. The ASA Difficult Airway Algorithm: New thoughts and considerations, in *Handbook of Difficult Airway Management*. Edited by Hagberg C. Philadelphia, Churchill Livingstone, 2000, pp. 31–48.

8. Benumof JL. Conventional (laryngoscopic), orotracheal, and nasotracheal intubation (single-lumen tube), in *Airway Management: Principles and Practice*. Edited by Benumof JL. St. Louis, Mosby, 1996, pp. 261–276.

9. Cormack RS, Lehane J. Difficult tracheal intubation in obstetrics. Anaesthesia 1984; 39: 1105–1111.

10. Crosby ET, Cooper RM, Douglas MJ, Doyle DJ, Hung OR, Labrecque P, Muir H, Murphy MF, Preston RP, Rose DK, Roy L. The unanticipated difficult airway with recommendations for management. Can J Anaesth 1998; 45: 757–776.

11. Levitan R. Rescuing intubation. Simple techniques to improve airway visualization. JEMS 2001; 26: 36–42, 44–46, 48–49.

12. Levitan R, Mechem C, Ochroch E, Shofer F, Hollander J. Head-elevated laryngoscopy position: Improving laryngeal exposure during laryngoscopy by increasing head elevation. Ann Emerg Med 2003; 41: 322–330.

13. Rich J. Use of an elevation pillow to produce the head-elevated laryngoscopy position for airway management in morbidly obese and large-framed patients (letter). Anesth Analg 2004; 98: 264–265.

14. Wilson W. Difficult intubation, in *Complications in Anesthesia*. Edited by Atlee J. Philadelphia, W.B. Saunders, 1999, pp. 138–147.

15. Practice guidelines for management of the difficult airway: An updated report by the American Society of Anesthesiologists Task Force on Management of the Difficult Airway. Anesthesiology 2003; 98: 1269–1277.

16. Rocke DA, Murray WB, Rout CC, Gouws E. Relative risk analysis of factors associated with difficult intubation in obstetric anesthesia. Anesthesiology 1992; 77: 67–73.

17. Samsoon GL, Young JR. Difficult tracheal intubation: A retrospective study. Anaesthesia 1987; 42: 487–490.

18. Wheeler M, Ovassapian A. Prediction and evaluation of the difficult airway, in *Handbook of Difficult Airway Management*. Edited by Hagberg C. Philadelphia, Churchill Livingstone, 2000, pp. 15–30.

19. Adnet F, Jouriles NJ, Le Toumelin P, Hennequin B, Taillandier C, Rayeh F, Couvreur J, Nougiere B, Nadiras P, Ladka A, Fleury M. Survey of out-of-hospital emergency intubations in the French prehospital medical system: A multicenter study. Ann Emerg Med 1998; 32: 454–460.

20. Benumof JL. Definition and incidence of the difficult airway, in *Airway Management: Principles and Practice*. Edited by Benumof JL. St. Louis, Mosby, 1996, pp. 121–125.

21. Sakles JC, Laurin EG, Rantapaa AA, Panacek EA. Airway management in the emergency department: A one-year study of 610 tracheal intubations. Ann Emerg Med 1998; 31: 325–332.

22. Tayal V, Riggs R, Marx J, Tomaszewski C, Schneider R. Rapid-sequence intubation at an emergency medicine residency: Success rate and adverse events during a two-year period. Acad Emerg Med 1999; 6: 31–37.

23. Wang HE, Sweeney TA, O'Connor RE, Rubinstein H. Failed prehospital intubations: An analysis of emergency department courses and outcomes. Prehosp Emerg Care 2001; 5: 134–141.

24. Jones J, Murphy M, Dickson R, Somerville G, Brizendine E. Emergency physician-verified out-of-hospital intubation: Miss rates by paramedics. Acad Emerg Med 2004; 11: 707–709.

25. Katz S, Falk J. Misplaced endotracheal tubes by paramedics in an urban emergency medical services system. Ann Emerg Med 2001; 37: 32–37.

26. American Heart Association guidelines for cardiopulmonary resuscitation and emergency cardiovascular care. Circulation 2005; 112: IV-1–IV-211.

27. Barnes T, MacDonald D, Nolan J, Otto C, Pepe P, Sayre M, Shuster M, Zaritsky A. Airway devices. Ann Emerg Med 2001; 37: S145–S151.

28. de Latorre F, Nolan J, Robertson C, Chamberlain D, Baskett P. European Resuscitation Council Guidelines 2000 for Adult Advanced Life Support. A statement from the Advanced Life Support Working Group(1) and approved by the Executive Committee of the European Resuscitation Council. Resuscitation 2001; 48: 211–221.

29. Rich J. Street Level Airway Management (SLAM): If your patient can't breathe—nothing else matters. Anesthesia Today 2005; 16: 13–22.

30. Rich J. Recognition and management of the difficult airway with special emphasis on the intubating LMA-Fastrach/whistle technique: A brief review with case reports. BUMC Proceedings 2005; 18: 220–227.

31. Rich J, Mason A, Bey T, Krafft P, Frass M. The critical airway, rescue ventilation and the Combitube: Part 1 (available at http://www.airwayeducation.com/PDFs/AANA_ARTICLE_2-04.pdf). AANA J 2004; 72: 17–27.

32. Stone D, Gal T. Airway management, in *Anesthesia,* Fifth Edition. Edited by Miller R. Philadelphia, Churchill Livingstone, 2000, pp. 1414–1451.

33. Cranton G. Personal communication. Largo, FL, July 16, 2005.

34. Jackson C, Jackson C. Direct laryngoscopy, in *Bronchoscopy, Esophagoscopy and Gastroscopy.* Philadelphia, Saunders, 1934, pp. 95–112.

35. Rich J. SLAM Airway Training Institute's Airway Products Catalogue, 2003. http://www.airwayeducation.com/products/products.asp

36. Dorsch J, Dorsch S. Endotracheal equipment, in *Understanding Anesthesia Equipment.* Baltimore, Williams & Wilkins, 1980, pp. 244–281.

37. Smith C. Cervical spine injury and tracheal intubation: A never ending conflict (available at http://www.airwayeducation.com/PDFs/SpringSummer_2000.pdf). TraumaCare 2000; 10(1): 20–26.

38. Heath KJ. The effect of laryngoscopy of different cervical spine immobilisation techniques. Anaesthesia 1994; 49: 843–845.

39. Mason A. The laryngeal mask airway (LMA) & intubating laryngeal mask airway (ILMA), in *Prehospital Trauma Care, Royal College of Anaesthetists—May 13, 2002.* London, UK, 2002.

40. MacIntosh P. New laryngoscope. Lancet 1943; 1: 205.

41. Finucane B, Santora A. *Techniques of Intubation, Principles of Airway Management,* Third Edition. New York, Springer, 2003, pp. 182–213.

42. Ovassapian A, Meyer R. Airway management, in *Principles and Practice of Anesthesiology.* Edited by Longnecker D, Tinker J. St Louis, Mosby-Year Book, 1998, pp. 1064–1102.

43. Stehling L. Management of the airway, in *Clinical Anesthesia,* Second Edition. Edited by Barash P, Cullen B, Stoelting R. Philadelphia, Lippincott-Raven, 1996, pp. 685–708.

44. Horton W, Fahy L, Charters P. Factor analysis in difficult tracheal intubation: Laryngoscopy-induced airway obstruction. British Journal of Anaesthesia 1990; 65: 801–805.

45. Domino K, Posner K, Caplan R, Cheney F. Airway injury during anesthesia: A closed claims analysis. Anesthesiology 1999; 91: 1703–1711.

46. Latto I. Management of difficult intubation, in *Difficulties in Tracheal Intubation.* Edited by Latto I, Vaughan R. London, WB Saunders Company Ltd, 1997, pp. 107–160.

47. Knill RL. Difficult laryngoscopy made easy with a "BURP." Can J Anaesth 1993; 40: 279–282.

48. Caplan RA, Posner KL, Ward RJ, Cheney FW. Adverse respiratory events in anesthesia: A closed claims analysis. Anesthesiology 1990; 72: 828–833.

49. Finucane BT, Santora AH. *Complications of Endotracheal Intubation, Principles of Airway Management, Second Edition*. St. Louis, Mosby, 1996, pp. 227–250.

50. Mallampati R. Airway management, in *Clinical Anesthesia*. Edited by Paul G. Barash, Stoelting R. Philadelphia, Lippincott-Raven, 1997, pp. 573–594.

51. Skinner MW, Waldron RJ, Anderson MB. Normal laryngoscopy and intubation, in *Airway Management*. Edited by Hanowell LH, Waldron RJ, Hwang AEJCF. Philadelphia, Lippincott-Raven, 1996, pp. 81–96.

52. Troop C. Simple techniques to rescue intubation, in *SLAM Dallas 2005: Emergency Airway Provider Course*. Edited by Rich J. Dallas, Texas, SLAM Airway Training Institute, 2005, pp. 69–83.

53. MacIntosh R. An aid to oral intubation. British Medical Journal 1949; 1: 28.

54. Cormack R, Carli F, Williams K. Unexpected difficult laryngoscopy. British Journal of Anaesthesia 1991; 67: 501.

55. SIMS Portex Tracheal Tube Introducer 15 FR: Package Insert. Keene, NH, SIMS Portex, Inc, 1999.

56. Dogra S, Falconer R, Latto IP. Successful difficult intubation: Tracheal tube placement over a gum-elastic bougie. Anaesthesia 1990; 45: 774–776.

57. Cupitt J. Microbial contamination of gum elastic bougies. Anaesthesia 2000; 55: 466–468.

58. Jackson C, Jackson C. Position of the patient for peroral endoscopy, in *Bronchoscopy, Esophagoscopy and Gastroscopy: A Manual of Peroral Endoscopy and Laryngeal Surgery*, Third Edition. Philadelphia, Saunders, 1934, pp. 85–94.

59. Wayne MA, Friedland E. Prehospital use of succinylcholine: A 20-year review. Prehosp Emerg Care 1999; 3: 107–109.

60. Benumof JL. Preoxygenation: Best method for both efficacy and efficiency. Anesthesiology 1999; 91: 603–605.

61. Li J, Murphy-Lavoie H, Bugas C, Martinez J, Preston C. Complications of emergency intubation with and without paralysis. Am J Emerg Med 1999; 17: 141–143.

Chapter 5

1. Rocke DA, Murray WB, Rout CC, Gouws E. Relative risk analysis of factors associated with difficult intubation in obstetric anesthesia. Anesthesiology 1992; 77: 67–73.

2. Samsoon GL, Young JR. Difficult tracheal intubation: A retrospective study. Anaesthesia 1987; 42: 487–490.

3. Wheeler M, Ovassapian A. Prediction and evaluation of the difficult airway, in *Handbook of Difficult Airway Management*. Edited by Hagberg C. Philadelphia, Churchill Livingstone, 2000, pp. 15–30.

4. Levitan R, Ochroch EA. Airway management and direct laryngoscopy. A review and update. Crit Care Clin 2000; 16: 373–388.

5. Adnet F, Jouriles NJ, Le Toumelin P, Hennequin B, Taillandier C, Rayeh F, Couvreur J, Nougiere B, Nadiras P, Ladka A, Fleury M. Survey of out-of-hospital emergency intubations in the French prehospital medical system: A multicenter study. Ann Emerg Med 1998; 32: 454–460.

6. Benumof JL. Definition and incidence of the difficult airway, in *Airway Management: Principles and Practice*. Edited by Benumof JL. St. Louis, Mosby, 1996, pp. 121–125.

7. Sakles JC, Laurin EG, Rantapaa AA, Panacek EA. Airway management in the emergency department: A one-year study of 610 tracheal intubations. Ann Emerg Med 1998; 31: 325–332.

8. Tayal V, Riggs R, Marx J, Tomaszewski C, Schneider R. Rapid-sequence intubation at an emergency medicine residency: Success rate and adverse events during a two-year period. Acad Emerg Med 1999; 6: 31–37.

9. Stewart R, Paris P, Winter P, Pelton G, Cannon G. Field endotracheal intubation by paramedical personnel: Success rates and complications. Chest 1984; 85: 341–345.

10. Katz S, Falk J. Misplaced endotracheal tubes by paramedics in an urban emergency medical services system. Ann Emerg Med 2001; 37: 32–37.

11. Wang HE, Kupas DF, Paris PM, Bates RR, Yealy DM. Preliminary experience with a prospective, multi-centered evaluation of out-of-hospital endotracheal intubation. Resuscitation 2003; 58: 49–58.

12. Jones J, Murphy M, Dickson R, Somerville g, Brizendine E. Emergency physician-verified out-of-hospital intubation: Miss rates by paramedics. Acad Emerg Med 2004; 11: 707–709.

13. Weber S. Traumatic complications of airway management. Anesthesiol Clin North America 2002; 20: v–vi, 265–274.

14. Henderson J, Popat M, Latto I, Pearce A. Difficult Airway Society guidelines for management of the unanticipated difficult intubation. Anaesthesia 2004; 59: 675–694.

15. Peterson G, Posner K, Domino K, Lee L, Caplan R, Cheney F. Management of the difficult airway in closed malpractice claims, 2003.

16. Wang HE, Sweeney TA, O'Connor RE, Rubinstein H. Failed prehospital intubations: An analysis of emergency department courses and outcomes. Prehosp Emerg Care 2001; 5: 134–141.

17. American Heart Association guidelines for cardiopulmonary resuscitation and emergency cardiovascular care. Circulation 2005; 112: IV-1–IV-211.

18. Barnes T, MacDonald D, Nolan J, Otto C, Pepe P, Sayre M, Shuster M, Zaritsky A. Airway devices. Ann Emerg Med 2001; 37: S145–S151.

19. de Latorre F, Nolan J, Robertson C, Chamberlain D, Baskett P. European Resuscitation Council Guidelines 2000 for Adult Advanced Life Support. A statement from the Advanced Life Support Working Group(1) and approved by the Executive Committee of the European Resuscitation Council. Resuscitation 2001; 48: 211–221.

20. Rich J. Street Level Airway Management (SLAM): If your patient can't breathe—nothing else matters. Anesthesia Today 2005; 16: 13–22.

21. Rich J. Recognition and management of the difficult airway with special emphasis on the intubating LMA-Fastrach/whistle technique: A brief review with case reports. BUMC Proceedings 2005; 18: 220–227.

22. Rich J, Mason A, Bey T, Krafft P, Frass M. The critical airway, rescue ventilation and the Combitube: Part 1 (available at http://www.airwayeducation.com/PDFs/AANA_ARTICLE_2-04.pdf). AANA J 2004; 72: 17–27.

23. Rich J, Mason A, Ramsay M. AANA Journal Course: Update for Nurse Anesthetists. The SLAM Emergency Airway Flowchart: A new guide for advanced airway practitioners (available at http://www.airwayeducation.com/PDFs/flowchart_AANA_journal_course.pdf). AANA J 2004; 72: 431–439.

24. Salem MR, Baraka A. Confirmation of tracheal intubation, in *Airway Management: Principles and Practice*. Edited by Benumof JL. St. Louis, Mosby, 1996, pp. 531–560.

25. Ornato J, Callaham M. International Guidelines 2000: The story and the science. Ann Emerg Med 2001; 37(4 suppl): S3–S4.

26. Anderson K, Schultz-Lebahn T. Oesophageal intubation can be undetected by auscultation of the chest. Acta Anaesthesiologica Scandinavica 1994; 38: 580–582.

27. Anderson K, Hald A. Assessing the position of the tracheal tube: The reliability of different methods. Anaesthesia 1989; 44: 984–985.

28. Howells T, Riethmuller R. Signs of endotracheal intubation. Anaesthesia 1980; 35: 984–986.

29. O'Flaherty D, Adams A. The end-tidal carbon dioxide detector: Assessment of a new method to distinguish oesophageal from tracheal intubation. Anaesthesia 1990; 45: 653–655.

30. Williams K, Nuff J. The oesophageal detector device: A prospective trial in 100 patients. Anaesthesia 1989; 44: 984–985.

31. Caplan RA, Posner KL, Ward RJ, Cheney FW. Adverse respiratory events in anesthesia: A closed claims analysis. Anesthesiology 1990; 72: 828–833.

32. Caplan RA, Posner KL. Medical-legal considerations: The ASA closed claims project, in *Airway Management: Principles and Practice*. Edited by Benumof JL. St. Louis, Mosby, 1996, pp. 944–955.

33. Nunn J. The oesophageal detector device (letter). Anaesthesia 1988; 43: 804.

34. O'Leary J, Pollard B, Ryan M. A method of detecting oesophageal intubation or confirming tracheal intubation. Anaesthesia Intensive Care 1988; 16: 299–301.

35. Pollard B. Oesophageal detector device (letter). Anaesthesia 1988; 43: 713–714.

36. Wafai Y, Salem MR, Czinn EA, Barbella J, Baraka A. The self-inflating bulb in detecting esophageal intubation: effect of bulb size and technique used. Anesthesiology 1993; 79: A496.

37. Wafai Y, Salem MR, Joseph NJ, Baraka A. The self-inflating bulb for confirmation of tracheal intubation: Incidence and demography of false negatives. Anesthesiology 1994; 81: A1303.

38. Wee M. The oesophageal detector device: Assessment of a method to distinguish oesophageal from tracheal intubation. Anaesthesia 1988; 43: 27–29.

39. Wee M. Comments on the oesophageal detector device (letter). Anaesthesia 1989; 44: 930–931.

40. Bozeman WP, Hexter D, Liang HK, Kelen GD. Esophageal detector device versus detection of end-tidal carbon dioxide level in emergency intubation. Ann Emerg Med 1996; 27: 595–599.

41. Sum-Ping ST, Mehta MP, Anderton JM. A comparative study of methods of detection of esophageal intubation. Anesth Analg 1989; 69: 627–632.

42. Baraka A, Salem R. The Combitube oesophageal-tracheal double lumen airway for difficult intubation. Canadian Journal of Anaesthesia 1993; 40: 1222–1223.

43. Zaleski L, Abello D, Gold MI. The esophageal detector device: Does it work? Anesthesiology 1993; 79: 244–247.

44. Butler B, Little T, Drtil S. Esophageal-tracheal Combitube, colorimetric carbon dioxide detection, and the esophageal detector device (letter-reply). Journal of Clinical Monitoring 1996; 12: 203.

45. Benumof J. The ASA Difficult Airway Algorithm: New thoughts and considerations, in *Handbook of Difficult Airway Management*. Edited by Hagberg C. Philadelphia, Churchill Livingstone, 2000, pp. 31–48.

46. Salem MR, Wafai Y, Joseph NJ, Baraka A, Czinn EA. Efficacy of the self-inflating bulb in detecting esophageal intubation: Does the presence of a nasogastric tube or cuff deflation make a difference? Anesthesiology 1994; 80: 42–48.

47. Salem M, Wafai Y, Baraka A, et al. Use of the self-inflating bulb for detecting esophageal intubation after "esophageal ventilation." Anesth Analg 1993; 77: 1227–1231.

48. Baraka A, Khoury PJ, Siddik SS, Salem MR, Joseph NJ. Efficacy of the self-inflating bulb in differentiating esophageal from tracheal intubation in the parturient undergoing cesarean section. Anesth Analg 1997; 84: 533–537.

49. Baraka A, Choueiry P, Salem M. The esophageal detector device in the morbidly obese (letter). Anesthesia and Analgesia 1993; 77: 400.

50. Baraka A. The oesophageal detector device (letter). Anaesthesia 1991; 45: 697.

51. Calder I, Smith M, Newton M. The oesophageal detector device (letter). Anaesthesia 1989; 44: 705.

52. Haynes S, Morten N. Use of the oesophageal detector device in children under one year of age. Anaesthesia 1991; 45: 1067–1069.

53. Lang D, Wafai Y, Salem M. Efficacy of the self-inflating bulb in confirming tracheal intubation in the morbidly obese. Anesthesiology 1996; 85: 246–253.

54. Heidegger T, Heim C. Esophageal detector device: Not always reliable. Annals of Emergency Medicine 1996; 28: 582.

55. Mathias J. Oesohageal detector device. Anaesthesia 1989; 44: 931.

56. Ardagh M, Moodie K. The esophageal detector device can give false positives for tracheal intubation. Journal of Emergency Medicine 1998; 16: 747–749.

57. Loeb R, Santos W. Monitoring ventilation, in *Airway Management*. Edited by Hanowell L, Waldron R, Hwang J. Philadelphia, Lippincott-Raven, 1996, pp. 15–38.

58. Zbinden S, Schupfer G. Detection of oesophageal intubation: The cola complication. Anaesthesia 1989; 44: 81.

59. Frakes M. Measuring end-tidal carbon dioxide: Clinical applications and usefulness. Critical Care Nurse 2001; 21: 23–37.

60. O'Callaghan J, Williams R. Confirmation of tracheal intubation using a chemical device (abstract). Canadian Journal of Anaesthesia 1988; 33: S59.

61. Thomas S, Wedel S, Wayne M. Oxygenation, ventilation, and monitoring, in *Prehospital Trauma Care*. Edited by Soreide E, Grande C. New York, Marcel Dekker, 2001, pp. 255–272.

62. Jones B, Dorsey M. Sensitivity of a disposable end-tidal carbon dioxide detector. Journal of Clinical Monitoring 1991; 7: 268–270.

63. Bhende M, Allen WJ. Evaluation of a Capno-Flo^{TM} resuscitator during transport of critically ill children. Pediatr Emerg Care 2002; 18: 414–416.

64. Birmingham P, Cheney F, Ward R. Esophageal intubation: A review of detection techniques. Anesth Analg 1986; 65: 886–891.

65. Butler B, Little T, Drtil S. Combined use of the esophageal-tracheal Combitube with a colorimetric carbon dioxide detector for emergency intubation/ventilation. Journal of Clinical Monitoring 1995; 11: 311–316.

66. Package insert: Capno-flo Pulmonary Manual Resuscitator with CO_2 level monitor. Kirk Specialty Systems, 1625 Crescent Circle, Suite 225, Carrollton, TX 75006.

67. Maleck W, Koetter K. Esophageal-tracheal Combitube, colorimetric carbon dioxide detection, and the esophageal detector device (letter). Journal of Clinical Monitoring 1996; 12: 203.

68. Bhende M, Thompson A, Cook D, et al. Validity of a disposable end-tidal CO_2 detector in verifying endotracheal tube placement in infants and children. Ann Emerg Med 1992; 21: 142–145.

69. Foutch R, Magelssen M, McMillan J. The esophageal detector device: A rapid and accurate method for assessing tracheal versus esophageal intubation in a porcine model (available at http://www.ncbi.nlm.nih.gov/entrez/query.fcgi?). Ann Emerg Med 1998; 21: 1073–1076.

70. Kaspner C, Deem S. The self-inflating bulb to detect esophageal intubation during emergency airway management. Anesthesiology 1998; 88: 898–902.

71. Li J. Capnography alone is imperfect for endotracheal tube placement confirmation during emergency intubation. J Emerg Med 2001; 20: 223–229.

72. Frakes M. Transport, in *Capnography: Clinical aspects*. Edited by Gravenstein J, Paulus D. Cambridge, UK, Cambridge University Press, 2004, pp. 65–72.

73. Evans A, Winslow E. Oxygen saturation and hemodynamic response in critically ill, mechanically ventilated adults during intrahospital transport. Am J Crit Care 1995; 4: 106–111.

74. Hurst JM, Davis K Jr. Johnson D, Branson R, Campbell R, Branson P. Risk, cost and complications during in-hospital transport of critically ill patients: A prospective cohort study. J Trauma 1992; 33: 582–585.

75. Indek M, Peterson S, Smith J, Brotman S. Risk, cost, and benefit of transporting ICU patients for special studies. J Trauma 1988; 28: 1020–1025.

76. Waydhas C, Schneck G. Deterioration of respiratory function after intrahospital transport of critically ill surgical patients. Intensive Care Med 1995; 21: 784–789.

77. Beker A, Ipekoglu Z, Tureyen K, Bilgin H, Korfali G, Kofali E. Secondary insults during intrahospital transport of neurosurgical intensive care patients. Neurosurg Rev 1998; 21: 98–101.

78. Braman S, Dunn S, Amico C, Millman R. Complications of intrahospital transport in critically ill patients. Ann Intern Med 1987; 107: 469–473.

79. Gervais H, Eberle B, Konietzke D, Hennes H, Dick W. Comparison of blood gases of ventilated patients during transport. Crit Care Med 1987; 15: 761–763.

80. Martin S, Agudelo W, Oschner M. Monitoring hyperventilation in patients with closed head injury during air transport. Air Med Jan 1997; 16(1): 15–17.

81. Mason A, Rich J, Ramsay M. Mason's PU-92 concept. Rapid recognition and treatment of the crash airway. TraumaCare 2003; 13: 46.

82. Miner J, Heegaard W, Lummer D. End-tidal carbon dioxide monitoring during procedural sedation. Acad Emerg Med 2002; 9: 275–280.

83. Vargo J, Zuccaro G, Dumont J, Conwell D, Morrow J, Shay S. Automated graphic assessment of respiratory activity is superior to pulse oximetry and visual assessment for the detection of early respiratory depression during therapeutic upper endoscopy. Gastrointest Endosc 2002; 55: 826–831.

84. Bhende H. Capnography in the pediatric emergency department. Pediatr Emerg Care 1999; 15: 64–69.

85. Benumof J. Interpretation of capnography. AANA J 1998; 66: 169–176.

86. Ward K, Yealy D. End-tidal carbon dioxide in emergency medicine, part 2: Clinical applications. Acad Emerg Med 1998; 5: 637–646.

87. Ward K, Yealy D. End-tidal carbon dioxide monitoring in emergency medicine, part 2: Clinical applications. Acad Emerg Med 1998; 5: 637–646.

88. Drew K, Brayton M, Ambrose A, Bernard G. End-tidal carbon dioxide monitoring for weaning patients: A pilot study. Dim Crit Care Nurse 1998; 17: 127–134.

89. Jones N, Robertson D, Kane J. Difference between end-tidal and arterial CO_2 in exercise. J Appl Physiol 1979; 47: 954–960.

90. Russell G, Graybeal J, Strout J. Stability of arterial to end-tidal carbon dioxide gradients during postoperative cardiorespiratory support. Can J Anaesth 1993; 49: 206–210.

91. Shankar K, Moseley H, Kumar Y, Vemula V. Arterial to end tidal carbon dioxide tension difference during caesarean section anesthesia. Anaesthesia 1986; 41: 689–702.

92. Shankar K, Moseley H, Kumar Y, Venula V, Krishnan A. Arterial to end-tidal carbon dioxide tension difference during anaesthesia for tubal ligation. Anaesthesia 1987; 42: 482–486.

93. Sahs R, Hankins D, Zietlow S. Capnography values versus laboratory analyzed blood sample values in flight (abstract). Air Med J 2000; 19: A2.

94. Belpomme V, Ricard-Hibon A, Devoir C, Dileseigres S, Devaud M, Chollet C, Marty J. Correlation of arterial PCO_2 and $PETCO_2$ in prehospital controlled ventilation. Am J Emerg Med 2005; 23: 852–859.

95. Bocka J, Overton D, Hauser A. Eletromechanical dissociation in human beings: An echocardiographic evaluation. Ann Emerg Med 1988; 17: 450–452.

96. Paridis N, Martin G, Goetting M, Rivers E, Feingold M, Nowark R. Aortic pressure during human cardiac arrest: Identification of pseudo-electromechanical dissociation. Chest 1992; 101: 123–128.

97. Isserles S, Breen P. Can changes in end-tidal pCO_2 measure changes in cardiac output? Anesth Analg 1991; 73: 808–814.

98. Sanders A, Ewy G, Bragg S, et al. Expired pCO_2 as a prognostic indicator of successful resuscitation from cardiac arrest. Ann Emerg Med 1985; 14.

99. White R, Asplin B. Out of hospital quantitative monitoring of end-tidal carbon dioxide pressure during CPR. Ann Emerg Med 1994; 23: 25–30.

100. Levine R, Wayne M, Miller C. End-tidal carbon dioxide and outcome of out-of-hospital cardiac arrest. New England Journal of Medicine 1997; 337: 301–306.

101. Callaham M, Barton C. Prediction of outcome of cardiopulmonary resuscitation from end-tidal carbon dioxide concentration. Crit Care Med 1990; 18: 358–362.

102. Egan's *Fundamentals of Respiratory Care,* Eighth Edition. Edited by Donald F. Egan, Craig L. Sconlan, Robert L. Wilkins, James K. Stoller, New York, Mosby, 2003.

103. Janice L. Zimmerman, MD, *Fundamental Critical Care Support,* Third Edition. Des Plaines, Ill, Society of Critical Care Medicine, 2001.

104. Pollack C. Mechanical ventilation and noninvasive ventilatory support, in *Emergency Medicine Concepts and Clinical Practice.* Edited by Rosen P. St Louis, Mosby, 1998, pp. 21–28.

105. Frakes M, Evans T. Ventilation modes and monitoring. J Resp Care Prac 2003; 16: 42–44.

Chapter 6

1. Benet L, Kroetz D, Sheiner L. Pharmacokinetics, in Goodman's & Gilman's *The Pharmacological Basis of Therapeutics.* Edited by Hardman J, Limbird L. New York, McGraw-Hill, 1996, pp. 3–27.

2. Ross E. Pharmacodynamics, in Goodman's & Gilman's *The Pharmacological Basis of Therapeutics.* Edited by Hardman J, Limbird L. New York, McGraw-Hill, 1996, pp. 29–41.

3. Van Hemelrijck J, White PF. Nonopoid intravenous anesthesia, in *Clinical Anesthesia.* Edited by Barash PG et al. Philadelphia, Lippincott-Raven, 1996, pp. 311–327.

4. Turmheim K. When drug therapy gets old: Pharmacokinetics and pharmacodynamics in the elderly. Exp Geront 2003; 38: 843–853.

5. Kanto J, Gepts E. Pharmacokinetic implications for the clinical use of propofol. Clin Pharmacokinet 1989; 17: 308–326.

6. Lange H, Stephan H, Zielman S, et al. Hepatic elimination of thiopental in heart surgery patients. Anaesthesist 1992; 41: 171–178.

7. Takla J. Determinants of splanchnic blood flow. Br J Anaesth 1997; 77: 50–58.

8. Wadbrook P. Advances in airway pharmacology: Emerging trends and evolving controversy. Emerg Med Clin North Am 2000; 18: 767–788.

9. White PF. Clinical pharmacology of intravenous induction drugs. Int Anaesthesiol Clin 1988; 26: 98–104.

10. Sparr JH, Giesinger H, Ulmer M, et al. Influence of induction technique on intubation conditions after rocuronium in adults: Comparison with rapid-sequence induction using thipentone and suxamethonium. Br J Anaesth 1996; 77: 339–342.

11. Jewett BA, Gibbs LM, Tarasiuk A, et al. Propofol and barbiturate depression of spinal nociceptive neurotransmission. Anesthesiology 1992; 77: 1059–1061.

12. Young CJ, Coalson D, Klock PA, et al. Analgesic and psychomotor effects of thiopental at subanesthetic concentrations in human volunteers. Acta Anaesthesiol Scand 1997; 41: 903–910.

13. Fuchs-Buder T, Sparr HJ, Ziegenfuss T. Thiopental or etomidate for rapid sequence induction with rocuronium. Br J Anaesth 1998; 80: 504–506.

14. Russo H, Bressolle F. Pharmacodynamics and pharmocokinetics of thiopental. Clin Pharmacokinet 1998; 35: 95–134.

15. Christensen JH, Andreasen F. Individual variation in response to thiopental. Acta Anaesthesiol Scand 1978; 22: 303–313.

16. Parviainen I, Uusaro A, Kalviainen R, et al. High-dose thiopental in the treatment of refractory status epilepticus in intensive care unit. Neurology 2002; 59: 1249–1251.

17. Ghouri AF, Mading W, Prabaker K. Accidental intraarterial drug injections via intravascular cathethers placed on the dorsum of the hand. Anesth Analg 2002; 95: 487–491.

18. Angel MF, Amiss ED, Amiss LR, et al. Deleterious effect of urokinase to treat experimental intraarterial thiopental injection injuries. Ann Plast Surg 1992; 28: 281–283.

19. Van Hamme MJ, Ghoneim MM, Ambre JJ. Pharmacokinetics of etomidate, a new intravenous anesthetic. Anaesthesiology 1978; 49: 274–277.

20. Mazerolles M, Senard JM, Verwaerde P, Tran MA, Montastruc JL, Virenque C, Montastruc P. Effects of pentobarbital and etomidate on plasma catecholamine levels and spectral analysis of blood pressure and heart rate in dogs. Fundam Clin Pharmacol 1996; 10: 298–303.

21. Bergen JM, Smith DC. A review of etomidate for rapid sequence intubation in the emergency department. J Emerg Med 1997; 15: 221–230.

22. Skinner HJ, Biswas A, Mahajan RP. Evaluation of intubating conditions with rocuronium and either propofol or etomidate for rapid sequence induction. Anaesthesia 1998; 53: 702–710.

23. Weiss-Bloom LJ, Reich DL. Hemodynamic responses to tracheal intubation following etomidate and fentanyl for anesthetic induction. Can J Anaesth 1992; 39: 780–785.

24. Kingsley C. Perioperative use of etomidate for trauma patients, in Use of Etomidate in Trauma, ITACCS Monograph. Edited by Smith C, Grande C. New York, McMahon Group, 1996, pp. 1–7.

25. Diago MC, Amado JA, Otero M, et al. Anti-adrenal action of a subanaesthetic dose of etomidate. Anaesthesia 1988; 43: 644–645.

26. Fellows IW, Byrne AJ, Allison SP. Adrenocortical suppression with etomidate. Lancet 1983; 2: 54–55.

27. Ledingham IM, Finlay WEI, Watt I, et al. Etomidate and adrenocortical function. Lancet 1983; 1: 1443.

28. Boidin MP, Erdmann WE, Faithfull NS. The role of ascorbic acid in etomidate toxicity. 1986; 3: 417–422.

29. Doenicke A: Etomidat-Propofol. Klin Anasthesiol Intensivther 1993; 42: 57–70.

30. Magee L, Goodsiff L, Matthews I, et al. Anaesthetic drugs and bacterial contamination. Eur J Anaesthesiol Suppl. 1995; 12: 41–43.

31. Kanto JH. Propofol, the newest induction agent of anesthesia. Int J Clin Pharmacol Ther Toxicol 1988; 26: 41–57.

32. Grounds RM, Morgan M, Lumley J. Some studies on the properties of the intravenous anaesthestic, propofol ('Disoprivan')—review. Postgrad Med J 1985; 61: 90–95.

33. Jantzen JP. Cerebral neuroprotection and ketamine. Anaesthesist 1994; 43 (Suppl 2): S41–S47.

34. Kohrs R, Durieux ME. Ketamine: Teaching an old drug new tricks. Anesth Analg 1998; 87: 1186–1193.

35. Ivani G, Vercellino C, Tonetti F. Ketamine: A new look to an old drug. Minerva Anestesiol 2003; 69: 468–471.

36. L'Hommedieu CS, Arens JJ. The use of ketamine for the emergency intubation of patients with status asthmaticus. Ann Emerg Med 1987; 16: 568–571.

37. Christ G, Mundigler G, Merhaut C, Zehetgruber M, Kratochwill C, Heinz G, Siostrzonek P. Adverse cardiovascular effects of ketamine infusion in patients with catecholamine-dependent heart failure. Anaesth Intensive Care 1997; 25: 255–259.

38. Sprung J, Schuetz SM, Stewart RW, Moravec CS. Effects of ketamine on the contractility of failing and nonfailing human heart muscles in vitro. Anesthesiology 1998; 88: 1202–1210.

39. Nordt SP, Clark RF. Midazolam: A review of therapeutic uses and toxicity. J Emerg Med 1997; 15: 357–365.

40. Steene J. Midazolam and flumazenil use in trauma patients, in *The Use of Midazolam and Flumazenil in Trauma Anesthesia.* Edited by Smith C, Grande C. Baltimore, MD, University of Maryland Medical System, 1999, pp. 2–4.

41. Baber R, Hobbes A, Munro IA, Purcell G, Binstead L. Midazolam as an intravenous induction agent for general anaesthesia: A clinical trial. Anaesth Intensive Care 1982; Feb: 10(1): 29–35.

42. Classen DC, Pestotnik SL, Evans RS, et al. Intensive surveillance of midazolam use in hospitalized patients and the occurrence of cardiorespiratory arrest. Pharmacotherapy 1992; 12: 213–216.

43. Yaster M, Nicholls DG, Deshpande JK, et al. Midazolam-fentanyl intravenous sedation in children: Case report of respiratory arrest. Pediatrics 1990; 86: 463–467.

44. Fee JPH, Collier PS, Howard PJ, et al. Cimetidine and ranitidine increase midazolam bioavailability. Clin Pharmacol Ther 1987; 41: 80–84.

45. Smith CE, Lewis G, Donati F, Bevan DR. Dose-response relationship for succinylcholine in a patient with genetically determined low plasma cholinesterase activity. Anesthesiology 1989; 70: 156–158.

46. Naguib M, Samarkandi A, Riad W, et al. Optimal dose of succinylcholine revisited. Anesthesiology 2003; 99: 1045–1049.

47. Perry J, Lee J, Wells G. Rocuronium versus succinylcholine for rapid sequence induction intubation. Cochrane Database Syst Rev 2003; 1: CD002788.

48. Markewitz BA, Elstad MR. Succinylcholine-induced hyperkalemia following prolonged pharmacologic neuromuscular blockade. Chest 1997; 1997: 248–250.

49. Yentis SM. Suxamethonium and hyperkalaemia. Anaesth Intensive Care 1990; 18: 92–101.

50. Naguib M, Flood P, McArdle JJ, Brenner HR. Advances in neurobiology of the neuromuscular junction: Implications for the anesthesiologist. Anesthesiology 2002; 96: 202–231.

51. Zink BJ, Snyder HS, Raccio-Robak N. Lack of a hyperkalemic response in emergency department patients receiving succinylcholine. Acad Emerg Med 1995; 2: 974–978.

52. Brown MM, Parr MJ, Manara AR. The effect of suxamethonium on intracranial pressure and cerebral perfusion pressure in patients with severe head injuries following blunt trauma. Eur J Anaesthesiol 1996; 13: 474–477.

53. Cheng CA, Aun CS, Gin T. Comparison of rocuronium and suxamethonium for rapid tracheal intubation in children. Pediatr Anaesth 2002; 12: 140–145.

54. Doenicke AW, Czeslick E, Moss J, Hoernecke R. Onset time, endotracheal intubating conditions, and plasma histamine after cisatracurium and vecuronium administration. Anesth Analg 1998; 87: 434–438.

55. Shafer S, Varvel J. Pharmacokinetics, pharmacodynamics, and rational opiod selection. Anestheisology 1991; 74: 53–63.

56. Sivilotti M, Ducharme J. Randomized, double-blind study on sedatives and hemodynamics during rapid-sequence intubation in the emergency department: The SHRED Study. Ann Emerg Med 1998; 31: 313–324.

57. Bowdle TA. Adverse effects of opioid agonists and agonist-antagonists in anaesthesia. Drug Saf 1998; 19: 173–189.

58. O'Hare R, McAtamney D, Mirakhur RK, Hughes D, Carabine U. Bolus dose remifentanil for control of haemodynamic response to tracheal intubation during rapid sequence induction of anaesthesia. Br J Anaesth 1999; 82: 283–285.

59. Chraemmer-Jorgensen B, Hoilund-Carlsen PF, Marving J, Christensen V. Lack of effect of intravenous lidocaine on hemodynamic responses to rapid sequence induction of general anesthesia: A double-blind controlled clinical trial. Anesth Analg 1986; 65: 1037–1041.

Chapter 7

1. Rich J. Street Level Airway Management (SLAM): If your patient can't breathe—nothing else matters. Anesthesia Today 2005; 16: 13–22.

2. Rich J, Mason A, Ramsay M. The SLAM Emergency Airway Flowchart: A new guide for advanced airway practitioners (available at http://www.airwayeducation.com/PDFs/flowchart_AANA_journal_course.pdf). AANA J 2004; 72: 431–439.

3. Smith C, Walls R, Lockey D, Kuhnigk H. Advanced airway management and use of anesthetic drugs, in *The International Textbook on Prehospital Trauma Care*. Edited by Grande C, Soreide E. New York, Marcel Dekker Inc., 2001.

4. Wayne MA, Friedland E. Prehospital use of succinylcholine: A 20-year review. Prehosp Emerg Care 1999; 3: 107–109.

5. Li J, Murphy-Lavoie H, Bugas C, Martinez J, Preston C. Complications of emergency intubation with and without paralysis. Am J Emerg Med 1999; 17: 141–143.

6. Benumof JL. Preoxygenation: Best method for both efficacy and efficiency. Anesthesiology 1999; 91: 603–605.

7. Baraka AS, Taha SK, Aouad MT, El-Khatib MF, Kawkabani NI. Preoxygenation: Comparison of maximal breathing and tidal volume breathing techniques. Anesthesiology 1999; 91: 612–616.

8. Benumof JL, Dagg R, Benumof R. Critical hemoglobin desaturation will occur before return to an unparalyzed state following 1 mg/kg intravenous succinylcholine. Anesthesiology 1997; 87: 979–982.

9. Lawes EG, Campbell I, Mercer D. Inflation pressure, gastric insufflation and rapid sequence induction. Br J Anaesth 1987; 59: 315–318.

10. Sellick BA. Cricoid pressure to control regurgitation of stomach contents during induction of anaesthesia. Lancet 1961; 2: 404–406.

11. Mallampati SR. Recognition of the difficult airway, in *Airway Management: Principles and Practice*. Edited by Benumof JL. St. Louis, Mosby, 1996, pp. 126–142.

12. Stene J, Grande C, Barton C. Airway management for the trauma patient, in *Trauma Anesthesia*. Edited by Stene J, Grande C. Baltimore, Williams and Wilkins, 1991, pp. 64–99.

13. Brimacombe JR, Berry AM. Cricoid pressure. Can J Anaesth 1997; 44: 414–425.

14. Smith C, Boyer D. Ease of tracheal intubation using fiberoptic laryngoscopy in patients receiving cricoid pressure. Canadian Journal of Anaesthesia 2002; 49: 614–619.

15. Brimacombe J, White A, Berry A. Effect of cricoid pressure on ease of insertion of the laryngeal mask airway. Br J Anaesth 1993; 71: 800–802.

16. Kingsley C. Perioperative use of etomidate for trauma patients, in Use of Etomidate in Trauma, ITACCS Monograph. Edited by Smith C, Grande C. New York, McMahon Group, 1996, pp. 1–7.

17. Kingsley C. Perioperative management of thoracic trauma. Anesthesiology Clinics of North America 1999; 17: 183–195.

18. Smith C, Grande C, Wayne M. Rapid Sequence Intubation in Trauma, International Trauma Anesthesia and Critical Care Society. Edited by ITACCS Consensus Panel. Baltimore, 1998.

19. Gronert GA. Cardiac arrest after succinylcholine: Mortality greater with rhabdomyolysis than receptor upregulation. Anesthesiology 2001; 94: 523–529.

20. Bevan D. Complications of muscle relaxants. Seminars in anesthesia 1995; 14: 63.

21. Grande C, Smith C, Stene J. Trauma anesthesia, in *Principles and Practice of Anesthesiology*, Second Edition. Edited by Longnecker D, Tinker J, Morgan G, 1998, pp. 2138–2164.

22. Smith C. Rapid sequence induction in adults: Indications and concerns. Clinical Pulmonary Medicine 2001; 8: 147–165.

23. Tryfus S, Abrams K, Grande C. Airway management in neurological injuries, in *Trauma Anesthesia and Critical Care of Neurological Injury*. Edited by Abrams K, Grande C. Armonk, NY, Futura Publishing, 1997, pp. 121–151.

Chapter 8

1. Li J, Murphy-Lavoie H, Bugas C, Martinez J, Preston C. Complications of emergency intubation with and without paralysis. Am J Emerg Med 1999; 17: 141–143.

2. Crosby ET, Cooper RM, Douglas MJ, Doyle DJ, Hung OR, Labrecque P, Muir H, Murphy MF, Preston RP, Rose DK, Roy L. The unanticipated difficult airway with recommendations for management. Can J Anaesth 1998; 45: 757–776.

3. Practice guidelines for management of the difficult airway: An updated report by the American Society of Anesthesiologists Task Force on Management of the Difficult Airway. Anesthesiology 2003; 98: 1269–1277.

4. Wilson W. Difficult intubation, in *Complications in Anesthesia*. Edited by Atlee J. Philadelphia, W.B. Saunders, 1999, pp. 138–147.

5. Rich J, Mason A, Bey T, Krafft P, Frass M. The critical airway, rescue ventilation and the Combitube: Part 1 (available at http://www.airwayeducation.com/PDFs/AANA_ARTICLE_2–04.pdf). AANA J 2004; 72: 17–27.

6. Guidelines 2000 for Cardiopulmonary Resuscitation and Emergency Cardiovascular Care—An International Consensus of Science, the American Heart Association in Collaboration with the International Liaison Committee on Resuscitation. Part 6: Advanced Cardiovascular Life Support. Section 3: Adjuncts for Oxygenation, Ventilation, and Airway Control. Resuscitation 2000 Aug. 23; 46 (1–3): 115–125.

7. Ornato J, Callaham M. International Guidelines 2000: The story and the science. Ann Emerg Med 2001; 37(4 suppl): S3–S4.

8. de Latorre F, Nolan J, Robertson C, Chamberlain D, Baskett P. European Resuscitation Council Guidelines 2000 for Adult Advanced Life Support. A statement from the Advanced Life Support Working Group(1) and approved by the Executive Committee of the European Resuscitation Council. Resuscitation 2001; 48: 211–221.

9. Benumof J. The ASA Difficult Airway Algorithm: New thoughts and considerations, in *Handbook of Difficult Airway Management*. Edited by Hagberg C. Philadelphia, Churchill Livingstone, 2000, pp. 31–48.

10. Brain A. The laryngeal mask—a new concept in airway management. Brit J Anaes 1983; 55: 801–805.

11. Heinrichs W, Weiler N, Latorre F, Eberie B. Respiratory mechanics, gastric insufflation pressure and air leakage of the laryngeal mask airway (abstract). Anesthesiology 1995; 83: A 1227.

12. Pennant J, Walker M. Comparison of the endotracheal tube and laryngeal mask in airway management by paramedical personnel. Anesth Analg 1992; 53: 531–534.

13. Davies P, Tigh S, Greenslade G, et al. Laryngeal mask airway and tracheal tube insertion by unskilled personnel. Lancet 1990; 336: 997–999.

14. Stone CK, Thomas SH. Is oral endotracheal intubation efficacy impaired in the helicopter environment? Air Med J 1994; 13: 319–321.

15. Reinhart DJ, Simmons G. Comparison of placement of the laryngeal mask airway with endotracheal tube by paramedics and respiratory therapists. Ann Emerg Med 1994; 24: 260–263.

16. Maltby, JR. The laryngeal mask airway in anaesthesia. Can J Anaesth 1994; 41: 930–960.

17. Brimacombe J, Berry A. The incidence of aspiration with the laryngeal mask airway: A meta-analysis of published literature. J Clin Anesth 1995; 7: 297–305.

18. Stone B, Leach A, Alexander C, et al. The use of the laryngeal mask airway by nurses during cardiopulmonary resuscitation—results of a multicentre trial. Anaesthesia 1994; 49: 3–7.

19. Lawes E, Baskett P. Pulmonary aspiration during unsuccessful cardiopulmonary resuscitation. Intensive Care Med 1987; 13: 379–382.

20. Lockey D, Coates T, Parr M. Aspiration in severe trauma. Anaesthesia 1999; 45: 1097–1098.

21. Preis C, Hartmann T, Zimpfer M. Laryngeal mask airway facilitates awake fibreoptic intubation in a patient with severe oropharyngeal bleeding. Anesth Analg 1998; 87: 728–729.

22. Berry A, Brimacombe J, McManus K, Goldblatt M. An evaluation of the factors influencing selection of the optimal size of laryngeal mask airway in normal adults. Anaesthesia. 1998; 53: 565–570.

23. Keller C, Puerhinger F, Brimacombe J. The influence of cuff volume on oropharyngeal leak pressure and fibreoptic position with the laryngeal mask airway. Br J Anaesth 1998; 81: 186–187.

24. Brimacombe J, Berry A. Laryngeal mask airway insertion. A comparison of the standard versus neutral position in normal patients with a view to its use in cervical spine instability. Anaesthesia 1993; 48: 670–671.

25. Brimacombe J, Keller C. Insertion of the LMA-Unique with and without digital intraoral manipulation by inexperienced personnel after manikin-only training. J Emerg Med 2004; 26: 1–5.

26. Mason A. Method of securing the laryngeal mask airway in pre-hospital care. Prehospital Immediate Care 1999; 3: 167–169.

27. Brimacombe J. Analysis of 1500 laryngeal mask uses by one anaesthetist in adults undergoing routine anaesthesia. Anaesthesia 1996; 51: 76–80.

28. Frass M. The Combitube: Esophageal/tracheal double lumen airway, in *Airway Management: Principles and Practice*. Edited by Benumof JL. St. Louis, Mosby, 1996, pp. 444–454.

29. Gaitini LA, Vaida SJ, Mostafa S, Yanovski B, Croitoru M, Capdevila MD, Sabo E, Ben-David B, Benumof J. The Combitube in elective surgery: A report of 200 cases. Anesthesiology 2001; 94: 79–82.

30. Krafft P, Nikolic A, Frass M. Esophageal rupture associated with the use of the Combitube (letter). Anesth Analg 1998; 87: 1457.

31. Panning B. Hemodynamic and catecholamine responses to insertion of the Combitube, laryngeal mask or tracheal intubation. Anesth Analg 2000; 90: 231.

32. Urtubia R, Aguila C, Cumsille M. Combitube. A study for proper use. Anesth Analg 2000; 90: 958–962.

33. Walz R, Davis S, Panning B. Is the Combitube a useful emergency airway device for anesthesiologists? (letter). Anesth Analg 1999; 88: 227–234.

34. Frass M, Frenzer R, Rauscha F, Weber H, Pacher R, Leithner C. Evaluation of esophageal tracheal Combitube in cardiopulmonary resuscitation. Crit Care Med 1987; 15: 609–611.

35. Bass RR, Allison EJ, Jr., Hunt RC. The esophageal obturator airway: A reassessment of use by paramedics. Ann Emerg Med 1982; 11: 358–360.

36. Frass M, Frenzer R, Ilias W, Lackner F, Hoflechner G, Losert U. The esophageal tracheal Combitube (ETC): Animal experiment results with a new emergency tube. Anasth Intensivther Notfallmed 1987; 22: 142–144.

37. Yardy N, Hancox D, Strang T. A comparison of two airway aids for emergency use by unskilled personnel. Anaesthesia 1999; 54: 181–183.

38. Mest DR. The esophageal-tracheal Combitube, in *Airway Management*. Edited by Hanowell LH, Waldron RJ, Hwang AEJCF. Philadelphia, Lippincott-Raven, 1996, pp. 213–222.

39. Frass M, Agro F, Rich J, Krafft P. The all-in-one concept for securing the airway and adequate ventilation. Seminars in Anesthesia, Perioperative Medicine and Pain 2001; 20: 202–211.

40. Frass M, Frenzer R, Zdrahal F, Hoflehner G, Porges P, Lackner F. The esophageal tracheal Combitube: Preliminary results with a new airway for CPR. Annals of Emergency Medicine 1987; 16: 768–772.

41. Knacke A. Fallbeispiel: Atemwegsmanagement bei eingeklemmtem Polytrauma-Patienten (case report: Prehospital airway management of a trapped person with polytrauma). Rettungsdienst 2001; 24: 994–996.

42. Ochs M, Davis D, Joyt D, Bailey D, Marshall L, Rosen P. Paramedic-performed rapid sequence intubation of patients with severe head injuries. Ann Emerg Med 2002; 40: 159–167.

43. Frass M, Johnson J, Atherton G, Fruhwald F, Traindl O, Schwaighofer B, Leithner C. Esophageal tracheal Combitube (ETC) for emergency intubation: Anatomical evaluation of ETC placement by radiography. Resuscitation 1989; 18: 95–102.

44. Rich J, Agro F, Frass M. The esophageal-tracheal Combitube for airway management in emergency situations, Internet Journal of Airway Management, Premier and Millenium Issue: Volume 1(January 2000 to December 2001). http://www.adais.at/ijam/volume01/specialarticlel.htm

45. Walz R, Bund M, Meier P, Panning, B. Esophageal rupture associated with the use of the Combitube (letter). Anesth Analg 1998; 87: 228.

46. Hartmann T, Krenn CG, Zoeggeler A, Hoerauf K, Benumof JL, Krafft P. The oesophageal-tracheal Combitube Small Adult. Anaesthesia 2000; 55: 670–676.

47. Hoerauf K, Harman T, Acimovic S, et al. Waste gas exposure to sevoflurane and nitrous oxide during anaesthesia using the oesophageal-tracheal Combitube small adult. Br J Anaesth 2001; 86: 124–126.

48. Wissler R. The esophageal-tracheal Combitube. Anesthesiology Review 1993; 4: 147–152.

49. Klein H, Williamson M, Sue-Ling H, Vucevic M, Quinn A. Esophageal rupture associated with the use of the Combitube. Anesth Analg 1997; 85: 937–939.

50. Vezina D, Trepanier C, Lessared M, Bussieres J. Esophageal and tracheal distortion by the esophageal-tracheal Combitube: A cadaver study. Can J Anaesth 1999; 46: 393–397.

51. Vezina D, Lessard MR, Bussieres J, Topping C, Trepanier CA. Complications associated with the use of the esophageal-tracheal Combitube. Can J Anaesth 1998; 45: 76–80.

52. Mason A, Rich J, Ramsay M. Mason's PU-92 concept: Rapid recognition and treatment of the crash airway. TraumaCare 2003; 13: 46.

53. Green K, Beger T. Proper use of the Combitube (letter). Anesthesiology 1994; 81: 513.

54. Suresh M, Wali A. Failed intubation in obstetrics: Airway management strategies. Anesthesiol Clin North America 1995; 16: 477–498.

55. Atherton GL, Johnson JC. Ability of paramedics to use the Combitube in prehospital cardiac arrest. Ann Emerg Med 1993; 22: 1263–1268.

56. Staudinger T, Brugger S, Watschinger B, Roggla M, Dielacher C, Lobl T, Fink D, Klauser R, Frass M. Emergency intubation with the Combitube: Comparison with the endotracheal airway. Annals of Emergency Medicine 1993; 22: 1573–1575.

57. Tanigawa K, Shigematsu A. Choice of airway devices for 12,020 cases of nontraumatic cardiac arrest in Japan. Prehospital Emergency Care 1998; 2: 96–100.

58. Blostein PA, Koestner AJ, Hoak S. Failed rapid sequence intubation in trauma patients: Esophageal tracheal Combitube is a useful adjunct. J Trauma 1998; 44: 534–537.

59. Ochs M, Vilke GM, Chan TC, Moats T, Buchanan J. Successful prehospital airway management by EMT-Ds using the Combitube. Prehosp Emerg Care 2000; 4: 333–337.

60. Frass M, Staudinger T, Losert H, Krafft P. Letter to the editor. Resuscitation 1999; 43: 79–81.

61. Frass M. Personal Communication. University of Vienna, Austria 1999.

62. Urtubia R, Frass M, Staudinger T, Krafft P. Modification of the Lipp maneuver for blind insertion of the esophageal-tracheal Combitube. Can J Anaesth 2005; 52: 216–217.

63. Highlights of the 2005 American Heart Association Guidelines for Cardiopulmonary Resuscitation and Emergency Cardiovascular Care. Currents in Emergency Cardiovascular Care Winter 2005–2006; 16: 1–28.

64. Anderson K, Hald A. Assessing the position of the tracheal tube: The reliability of different methods. Anaesthesia 1989; 44: 984–985.

65. Anderson K, Schultz-Lebahn T. Oesophageal intubation can be undetected by auscultation of the chest. Acta Anaesthesiologica Scandinavica 1994; 38: 580–582.

66. Salem MR, Baraka A. Confirmation of tracheal intubation, in *Airway Management: Principles and Practice*. Edited by Benumof JL. St. Louis, Mosby, 1996, pp. 531–560.

67. Hartmann T, Hoauf K, Faybik P, Lorenz V, Krafft P. Randomized controlled trial comparing Combitube SA™, laryngeal tube™, Proseal™ for ventilatory support during laparoscopic surgery (AIC07). Br J Anaesth 2002; 88: 31a.

68. Frass M, Frenzer R, Rauscha F, Schuster E, Glogar D. Ventilation with the esophageal tracheal Combitube in cardiopulmonary resuscitation: Promptness and effectiveness. Chest 1988; 93: 781–784.

69. Yurino M. Esophageal tracheal Combitube overcomes difficult intubation: Flexion deformity of the cervical spine due to rheumatoid arthritis. Journal of Anesthesia 1994; 8: 233–235.

70. Staudinger T, Tesinsky P, Klappacher G, Brugger S, Rintelen C, Locker G, Weiss K, Frass M. Emergency intubation with the Combitube in two cases of difficult airway management. Eur J Anaesthesiol 1995; 12: 189–193.

71. Della Puppa A, Pittoni G, Frass M. Tracheal esophageal Combitube: A useful airway for morbidly obese patients who cannot intubate or ventilate. Acta Anaesthesiol Scand 2002; 46: 911–913.

72. Frass M, Lackner F, Frenzer R, Hofbauer R. Analysis of 500 uses of the Combitube: Safety, efficacy, and maximum ventilatory pressures during routine surgery. Difficult Airway 2001; 2: 84–90.

73. Haynes BE, Pritting J. A rural emergency medical technician with selected advanced skills. Prehosp Emerg Care 1999; 3: 343–346.

74. Lefrancois D, Dufour D. Use of the esophageal tracheal Combitube™ by basic emergency medical technicians. Resuscitation 2002; 52: 77–83.

75. Rumball C, MacDonald D. The PTL, Combitube, laryngeal mask, and oral airway: A randomized pre-hospital comparative study of ventilatory device effectiveness and cost-effectiveness in 470 cases of cardiorespiratory arrest. Prehospital Emergency Care 1997; 1: 1–10.

76. Dunham CM, Barraco RD, Clark DE, Daley BJ, Davis FEI, Gibbs MA, Knuth T, Letartc PB, Luchette FA, Omert L, Weireter LJ, Wiles CEI. Guidelines for emergency tracheal intubation immediately after traumatic injury. J Trauma 2003; 55: 162–179.

77. Dunham C, Barraco R, Clark D, Daley B, Davis F, III, Gibbs M, Knuth T, Letarte P, Luchette F, Omert L, Weireter L, Wiles C. Guidelines for emergency tracheal intubation immediately following traumatic injury. J Trauma 2003 July; 55(3): 722–723.

78. Davis DP, Valentine C, Ochs M, Vilke GM, Hoyt DB. The Combitube as a salvage airway device for paramedic rapid sequence intubation. Ann Emerg Med 2003; 42: 697–704.

79. Tanigawa K, Tanaka K. Demographic differences in the resuscitation knowledge and skills of the Standard First Aid Class ambulance crews in Japan. Eur J Emerg Med 1998; 5: 41–46.

80. Rabitsch W, Krafft P, Lackner FX, Frenzer R, Hofbauer R, Sherif C, Frass M. Evaluation of the oesophageal-tracheal double-lumen tube (Combitube) during general anaesthesia. Wien Klin Wochenschr 2004; 116: 90–93.

81. Rich J, Mason A, Bey T, Krafft P, Frass M. The critical airway, rescue ventilation and the Combitube: Part 2 (available at http://www.airwayeducation.com/PDFs/AANA_ARTICLE_4–04.pdf). AANA J 2004; 72: 115–124.

82. Mallick A, Quinn AC, Bodenham AR, Vucevic M. Use of the Combitube for airway maintenance during percutaneous dilatational tracheostomy. Anaesthesia 1998; 53: 249–255.

83. Letheren M, Parry N, Slater R. A complication of percutaneous tracheostomy whilst using the Combitube for airway control. Eur J Anaesthesiol 1997; 81: 464–466.

84. Wiltschke C, Kment G, Swoboda H, Knobl P, Kornek GV, Globits S, Staudinger T, Frass M. Ventilation with the Combitube during tracheostomy. Laryngoscope 1994; 104: 763–765.

85. Gaitini L, Vaida S, Somri M, Fradis M, Ben-David B. Fiberoptic-guided exchange of esophageal-tracheal Combitube in spontaneously breathing versus mechanically ventilated patients. Anesth Analg 1999; 88: 193–196.

86. Ovassapian A, Liu L, Krejcie T. Fiberoptic tracheal intubation with Combitube in place. Anesth Analg 1993; 76: S315.

87. Krafft P, Roeggla M, Fridirch P, Locker G, Frass M, Benumof J. Bronchoscopy via a redesigned Combitube in the esophageal position. Anesthesiology 1997; 86: 1041–1045.

88. Ovassapian A. Double-lumen and Univent tube insertion under fiberoptic control, in *Atlas of the Difficult Airway*, Second Edition. Edited by Norton ML. St. Louis, Mosby, 1996, pp. 142–160.

89. Rabitsch W, Schellongowski P, Staudinger T, Hofbauer R, Dufek V, Eder B, Raab H, Thell R, Schuster E, Frass M. Comparison of a conventional tracheal airway with the Combitube in an urban emergency medical services system run by physicians. Resuscitation 2003; 57: 27–32.

90. Baskett PJ, Dow A, Nolan J, Maull K. Upper airway control, in *Practical Procedures in Anesthesia and Critical Care*. St. Louis, Mosby, 1995, pp. 68–84.

91. Mercer M, Gabbott D. Insertion of the Combitube airway with the cervical spine immobilised in a rigid cervical collar. Anaesthesia 1998; 53: 971–974.

92. Asai T, Latto P. Role of the laryngeal mask in patients with difficult tracheal intubation and difficult ventilation, in *Difficulties in Tracheal Intubation*, Second Edition. Edited by Latto IP, Vaughn RS. London, W.B. Saunders Ltd., 1997, pp. 177–196.

93. Parmet J, Colonna-Romano P, Horrow J, Miller F, Gonzales J, Rosenberg H. The laryngeal mask airway reliably provides rescue ventilation in cases of unanticipated difficult tracheal intubation along with difficult mask ventilation. Anesth Analg 1998; 87: 661–665.

94. Frass M, Frenzer R, Zahler J, Ilias W, Leithner C. Ventilation via the esophageal tracheal Combitube in a case of difficult intubation. Journal of Cardiothorasic Anesthesia 1987; 1: 565–568.

95. Bigenzahn W, Pesau B, Frass M. Emergency ventilation using the Combitube in cases of difficult intubation. Eur Arch Otorhinolaryngol 1991; 248: 129–131.

96. Eichinger S, Schreiber W, Heinz T, Kier P, Dufek V, Goldin M, Leithner C, Frass M. Airway management in a case of neck impalement: Use of the oesophageal tracheal Combitube airway. British Journal of Anaesthesia 1992; 68: 534–535.

97. Klauser R, Roggla G, Pidlich J, Leithner C, Frass M. Massive upper airway bleeding after thrombolytic therapy: Successful airway management with the Combitube. Annals of Emergency Medicine 1992; 21: 431–433.

98. Banyai M, Falger S, Roggla M, Brugger S, Staudinger T, Klauser R, Muller-Spoljaritsch C, Vychytil A, Erlacher L, Sterz F, et al. Emergency intubation with the Combitube in a grossly obese patient with bull neck. Resuscitation 1993; 26: 271–276.

99. Baraka A, Salem R. The Combitube oesophageal-tracheal double lumen airway for difficult intubation. Canadian Journal of Anaesthesia 1993; 40: 1222–1223.

100. Wagner A, Roeggla M, Roeggla G, Weiss K, Marosi C, Locker G, Knapp S, Staudinger T, Metnitz P, Frass M. Emergency intubation with the Combitube in a case of severe facial burn (letter). American Journal of Emergency Medicine 1995; 13: 681–683.

101. Liao D, Shalit M. Successful intubation with the Combitube in acute asthmatic respiratory distress by a parkmedic. Journal of Emergency Medicine 1996; 14: 561–563.

102. Kulozik U, Georgi R, Krier C. Intubation with the Combitube™ in massive hemorrhage from the locus Kieselbachii. Anasthesiologie, Intensivmedizin, Notfallmedizin, Schmerztherapie 1996; 31: 191–193.

103. Mercer M. Respiratory failure after tracheal extubation in a patient with halo frame cervical spine immobilization—rescue therapy using the Combitube airway. Br J Anaesth 2001; 86: 886–891.

104. Klein U, Rich J, Seifert A, Tesinsky P. Use of the Combitube as a rescue airway during a case of "can't ventilate—can't intubate (CVCI)" in the operating room when a laryngeal mask failed. Difficult Airway 2000; 3: 5–7.

105. Brain A. The laryngeal mask airway—a possible new solution to airway problems in the emergency situation. Arch Emerg Med 1984: 229–232.

106. Levitan RM, Kush S, Hollander JE. Devices for difficult airway management in academic emergency departments: Results of a national survey. Ann Emerg Med 1999; 33: 694–698.

107. Rosenblatt WH, Wagner PJ, Ovassapian A, Kain ZN. Practice patterns in managing the difficult airway by anesthesiologists in the United States. Anesth Analg 1998; 87: 153–157.

108. Rich J, Mason A, Ramsay M, Beeson J, Hancock R. The Universal Emergency Airway Algorithm: Flowchart: Preventing accidents associated with emergency airway management (abstract). AANA J 2003: 71: 462. Abstract A 33.

109. Walls R. The emergency airway algorithms, in *Manual of Emergency Airway Management*. Edited by Walls R. Philadelphia, Lippincott Williams & Wilkins, 2000, pp. 16–26.

110. Rich J, Mason A, Ramsay M, Beeson J, Hancock R. The Universal Emergency Airway Flowchart: Preventing accidents associated with emergency airway management (abstract A 33). AANA J 2003; 71: 462.

111. Rich J. SLAM Emergency Airway Flowchart: Universal considerations for the emergency airway. TraumaCare 2003; 13: 46–47.

112. Stone B, Chantler P, Baskett P. The incidence of regurgitation during cardiopulmonary resuscitation: A comparison between the bag valve mask and laryngeal mask airway. Resuscitation 1998; 38: 3–6.

113. Mercer M. An assessment of the airway from aspiration of oropharyngeal contents using the Combitube airway. Resuscitation 2001; 51: 135–138.

114. Barnes T, MacDonald D, Nolan J, Otto C, Pepe P, Sayre M, Shuster M, Zaritsky A. Airway devices. Ann Emerg Med 2001; 37: S145–S151.

115. Adult Advanced Cardiac Life Support. JAMA 1992; 268: 2199–2241.

116. Practice guidelines for management of the difficult airway. A report by the American Society of Anesthesiologists Task Force on management of the difficult airway. Anesthesiology 1993; 78: 597–602.

117. Benumof JL. The American Society of Anesthesiologists' management of the difficult airway algorithm and explanation-analysis of the algorithm, in *Airway Management: Principles and Practice*. Edited by Benumof JL. St. Louis, Mosby, 1996, pp. 143–158.

Chapter 9

1. Murrin KR. Causes of difficult intubation and intubation procedures, in *Difficulties in Tracheal Intubation, Second Edition*. Edited by Latto IP, Vaughn RS. London, W.B. Saunders, 1997, pp. 89–160.

2. Nolan JP, Wilson ME. An evaluation of the gum elastic bougie. Intubation times and incidence of sore throat. Anaesthesia 1992; 47: 878–881.

3. Rich J. Street Level Airway Management (SLAM): If your patient can't breathe—nothing else matters. Anesthesia Today 2005; 16: 13–22.

4. Rich J. Recognition and management of the difficult airway with special emphasis on the intubating LMA-Fastrach/whistle technique: A brief review with case reports. BUMC Proceedings 2005; 18: 220–227.

5. Katz S, Falk J. Misplaced endotracheal tubes by paramedics in an urban emergency medical services system. Ann Emerg Med 2001; 37: 32–37.

6. Knacke A. Fallbeispiel: Atemwegsmanagement bei eingeklemmtem Polytrauma-Patienten (case report: Prehospital airway management of a trapped person with polytrauma). Rettungsdienst 2001; 24: 994–996.

7. Mason AM. Use of the intubating laryngeal mask airway in pre-hospital care: A case report. Resuscitation 2001; 51: 91–95.

8. Mason A. The laryngeal mask airway (LMA) & intubating laryngeal mask airway (iLMA) in pre-hospital trauma care, Royal College of Anaesthetists—May 13, 2002. London, UK, 2002.

9. Peterson G, Domino K, Caplan R, Posner L, Lee L, Cheney F. Management of the difficult airway: a closed claims analysis. Anesthesiology 2005 Jul 103(1): 33–39.

10. Rich J, Mason A, Bey T, Krafft P, Frass M: The critical airway, rescue ventilation and the Combitube: Part 1 (available at http://www.airwayeducation.com/PDFs/AANA_ARTICLE_2-04.pdf). AANA J 2004; 72: 17–27.

11. Rich J, Mason A, Bey T, Krafft P, Frass M: The critical airway, rescue ventilation and the Combitube: Part 2 (available at http://www.airwayeducation.com/PDFs/AANA_ARTICLE_4-04.pdf). AANA J 2004; 72: 115–124.

12. Crosby ET, Cooper RM, Douglas MJ, Doyle DJ, Hung OR, Labrecque P, Muir H, Murphy MF, Preston RP, Rose DK, Roy L. The unanticipated difficult airway with recommendations for management. Can J Anaesth 1998; 45: 757–776.

13. Rich J, Mason A, Ramsay M. AANA Journal Course: Update for Nurse Anesthetists. The SLAM Emergency Airway Flowchart: A new guide for advanced airway practitioners (available at http://www.airwayeducation.com/PDFs/flowchart_AANA_journal_course.pdf). AANA J 2004; 72: 431–439.

14. Cormack RS, Lehane J. Difficult tracheal intubation in obstetrics. Anaesthesia 1984; 39: 1105–1111.

15. Henderson J, Popat M, Latto I, Pearce A. Difficult Airway Society guidelines for management of the unanticipated difficult intubation. Anaesthesia 2004; 59: 675–694.

16. Smith C. Cervical spine injury and tracheal intubation: A never ending conflict (available at http://www.airwayeducation.com/PDFs/SpringSummer_2000.pdf). TraumaCare 2000; 10(1): 20–26.

17. Rocke DA, Murray WB, Rout CC, Gouws E. Relative risk analysis of factors associated with difficult intubation in obstetric anesthesia. Anesthesiology 1992; 77: 67–73.

18. Stone B, Chantler P, Baskett P. The incidence of regurgitation during cardiopulmonary resuscitation: A comparison between the bag valve mask and laryngeal mask airway. Resuscitation 1998; 38: 3–6.

19. Baskett P. The use of the laryngeal mask airway by nurses during cardiopulmonary resuscitation. Multicentre trial. Anaesthesia 1994; 49: 3–7.

20. Benumof JL, Scheller MS. The importance of transtracheal jet ventilation in the management of the difficult airway. Anesthesiology 1989; 71: 769–778.

21. Benumof J. The ASA Difficult Airway Algorithm: New thoughts and considerations, in *Handbook of Difficult Airway Management*. Edited by Hagberg C. Philadelphia, Churchill Livingstone, 2000, pp. 31–48.

22. Sanchez A, Morrison D. Preparation of the patient for awake intubation, in *Handbook of Difficult Airway Management*. Edited by Hagberg C. Philadelphia, Churchill Livingstone, 2000, pp. 49–82.

23. Benumof JL. Management of the difficult adult airway. With special emphasis on awake tracheal intubation. Anesthesiology 1991; 75: 1087–1110.

24. Beck G. Blind nasal intubation. Emerg Med Serv 2002; 31: 79.

25. Ferson DZ, Rosenblatt WH, Johansen MJ, Osborn I, Ovassapian A. Use of the intubating LMA-Fastrach in 254 patients with difficult-to-manage airways. Anesthesiology 2001; 95: 1175–1181.

26. Sanchez A, Pallares V. Retrograde intubation technique, in *Airway Management: Principles and Practice*. Edited by Benumof JL. St. Louis, Mosby, 1996, pp. 320–341.

27. Minkowitz H. Airway gadgets, in *Handbook of Difficult Airway Management*. Edited by Hagberg C. Philadelphia, Churchill Livingstone, 2000, pp. 149–169.

28. Ovassapian A, Wheeler M. Flexible fiberoptic tracheal intubation, in *Handbook of Difficult Airway Management*. Edited by Hagberg C. Philadelphia, Churchill Livingstone, 2000, pp. 83–114.

29. Cooper R, Pacey J, Bishop M, McCluskey S. Early clinical experience with a new videolaryngoscope (GlideScope) in 728 patients. Can J Anaesth 2005; 52: 191–198.

30. Agro F, Cataldo R, Carassiti M, Costa F. The seeing stylet: A new device for tracheal intubation. Resuscitation 2000; 44: 177–180.

31. Sanchez A, Trivedi NS, Morrison DE. Preparation of the patient for awake intubation, in *Airway Management: Principles and Practice*. Edited by Benumof JL. St. Louis, Mosby, 1996, pp. 159–182.

32. Rich J. Dexmedetomidine as a sole sedating agent with local anesthesia in a high-risk patient for axillofemoral bypass graft: A case report. AANA J 2005; 73: 357–360.

33. Beck G. Whistle assisted blind nasal intubation, SLAM 2000 Emergency & Rescue Airway Conference. Edited by Rich J. Dallas, Texas, SLAM Airway Training Institute, 2000, pp. 73–75.

34. Osborn I. The intubating laryngeal mask airway (ILMA) is assisted by an old device. Anesth Analg 2000; 91: 1561–1562.

35. Cook Airway Exchange Catheters with Rapi-fit™ adapters. Suggested Instructions for Use—Cook Critical Care C-t-CAE394. Bloomington, IN, Cook Critical Care, 1990.

36. Benumof JL, Cooper SD. Remember the gum-elastic bougie at extubation: Perhaps not so memorable? Journal of Clinical Anesthesia 1994; 6: 169–170.

37. Out-of-hospital use of intubating laryngeal mask airway for difficult intubation caused by cervical dislocation. Combes X, Jabre P, Ferrand E, Margenent A, Marty J. Emerg Med J 2007 May; 24(3); e27.

38. de Latorre F, Nolan J, Robertson C, Chamberlain D, Baskett P. European Resuscitation Council Guidelines 2000 for Adult Advanced Life Support. A statement from the Advanced Life Support Working Group(1) and approved by the Executive Committee of the European Resuscitation Council. Resuscitation 2001; 48: 211–221.

39. Wali A. Strategies to overcome failed intubation an obstetrics, SLAM society annual meeting, June 3, 2007, Dallas, TX, 2007.

40. Wali A. Strategies to overcome failed intubation an obstetrics, SLAM society annual meeting, June 3, 2007, Dallas, TX, 2007.

41. Lyons G. Failed intubation. Six years' experience in a teaching maternity unit. Anaesthesia 1985; 40: 759–762.

42. Samsoon GL, Young JR. Difficult tracheal intubation: A retrospective study. Anaesthesia 1987; 42: 487–490.

43. Glassenberg R. General anesthesia and maternal mortality. Semin Perinatol 1991; 15: 386–396.

44. Brodsky JB, Lemmens HJ, Brock-Utne JG, Saidman LJ, Levitan R. Anesthetic considerations for bariatric surgery: Proper positioning is important for laryngoscopy. Anesth Analg 2003; 96: 1841–1842; author reply, 1842.

45. Benumof JL. Conventional (laryngoscopic) orotracheal and nasotracheal intubation (single-lumen tube), in *Airway Management: Principles and Practice*. Edited by Benumof JL. St. Louis, Mosby, 1996, pp. 261–276.

46. Knill RL. Difficult laryngoscopy made easy with a "BURP." Can J Anaesth 1993; 40: 279–282.

47. Benson PF. The gum-elastic bougie: A life saver. Anesth Analg 1992; 74: 318.

48. Dogra S, Falconer R, Latto IP. Successful difficult intubation: Tracheal tube placement over a gum-elastic bougie. Anaesthesia 1990; 45: 774–776.

49. Datta S, Briwa J. Modified laryngoscope for endotracheal intubation of obese patients. Anesth Analg 1981; 60: 120–121.

50. Rosen M. Difficult and failed intubation in obstetrics, in *Difficulties in Tracheal Intubation*. Edited by Ian Latto Ralph Vaughan. London, Bailliere Tindall, 1996, pp. 152–155.

51. Tunstall ME. Failed intubation in the parturient. Can J Anaesth 1989; 36: 611–613.

52. An updated report by the American Society of Anesthesiologists Task Force on management of the difficult airway. Practice guidelines for management of the difficult airway. Anesthesiology 2003; 98: 1269–1277.

Chapter 10

1. Practice guidelines for management of the difficult airway: An updated report by the American Society of Anesthesiologists Task Force on management of the difficult airway. Anesthesiology 2003; 98: 1269–1277.

2. Rich J. Street Level Airway Management (SLAM): If your patient can't breathe—nothing else matters. Anesthesia Today 2005; 16: 13–22.

3. Rich J, Mason A, Ramsay M. AANA Journal Course: Update for Nurse Anesthetists. The SLAM Emergency Airway Flowchart: A new guide for advanced airway practitioners (available at http://www.airwayeducation.com/PDFs/flowchart_AANA_journal_course.pdf). AANA J 2004; 72: 431–439.

4. Thierbach A, Lipp M. Airway management in trauma patients. Anesth Clinics of North America 1999; 17: 63–81.

5. Mandavia DP, Qualls S, Rokos I. Emergency airway management in penetrating neck injury. Ann Emerg Med 2000; 35: 221–225.

6. McGuire G, el-Beheiry H. Complete upper airway obstruction during awake fibreoptic intubation in patients with unstable cervical spine fractures. Can J Anaesth 1999; 46: 176–178.

7. Rosen CL, Wolfe RE, Chew SE, Branney SW, Roe EJ. Blind nasotracheal intubation in the presence of facial trauma. J Emerg Med 1997; 15: 141–145.

8. Holzapfel L, Chastang C, Demingeon G, Bohe J, Piralla B, Coupry A. A randomized study assessing the systematic search for maxillary sinusitis in nasotracheally mechanically ventilated patients. Influence of nosocomial maxillary sinusitus on the occurrence of ventilator-associated pneumonia. Am J Respir Crit Care Med 1999; 159: 695–701.

9. Kim Y, Lee S, Noh G, Cho S, Yeom J, Shin W, Lee D, Ryu J, Park Y, Cha K, Lee S. Thermosoftening treatment of the nasotracheal tube before intubation can reduce epistaxis and nasal damage. Anesth Analg 2000; 9: 698–701.

10. Dhar P, Osborn I, Brimacombe J, Meenan M, Linton P. Blind orotracheal intubation with the intubating laryngeal mask versus fiberoptic guided orotracheal intubation with the Ovassapian airway. A pilot study of awake patients. Anaesth Intensive Care 2001; 29: 252–254.

11. Williams RT, Harrison RE. Prone tracheal intubation simplified using an airway intubator. Can Anaesth Soc J 1981; 28: 288–289.

12. Wedel D, Horlocker T. Nerve blocks, in *Miller's Anesthesiology*. Edited by Miller R. Philadelphia, Elsevier, 2005, pp. 1685–1717.

13. Adachi YU, Satomoto M, Higuchi H. Fiberoptic orotracheal intubation in the left semilateral position. Anesth Analg 2002; 94: 477–478.

14. Levitan RM, Kush S, Hollander JE. Devices for difficult airway management in academic emergency departments: Results of a national survey. Ann Emerg Med 1999; 33: 694–698.

15. Gaitini L, Vaida S, Somri M, Fradis M, Ben-David B. Fiberoptic-guided exchange of esophageal-tracheal Combitube in spontaneously breathing versus mechanically ventilated patients. Anesth Analg 1999; 88: 193–196.

16. Krafft P, Roeggla M, Fridirch P, Locker G, Frass M, Benumof J. Bronchoscopy via a redesigned Combitube in the esophageal position. Anesthesiology 1997; 86: 1041–1045.

17. Salem MR, Baraka A. Confirmation of tracheal intubation, in *Airway Management: Principles and Practice*. Edited by Benumof JL. St. Louis, Mosby, 1996, pp. 531–560.

18. Smith C. Cervical spine injury and tracheal intubation: A never ending conflict (available at http://www.airwayeducation.com/PDFs/SpringSummer_2000.pdf). TraumaCare 2000; 10(1): 20–26.

19. Bivins HG, Ford S, Bezmalinovic Z, Price HM, Williams JL. The effect of axial traction during orotracheal intubation of the trauma victim with an unstable cervical spine. Ann Emerg Med 1988; 17: 25–29.

20. Grande C, Barton C, Stene J. Emergency airway management in trauma patients with a suspected cervical spine injury: In response. Anesth Analg 1989; 68: 416–418.

21. Criswell JC, Parr MJ, Nolan JP. Emergency airway management in patients with cervical spine injuries. Anaesthesia 1994; 49: 900–903.

22. Desjardins G, Varon AJ. Airway management for penetrating neck injuries: The Miami experience. Resuscitation 2001; 48: 71–75.

23. Miller GT. LMA fastrach. EMS discovers the intubating laryngeal mask airway. J Emerg Med Serv JEMS 2002; 27: 68–74.

24. Pollack CV, Jr. The laryngeal mask airway: A comprehensive review for the emergency physician. J Emerg Med 2001; 20: 53–66.

25. Genzwurker H, Hundt A, Finteis T, Ellinger K. Comparison of different laryngeal mask airways in a resuscitation model. Anasthesiol Intensivmed Notfallmed Schmerzther 2003; 38: 94–101.

26. van Vlymen JM, Coloma M, Tongier WK, White PF. Use of the intubating laryngeal mask airway: Are muscle relaxants necessary? Anesthesiology 2000; 93: 340–345.

27. Osborn I, Soper R. It's a disposable LMA, just cut it shorter—for fiberoptic intubation. Anesth Analg 2003; 97: 299–300.

28. Silk JM, Hill HM, Calder I. Difficult intubation and the laryngeal mask. Eur J Anaesthesiol Suppl 1991; 4: 47–51.

29. Kitamura S, Yamada M, Morikawa M, Kamikawa K, Kono K. Fiberoptic intubation via laryngeal mask airway under general anesthesia in the patients with halo vest. Masui 2003; 52: 505–508.

30. Foley L, Ochroch E. Bridges to establish an emergency airway and alternate intubating techniques. Crit Care Clin 2000; 16: 429–444.

31. Wu TL, Chou HC. A new laryngoscope: The combination intubating device. Anesthesiology 1994; 81: 1085–1087.

32. Smith CE, Pinchak AB, Sidhu TS, Radesic BP, Pinchak AC, Hagen JF. Evaluation of tracheal intubation difficulty in patients with cervical spine immobilization: Fiberoptic (WuScope) versus conventional laryngoscopy. Anesthesiology 1999; 91: 1253–1259.

33. Smith CE, Sidhu TS, Lever J, Pinchak AB. The complexity of tracheal intubation using rigid fiberoptic laryngoscopy (WuScope). Anesth Analg 1999; 89: 236–239.

34. Smith CE, Kareti M. Fiberoptic laryngoscopy (WuScope) for double-lumen endobronchial tube placement in two difficult-intubation patients. Anesthesiology 2000; 93: 906–907.

35. Hastings RH, Vigil AC, Hanna R, Yang BY, Sartoris DJ. Cervical spine movement during laryngoscopy with the Bullard, Macintosh, and Miller laryngoscopes. Anesthesiology 1995; 82: 859–869.

36. Saunders P, Giesecke A. Clinical assessment of the adult Bullard laryngoscope. Canadian Journal of Anaesthesia 1989; 36: 118–119.

37. Watts AD, Gelb AW, Bach DB, Pelz DM. Comparison of the Bullard and Macintosh laryngoscopes for endotracheal intubation of patients with a potential cervical spine injury. Anesthesiology 1997; 87: 1335–1342.

38. MacQuarrie K, Hung O, Law J. Tracheal intubation using Bullard laryngoscope for patients with a simulated difficult airway. Can J Anaesth 1999; 46: 760–765.

39. Weiss M, Schwarz U, Gerber AC. Difficult airway management: Comparison of the Bullard laryngoscope with the video-optical intubation stylet. Can J Anaesth 2000; 47: 280–284.

40. Shulman B, Connelly NR. The adult Bullard laryngoscope as an alternative to the Wis-Hipple 1(1/2) in paediatric patients. Paediatr Anaesth 2000; 10: 41–45.

41. Cooper RM. Use of a new videolaryngoscope (GlideScope) in the management of a difficult airway. Can J Anaesth 2003; 50: 611–613.

42. Dacar D. University of Graz, Austria, 2003.

Chapter 11

1. Agro F, Totonelli A, Gherardi S. Planned lightwand intubation in a patient with a known difficult airway. Can J Anaesth 2004; 51: 1051–1052.

2. Macintosh R, Richard H. Illuminated introducer for endotracheal tubes. Anaesthesia 1957; 12: 223–225.

3. Berman R. Current comment. Anesthesiology. 1959; 20: 383.

4. Yamamura H, Yamamoto T, Kamiyama M. Device for blind nasal intubation. Anesthesiology 1959; 20: 221.

5. Rayburn R. Lightwand intubation. Anaesthesia 1979; 34: 677–678.

6. Hung OR. Lightwand intubation. A new lightwand device. Can J Anaesth 1995; 42: 820–825.

7. Davis L, Cook-Sather S, Schreiner M. Lighted stylet tracheal intubation: Review. Anesth Analg 2000; 90: 745–756.

8. Stewart R, LaRosee A, Kaplan R, et al. Correct positioning of an endotracheal tube using a flexible lighted stylet. Crit Care Med 1990; 18: 97–99.

9. Hartman RA, Castro T, Jr., Matson M, Fox DJ. Rapid orotracheal intubation in the clenched-jaw patient: A modification of the lightwand technique. J Clin Anesth 1992; 4: 245–246.

10. Yoshitaka I, Kazunori K, Shigematsu A. Anesth Analg 2002; 94: 667–671.

11. Vollmer TP, Stewart RD, Paris PM, Ellis D, Berkebile PE. Use of a lighted stylet for guided orotracheal intubation in the prehospital setting. Ann Emerg Med 1985; 14: 324–328.

12. Berns S, Patel R, Chamberlain R. Oral intubation using a lighted stylet vs. direct laryngoscopy in older children with cervical immobilization. Acad Emerg Med 1996; 3: 1.

13. Cote C, Ryan J, Todres I, et al. The normal airway, *A Practice of Anesthesia for Infants and Children*. Edited by N.G. Goudsouzian. Philadelphia, W.B. Saunders Co., 1993: 65–66.

14. Fisher QA, Tunkel DE. Lightwand intubation of infants and children. J Clin Anesth 1997; 9: 275–279.

15. Foster C. An aid to blind nasal intubation in children (letter). Anaesthesia 1977; 32: 1038.

16. Fox DJ, Matson MD. Management of the difficult pediatric airway in an austere environment using the lightwand. J Clin Anesth 1990; 2: 123–125.

17. Holzman R, Nargozian C, Florence F. Lightwand intubation in children with abnormal upper airways. Anesthesiology 1988; 69: 784–787.

18. Krucylak C, Schreiner M. Orotracheal intubation of an infant with hemifacial microsomia using a modified lighted stylet. Anesthesiology 1992; 77: 826–827.

19. Heller R, Cotton R. Early experience with illuminated endotracheal tubes in premature and term infants. Pediatrics 1985; 75: 664–666.

20. Chan PL, Lee TW, Lam KK, Chan WS. Intubation through intubating laryngeal mask with and without a lightwand: A randomized comparison. Anaesth Intensive Care 2001; 29: 255–259.

21. Dimitriou V, Voyagis GS, Brimacombe JR. Flexible lightwand-guided tracheal intubation with the intubating laryngeal mask Fastrach in adults after unpredicted failed laryngoscope-guided tracheal intubation. Anesthesiology 2002; 96: 296–299.

22. Fan KH, Hung OR, Agro F. A comparative study of tracheal intubation using an intubating laryngeal mask (Fastrach) alone or together with a lightwand (Trachlight). J Clin Anesth 2000; 12: 581–585.

23. Kihara S, Watanabe S, Taguchi N, et al. A comparison of blind and lightwand-guided tracheal intubation through the intubating laryngeal mask. Anaesthesia 2000; 55: 427–431.

24. Hung O, Al-Qatari M. Light guided retrograde intubation. Can J Anaesth 1997; 44: 877–882.

25. Lupien AE, Taylor C. Hybrid intubation technique for the management of a difficult airway: A case report. AANA J 1995; 63: 50–52.

26. Agro F, Guerardi S, Casale M. The lightwand: A useful aid in the difficult tracheostomy. Can J Anaesth 2002; 49: 1000–1001.

27. Favaro R, Tordiglione P, Lascio FD, et al. Effective nasotracheal intubation using a modified transillumination technique. Can J Anaesth 2002; 49: 91–95.

28. Iseki K, Murakawa M, Choichiro T, et al. Use of a modified lightwand for nasal intubation. Anesthesiology 1999; 90: 635.

29. Dimitriou V, Voyagis G, Iatrou C, et al. Flexible lightwand-guided intubation using the intubating laryngeal mask airway in the supine, right and left lateral positions in healthy patients by experienced users. Anesth Analg 2003; 96: 896–898.

30. Saha A, Higgins M, Walker G, et al. Comparison of awake endotracheal intubation in patients with cervical spine disease: The lighted intubating stylet versus the fiberoptic bronchoscope. Anesth Analg 1998; 87: 477–479.

31. Stone D, Stirt J, Kaplan M, et al. A complication of lightwand-guided nasotracheal intubation. Anesthesiology 1984; 61: 780–781.

32. Stalter B, Currier D. Endotracheal tube foreign body after intubation with a Vital Signs, Inc. lightwand (letter). Anesthesiology 2003; 99: 514–515.

33. Debo RF, Colonna D, Dewerd G, Gonzalez C. Cricoarytenoid subluxation: Complication of blind intubation with a lighted stylet. Ear Nose Throat J 1989; 68: 517–520.

34. Nishiyama T, Takashi M, Kazuo H. Optimal length and angle of a new lightwand device (Trachlight). J Clin Anesth 1999; 11: 332–335.

35. Chen T, Tsai S, Lin C, et al. Does the suggested lightwand bent length fit every patient? The relation between bent length and patient's thyroid prominence-to-mandibular-angle distance. Anesthesiology 2003; 98: 1070–1076.

36. Inoue Y. Lightwand intubation can improve airway management. Can J Anaesth 2004; 51: 1052–1053.

Chapter 12

1. Rich J, Mason A, Ramsay M. AANA Journal Course: Update for Nurse Anesthetists. The SLAM Emergency Airway Flowchart: A new guide for advanced airway practitioners (available at http://www.airwayeducation.com/PDFs/flowchart_AANA_journal_course.pdf). AANA J 2004; 72: 431–439.

2. Mulder DS, Marelli D. The 1991 Fraser Gurd Lecture: Evolution of airway control in the management of injured patients. J Trauma 1992; 33: 856–862.

3. Feller-Kopman D. Acute complications of artificial airways. Clin Chest Med 2003; 24: 445–455.

4. Jackson C. Tracheostomy. Laryngoscope 1909; 19: 285.

5. Jackson C. High tracheostomy and other errors: The chief cause of laryngeal stenosis. Surg Gynecol Obstet 1921; 32: 392.

6. Brantigan CO, Grow JB, Sr. Cricothyroidotomy: Elective use in respiratory problems requiring tracheotomy. J Thorac Cardiovasc Surg 1976; 71: 72–81.

7. Brantigan C, Grow J. Cricothyroidotomy revisited again. Ear Nose and Throat Journal 1980; 59: 26–38.

8. Toye F, Weinstein J. Clinical experience with percutaneous tracheostomy and cricothyroidotomy in 100 patients. J Trauma 1986; 26: 1034–1040.

9. Walls RM. Cricothyroidotomy. Emerg Med Clin North Am 1988; 6: 725–736.

10. McCarthy MC, Ranzinger MR, Nolan DJ, Lambert CS, Castillo MH. Accuracy of cricothyroidotomy performed in canine and human cadaver models during surgical skills training. J Am Coll Surg 2002; 195: 627–629.

11. Koppel JN, Reed AP. Formal instruction in difficult airway management. A survey of anesthesiology residency programs. Anesthesiology 1995; 83: 1343–1346.

12. Ezri T, Szmuk P, Warters RD, Katz J, Hagberg CA. Difficult airway management practice patterns among anesthesiologists practicing in the United States: Have we made any progress? J Clin Anesth 2003; 15: 418–422.

13. Hagberg CA, Greger J, Chelly JE, Saad-Eddin HE. Instruction of airway management skills during anesthesiology residency training. J Clin Anesth 2003; 15: 149–153.

14. Hockberger RS, Binder LS, Graber MA, Hoffman GL, Perina DG, Schneider SM, Sklar DP, Strauss RW, Viravec DR, Koenig WJ, Augustine JJ, Burdick WP, Henderson WV, Lawrence LL, Levy DB, McCall J, Parnell MA, Shoji KT. The model of the clinical practice of emergency medicine. Ann Emerg Med 2001; 37: 745–770.

15. Hayden SR, Panacek EA. Procedural competency in emergency medicine: The current range of resident experience. Acad Emerg Med 1999; 6: 728–735.

16. Wong DT, Prabhu AJ, Coloma M, Imasogie N, Chung FF. What is the minimum training required for successful cricothyroidotomy? A study in mannequins. Anesthesiology 2003; 98: 349–353.

17. Swanson ER, Fosnocht DE. Effect of an airway education program on prehospital intubation. Air Med J 2002; 21: 28–31.

18. Rich J, Mason A, Bey T, Krafft P, Frass M. The critical airway, rescue ventilation and the Combitube: Part 1 (available at http://www.airwayeducation.com/PDFs/AANA_ARTICLE_2–04.pdf). AANA J 2004; 72: 17–27.

19. Barkin Rm, Rusen P. *Emergency Pediatrics: A Guide to Ambulatory Care*, Sixth Edition. St. Louis, Mosby, Inc., 2003, p. 23.

20. Blanda M, Gallo UE. Emergency airway management. Emerg Med Clin North Am 2003; 21: 1–26.

21. Blostein PA, Koestner AJ, Hoak S. Failed rapid sequence intubation in trauma patients: Esophageal tracheal Combitube is a useful adjunct. J Trauma 1998; 44: 534–537.

22. Mason AM. Use of the intubating laryngeal mask airway in pre-hospital care: A case report. Resuscitation 2001; 51: 91–95.

23. Mason A. The Laryngeal Mask Airway (LMA) & Intubating Laryngeal Mask Airway (ILMA) in Prehospital Trauma Care, Royal College of Anaesthetists—May 13, 2002. London, UK, 2002.

24. Browner B, Jupiter J, Leuine A, Trafton P, Geen N, Susiontkowski: M. *Skeletal Trauma: Basic Science, Management and Reconstruction*, Third Edition. Elsevier, 2003, p. 123.

25. Roberts J, Hedges J. *Clinic Procedures in Emergency Medicine*, Fourth Edition. Elsevier, 2004, pp. 117–124.

26. Klein U, Rich J, Seifert A, Tesinsky P. Use of the Combitube as a rescue airway during a case of "can't ventilate–can't intubate (CVCI)" in the operating room when a laryngeal mask failed. Difficult Airway 2000; 3: 5–7.

27. Cummings C, Haughey B, Thomas J, Harker L, Flint P. *Otolaryngology: Head and Neck Surgery*, Fourth Edition. Edited by St. Louis Mosby, 2005, pp. 2448–2450.

28. Benumof JL. Management of the difficult adult airway. With special emphasis on awake tracheal intubation. Anesthesiology 1991; 75: 1087–1110.

29. Gaufberg SV, Workman TP. New needle cricothyroidotomy setup. Am J Emerg Med 2004; 22: 37–39.

30. Marr JK, Yamamoto LG. Gas flow rates through transtracheal ventilation catheters. Am J Emerg Med 2004; 22: 264–266.

31. Butler KH, Clyne B. Management of the difficult airway: Alternative airway techniques and adjuncts. Emerg Med Clin North Am 2003; 21: 259–289.

32. Abbrecht PH, Kyle RR, Reams WH, Brunette J. Insertion forces and risk of complications during cricothyroid cannulation. J Emerg Med 1992; 10: 417–426.

33. Vodadoria B, et al. Comparison of four different emergency airway access equipment sets on a human patient simulator. Anesth 2004; 59: 73–79.

34. Brofeldt BT, Panacek EA, Richards JR. An easy cricothyrotomy approach: The rapid four-step technique. Acad Emerg Med 1996; 3: 1060–1063.

35. Davis DP, Bramwell KJ, Hamilton RS, Chan TC, Vilke GM. Safety and efficacy of the Rapid Four-Step Technique for cricothyrotomy using a Bair Claw. J Emerg Med 2000; 19: 125–129.

36. Holmes JF, Panacek EA, Sakles JC, Brofeldt BT. Comparison of 2 cricothyrotomy techniques: Standard method versus rapid 4-step technique. Ann Emerg Med 1998; 32: 442–446.

37. Davis DP, Bramwell KJ, Vilke GM, Cardall TY, Yoshida E, Rosen P. Cricothyrotomy technique: Standard versus the Rapid Four-Step Technique. J Emerg Med 1999; 17: 17–21.

38. Schaumann N, Lorenz V, Schellongowski P, Staudinger T, Locker GJ, Burgmann H, Pikula B, Hofbauer R, Schuster E, Frass M. Evaluation of Seldinger technique emergency cricothyroidotomy versus standard surgical cricothyroidotomy in 200 cadavers. Anesthesiology 2005; 102: 7–11.

39. Jacobson LE, Gomez GA, Sobieray RJ, Rodman GH, Solotkin KC, Misinski ME. Surgical cricothyroidotomy in trauma patients: Analysis of its use by paramedics in the field. J Trauma 1996; 41: 15–20.

40. Taussig L, Landau L. Pediatric Respiratory Medicine, First Edition. St. Louis, Mosby I, 1999.

41. Francois B, Clavel M, Desachy A, Puyraud S, Roustan J, Vignon P. Complications of tracheostomy performed in the ICU: Subthyroid tracheostomy vs surgical cricothyroidotomy. Chest 2003; 123: 151–158.

42. Sue RD, Susanto I. Long-term complications of artificial airways. Clin Chest Med 2003; 24: 457–471.

43. Gleeson MJ, Pearson RC, Armistead S, Yates AK. Voice changes following cricothyroidotomy. J Laryngol Otol 1984; 98: 1015–1019.

44. Holst M, Hertegard S, Persson A. Vocal dysfunction following cricothyroidotomy: A prospective study. Laryngoscope 1990; 100: 749–755.

45. Boyd AD, Romita MC, Conlan AA, Fink SD, Spencer FC. A clinical evaluation of cricothyroidotomy. Surg Gynecol Obstet 1979; 149: 365–368.

Chapter 13

1. Dutton R, McCunn M. Anesthesia for trauma, in *Miller's Anesthesia*. Edited by Miller R. Philadelphia: Churchill Livingstone. 2005: 2451–2459.

2. Chen AY, Stewart MG, Raup G. Penetrating injuries of the face. Otolaryngol Head Neck Surg 1996; 115: 464–470.

3. Merritt RM, Williams MF. Cervical spine injury complicating facial trauma: Incidence and management. Am J Otolaryngol 1997; 18: 235–238.

4. Chesshire NJ, Knight DJW. The anaesthetic management of facial trauma and fracture. BJA CEPD Reviews 2001; 1: 108–112.

5. Kannan S, Chestnutt N, McBride G. Intubating LMA guided awake fibreoptic intubation in severe maxillo-facial injury. Can J Anaesth 2000; 47: 989–991.

6. Neal MR, Groves J, Gell IR. Awake fibreoptic intubation in the semi-prone position following facial trauma. Anaesthesia 1996; 51: 1053–1054.

7. Patteson SK, Epps JL, Hall J. Simultaneous oral and nasal tracheal intubation utilizing a fiberoptic scope in a patient with facial trauma. J Clin Anesth 1996; 8: 258–259.

8. Marlow TJ, Goltra DD, Jr., Schabel SI. Intracranial placement of a nasotracheal tube after facial fracture: A rare complication. J Emerg Med 1997; 15: 187–191.

9. Rosen CL, Wolfe RE, Chew SE, Branney SW, Roe EJ. Blind nasotracheal intubation in the presence of facial trauma. J Emerg Med 1997; 15: 141–145.

10. Walls M. Blind nasotracheal intubation in the presence of facial trauma—is it safe? J Emerg Med 1997; 15: 243–244.

11. Rich J, Mason A, Bey T, Krafft P, Frass M. The critical airway, rescue ventilation and the Combitube: Part 2 (available at http://www.airwayeducation.com/PDFs/AANA_ARTICLE_4-04.pdf). AANA J 2004; 72: 115–124.

12. Leibovici D, Fredman B, Gofrit ON, Shemer J, Blumenfeld A, Shapira SC. Prehospital cricothyroidotomy by physicians. Am J Emerg Med 1997; 15: 91–93.

13. Kadish H, Schunk J, Woodward GA. Blunt pediatric laryngotracheal trauma: Case reports and review of the literature. Am J Emerg Med 1994; 12: 207–211.

14. Kaufman HJ, Ciraulo DL, Burns RP. Traumatic fracture of the hyoid bone: Three case presentations of cardiorespiratory compromise secondary to missed diagnosis. Am Surg 1999; 65: 877–880.

15. Keogh IJ, Rowley H, Russell J. Critical airway compromise caused by neck haematoma. Clin Otolaryngol 2002; 27: 244–245.

16. Vassiliu P, Baker J, Henderson S, Alo K, Velmahos G, Demetriades D. Aerodigestive injuries of the neck. Am Surg 2001; 67: 75–79.

17. Desjardins G, Varon AJ. Airway management for penetrating neck injuries: The Miami experience. Resuscitation 2001; 48: 71–75.

18. Demetriades D, Velmahos GG, Asensio JA. Cervical pharyngoesophageal and laryngotracheal injuries. World J Surg 2001; 25: 1044–1048.

19. van As AB, van Deurzen DF, Verleisdonk EJ. Gunshots to the neck: Selective angiography as part of conservative management. Injury 2002; 33: 453–456.

20. Hirshberg A, Wall MJ, Johnston RH, Jr., Burch JM, Mattox KL. Transcervical gunshot injuries. Am J Surg 1994; 167: 309–312.

21. Mussi A, Ambrogi MC, Ribechini A, Lucchi M, Menoni F, Angeletti CA. Acute major airway injuries: Clinical features and management. Eur J Cardiothorac Surg 2001; 20: 46–51. Discussion, 51–42.

Chapter 14

1. Todd M. Cervical spine anatomy, function, and diseases, American Society of Anesthesiologists Annual Meeting Refresher Course, 2003, pp. 1–7.

2. ACS. American College of Surgeons Committee on Trauma. Advanced trauma life support program for physicians, Student and Instructor Manual. Chicago 2004.

3. Bachulis BL, Long WB, Hynes GD, Johnson MC. Clinical indications for cervical spine radiographs in the traumatized patient. Am J Surg 1987; 153: 473–478.

4. Criswell JC, Parr MJ, Nolan JP. Emergency airway management in patients with cervical spine injuries. Anaesthesia 1994; 49: 900–903.

5. Wright SW, Robinson GG, 2nd, Wright MB. Cervical spine injuries in blunt trauma patients requiring emergent endotracheal intubation. Am J Emerg Med 1992; 10: 104–109.

6. Domeier RM, Evans RW, Swor RA, Hancock JB, Fales W, Krohmer J, Frederiksen SM, Shork MA. The reliability of prehospital clinical evaluation for potential spinal injury is not affected by the mechanism of injury. Prehosp Emerg Care 1999; 3: 332–337.

7. Scannell G, Waxman K, Tominaga G, Barker S, Annas C. Orotracheal intubation in trauma patients with cervical fractures. Arch Surg 1993; 128: 903–905; Discussion, 905–906.

8. Cadoux CG, White JD, Hedberg MC. High-yield roentgenographic criteria for cervical spine injuries. Ann Emerg Med 1987; 16: 738–742.

9. Beirne JC, Butler PE, Brady FA. Cervical spine injuries in patients with facial fractures: A 1-year prospective study. Int J Oral Maxillofac Surg 1995; 24: 26–29.

10. Neifeld GL, Keene JG, Hevesy G, Leikin J, Proust A, Thisted RA. Cervical injury in head trauma. J Emerg Med 1988; 6: 203–207.

11. Williams J, Jehle D, Cottington E, Shufflebarger C. Head, facial, and clavicular trauma as a predictor of cervical-spine injury. Ann Emerg Med 1992; 21: 719–722.

12. Hockberger R, Kirshenbaum K, Doris P. Spinal injuries, in *Emergency Medicine,* Fourth Edition. Edited by Rosen P, Barkin R. St Louis, Mosby, 1998, pp. 462–505.

13. Urdaneta F, Layon AJ. Respiratory complications in patients with traumatic cervical spine injuries: Case report and review of the literature. J Clin Anesth 2003; 15: 398–405.

14. Overview of changes for Seventh Edition, Advanced Trauma Life Support, American College of Surgeons Committee on Trauma, 2002.

15. Hastings RH, Marks JD. Airway management for trauma patients with potential cervical spine injuries. Anesth Analg 1991; 73: 471–482.

16. Lam A. Acute spinal cord ischemia: Implications for anesthetic management, in *Advances in Anesthesia.* Edited by Stoelting R. St Louis, Mosby Year Book, 1993, pp. 247–273.

17. Holley J, Jorden R. Airway management in patients with unstable cervical spine fractures. Ann Emerg Med 1989; 18: 1237–1239.

18. Marion D, Przybylski G. Injury to the vertebrae and spinal cord, in Trauma, Fourth Edition. Edited by Mattox K, Feliciano D, Moore E. New York, McGraw Hill, 2000, pp. 451–471.

19. Smith C. Cervical spine injury and tracheal intubation: A never ending conflict (available at http://www.airwayeducation.com/PDFs/SpringSummer_2000.pdf). TraumaCare 2000; 10(1): 20–26.

20. Hoffman JR, Mower WR, Wolfson AB, Todd KH, Zucker MI. Validity of a set of clinical criteria to rule out injury to the cervical spine in patients with blunt trauma. National Emergency X-Radiography Utilization Study Group. N Engl J Med 2000; 343: 94–99.

21. Pasquale M, Fabian TC. Practice management guidelines for trauma from the Eastern Association for the Surgery of Trauma. J Trauma 1998; 44: 941–956. Discussion, 956–957.

22. Marion D, Domeier R, Dunham C, Luchette F, Haid R. Determination of cervical stability in trauma patients, (2000 update of the 1997 EAST practice management guidelines for identifying cervical spine injuries following trauma). Available at http://www.east.org.

23. Reid DC, Henderson R, Saboe L, Miller JD. Etiology and clinical course of missed spine fractures. J Trauma 1987; 27: 980–986.

24. Sawin PD, Todd MM, Traynelis VC, Farrell SB, Nader A, Sato Y, Clausen JD, Goel VK. Cervical spine motion with direct laryngoscopy and orotracheal intubation. An in vivo cinefluoroscopic study of subjects without cervical abnormality. Anesthesiology 1996; 85: 26–36.

25. Mescino A, Devitt J, Koch J, Szalai J, Schwartz M. The safety of awake tracheal intubation in cervical spine injury. Can J Anaesth 1988; 35: 131–132.

26. Suderman VS, Crosby ET, Lui A. Elective oral tracheal intubation in cervical spine-injured adults. Can J Anaesth 1991; 38: 785–789.

27. Dangor A, Lam A. Perioperative management of patients with head and spinal cord trauma. Anesth Clinics of North America 1999; 17: 157–170.

28. Smith C. Rapid sequence induction in adults: Indications and concerns. Clinical Pulmonary Medicine 2001; 8: 147–165.

29. Crosby ET, Lui A. The adult cervical spine: Implications for airway management. Can J Anaesth 1990; 37: 77–93.

30. Hastings RH, Wood PR. Head extension and laryngeal view during laryngoscopy with cervical spine stabilization maneuvers. Anesthesiology 1994; 80: 825–831.

31. Heath KJ. The effect of laryngoscopy of different cervical spine immobilisation techniques. Anaesthesia 1994; 49: 843–845.

32. Nolan JP, Wilson ME. Orotracheal intubation in patients with potential cervical spine injuries: An indication for the gum elastic bougie. Anaesthesia 1993; 48: 630–633.

33. Smith CE, Pinchak AB, Sidhu TS, Radesic BP, Pinchak AC, Hagen JF. Evaluation of tracheal intubation difficulty in patients with cervical spine immobilization: Fiberoptic (WuScope) versus conventional laryngoscopy. Anesthesiology 1999; 91: 1253–1259.

34. Gabbott DA. Laryngoscopy using the McCoy laryngoscope after application of a cervical collar. Anaesthesia 1996; 51: 812–814.

35. Laurent SC, de Melo AE, Alexander-Williams JM. The use of the McCoy laryngoscope in patients with simulated cervical spine injuries. Anaesthesia 1996; 51: 74–75.

36. Ovassapian A, Mesnick PS. The art of fiberoptic intubation, in *Anesthesiology Clinics of North America*. Edited by Benumof JL. Philadelphia, W.B. Saunders, 1995, pp. 391–410.

37. Reed AP. Preparation of the patient for awake flexible fiberoptic bronchoscopy. Chest 1992; 101: 244–253.

38. Hastings RH, Vigil AC, Hanna R, Yang BY, Sartoris DJ. Cervical spine movement during laryngoscopy with the Bullard, Macintosh, and Miller laryngoscopes. Anesthesiology 1995; 82: 859–869.

39. Saunders P, Giesecke A. Clinical assessment of the adult Bullard laryngoscope. Canadian Journal of Anaesthesia 1989; 36: 118–119.

40. Watts AD, Gelb AW, Bach DB, Pelz DM. Comparison of the Bullard and Macintosh laryngoscopes for endotracheal intubation of patients with a potential cervical spine injury. Anesthesiology 1997; 87: 1335–1142.

41. Smith CE, Sidhu TS, Lever J, Pinchak AB. The complexity of tracheal intubation using rigid fiberoptic laryngoscopy (WuScope). Anesth Analg 1999; 89: 236–239.

42. Wu TL, Chou HC. A new laryngoscope: The combination intubating device. Anesthesiology 1994; 81: 1085–1087.

43. Smith CE, Kareti M. Fiberoptic laryngoscopy (WuScope) for double-lumen endobronchial tube placement in two difficult-intubation patients. Anesthesiology 2000; 93: 906–907.

44. Keller C, Brimacombe J, Keller K. Pressures exerted against the cervical vertebrae by the standard and intubating laryngeal mask airways: A randomized, controlled, cross-over study in fresh cadavers. Anesth Analg 1999; 89: 1296–1300.

45. Nakazawa K, Tanaka N, Ishikawa S, Ohmi S, Ueki M, Saitoh Y, Makita K, Amaha K. Using the intubating laryngeal mask airway (LMA-Fastrach) for blind endotracheal intubation in patients undergoing cervical spine operation. Anesth Analg 1999; 89: 1319–1321.

46. Inoue Y, Koga K, Shigematsu A. A comparison of two tracheal intubation techniques with Trachlight and Fastrach in patients with cervical spine disorders. Anesth Analg 2002; 94: 667–671.

47. Grande C, Smith C, Stene J. Trauma anesthesia, in *Principles and Practice of Anesthesiology*, Second Edition. Edited by Longnecker D, Tinker J, Morgan G. 1998, pp. 2138–2164.

48. Naguib M, Flood P, McArdle JJ, Brenner HR. Advances in neurobiology of the neuromuscular junction: Implications for the anesthesiologist. Anesthesiology 2002; 96: 202–231.

49. Benumof JL, Cooper SD. Quantitative improvement in laryngoscopic view by optimal external laryngeal manipulation. J Clin Anesth 1996; 8: 136–140.

50. Knill RL. Difficult laryngoscopy made easy with a "BURP." Can J Anaesth 1993; 40: 279–282.

51. Smith C, Boyer D. Ease of tracheal intubation using fiberoptic laryngoscopy in patients receiving cricoid pressure. Canadian Journal of Anaesthesia 2002; 49: 614–619.

52. Uchida T, Hikawa Y, Saito Y, Yasuda K. The McCoy levering laryngoscope in patients with limited neck extension. Can J Anaesth 1997; 44: 674–676.

53. Dunham C, Barraco R, Clark D, Daley B, Davis F, III, Gibbs M, Knuth T, Letarte P, Luchette F, Omert L, Weireter L, Wiles C. Guidelines for emergency tracheal intubation immediately following traumatic injury, 2002. Available from: http://www.east.org/tpg/intubation.pdf.

Chapter 15

1. Larkin JM, Brahos GJ, Moylan JA. Treatment of carbon monoxide poisoning: Prognostic factors. J Trauma 1976; 16: 111–114.

2. Grube BJ, Marvin JA, Heimbach DM. Therapeutic hyperbaric oxygen: Help or hindrance in burn patients with carbon monoxide poisoning? J Burn Care Rehabil 1988; 9: 249–252.

3. Weaver LK, Hopkins RO, Chan KJ, et al. Hyperbaric oxygen for acute carbon monoxide poisoning. N Engl J Med 2002; 347: 1057–1067.

4. Brannen AL, Still J, Haynes M, et al. A randomized prospective trial of hyperbaric oxygen in a referral burn center population. Am Surg 1997; 63: 205–208.

5. Gatling R. Acute supraglottic laryngeal edema. Contem Surg 1981; 18: 8588.

6. Bowers BL, Purdue GF, Hunt JL. Paranasal sinusitis in burn patients following nasotracheal intubation. Arch Surg 1991; 126: 1411–1412.

7. Cioffi WG, Jr., Rue LW, III, Graves TA, McManus WF, Mason AD, Jr., Pruitt BA, Jr. Prophylactic use of high-frequency percussive ventilation in patients with inhalation injury. Ann Surg 1991; 213: 575–580. Discussion, 580–582.

8. Cortiella J, Mlcak R, Herndon D. High frequency percussive ventilation in pediatric patients with inhalation injury. J Burn Care Rehabil 1999; 20: 232–235.

Chapter 16

1. Infosino A. Pediatric upper airway and congenital anomalies. Anesthesiol Clin North America 2002; 20: 747–766.

2. Cotton RT. Management and prevention of subglottic stenosis in infants and children, in *Pediatric Otolaryngology*, Third Edition. Philadelphia, PA, Saunders, 1996, pp. 1373–1389.

3. Hudgins PA, Siegel J, Jacobs I, Abramowsky CR. The normal pediatric larynx on CT and MR. AJNR Am J Neuroradiol 1997; 18: 239–245.

4. Fitz-Hugh GS, Powell JB, II. Acute traumatic injuries of the oropharynx, laryngopharynx, and cervical trachea in children. Otolaryngol Clin North Am 1970; 3: 375–393.

5. Bledsoe B, Porter R, Cherry R. Pediatrics, in *Paramedic Care: Principles and Practice*. Upper Saddle River, NJ, Prentice Hall, 2006, Vol. 5, pp. 38–137.

6. Highlights of the 2005 American Heart Association Guidelines for Cardiopulmonary Resuscitation and Emergency Cardiovascular care. Currents in emergency cardiovascular care, Winter: 2005–2006; 16: 1–28.

7. Hill JR, Rahimtulla KA. Heat balance and the metabolic rate of new-born babies in relation to environmental temperature; and the effect of age and of weight on basal metabolic rate. J Physiol 1965; 180: 239–265.

8. Benumof J. The laryngeal mask airway and the ASA difficult airway algorithm. Anesthesiology News 1996: 4–21.

9. Mallampati SR, Gatt SP, Gugino LD, Desai SP, Waraksa B, Freiberger D, Liu PL. A clinical sign to predict difficult tracheal intubation: A prospective study. Can Anaesth Soc J 1985; 32: 429–434.

10. Sullivan KJ, Kissoon N. Securing the child's airway in the emergency department. Pediatr Emerg Care 2002; 18: 108–121. Quiz, 122–124.

11. Berry F. Anesthesia for child with a difficult airway, in *Anesthesic Management of Difficult and Routine Pediatric Patients*. New York, Churchill Livingstone, 1990, pp. 167–198.

12. Markakis DA, Sayson SC, Schreiner MS. Insertion of the laryngeal mask airway in awake infants with the Robin sequence. Anesth Analg 1992; 75: 822–824.

13. Goldman LJ, Nodal C, Jimenez E. Successful airway control with the laryngeal mask in an infant with Beckwith-Wiedemann syndrome and hepatoblastoma for central line catheterization. Paediatr Anaesth 2000; 10: 445–458.

14. Chung CJ, Fordham LA, Mukherji SK. The pediatric airway: A review of differential diagnosis by anatomy and pathology. Neuroimaging Clin N Am 2000; 10: ix, 161–180.

15. Bledsoe B, Porter R, Cherry R. Airway management and ventilation, in *Paramedic Care: Principles and Practice*. Upper Saddle River, NJ, Pearson Prentice Hall, 2006, Vol. 1, pp. 504–611.

16. Omert L, Yeaney W, Mizikowski S, Protetch J. Role of the emergency medicine physician in airway management of the trauma patient. J Trauma 2001; 51: 1065–1068.

17. Volker D. Comparison of different airway management strategies to ventilate apnic, non-preoxygenated patients. Critical Care Medicine 2003; 31: 800–804.

18. Rich J, Mason A, Ramsay M. AANA Journal Course: Update for Nurse Anesthetists. The SLAM Emergency Airway Flowchart: A new guide for advanced airway practitioners (available at http://www.airwayeducation.com/PDFs/flowchart_AANA_journal_course.pdf). AANA J 2004; 72: 431–439.

19. Benumof JL. Management of the difficult adult airway. With special emphasis on awake tracheal intubation. Anesthesiology 1991; 75: 1087–1110.

20. Caplan R, Benumof J, Berry A, et al. Practice guidelines for management of the difficult airway. A report by the American Society of Anesthesiologists Task Force on Management of the Difficult Airway. Anesthesiology 1993; 78: 597–602.

21. Benumof JL. Difficult laryngoscopy: Obtaining the best view. Can J Anaesth 1994; 41: 361–365.

22. Benumof JL, Cooper SD. Quantitative improvement in laryngoscopic view by optimal external laryngeal manipulation. J Clin Anesth 1996; 8: 136–140.

23. Tobias JD, Higgins M. Capnography during transtracheal needle cricothyrotomy. Anesth Analg 1995; 81: 1077–1078.

24. Benumof J. The laryngeal mask airway (editorial). Anesthesiology 1992; 77: 843–846.

25. White P, Smith L. Laryngeal mask airway, in *Airway Management: Principles and Practice*. Edited by Benumof J. St. Louis, MO, C.V. Mosby, Inc., 1995, chap. 19.

26. Frass M. The Combitube, in *Airway Management: Principles and Practice*. Edited by Benumof J. St. Louis, MO, C. V. Mosby, Inc., 1995, chap. 22.

27. Lee B, Gausche-Hill M. Pediatric airway management. Clinical Pediatric Emergency Medicine 2001; 2: 91–106.

28. APLS: The pediatric emergency medicine course. 1993.

29. Craft T, Chambers P, Ward M, Goat V. Two cases of barotrauma associated with transtracheal jet ventilation. British Journal of Anaesthesia 1990; 64: 524–527.

30. Arndt G, Fender M, Hecht M. An evaluation of the air contrast cricothyrotomy system (ACCS) in a large swine model. Anesthesia and Analgesia 1995; 80: S14.

31. Strange G, Cooper A, Gausche-Hill M. APLS: The pediatric emergency medicine course instructor manual. 1998.

32. Carron JD, Derkay CS, Strope GL, Nosonchuk JE, Darrow DH. Pediatric tracheotomies: Changing indications and outcomes. Laryngoscope 2000; 110: 1099–1104.

33. Simma B, Spehler D, Burger R, Uehlinger J, Ghelfi D, Dangel P, Hof E, Fanconi S. Tracheostomy in children. Eur J Pediatr 1994; 153: 291–296.

34. Davis DP, Hoyt DB, Ochs M, Fortlage D, Holbrook T, Marshall LK, Rosen P. The effect of paramedic rapid sequence intubation on outcome in patients with severe traumatic brain injury. J Trauma 2003; 54: 444–453.

35. Gausche M, Lewis RJ, Stratton SJ, Haynes BE, Gunter CS, Goodrich SM, Poore PD, McCollough MD, Henderson DP, Pratt FD, Seidel JS. Effect of out-of-hospital pediatric endotracheal intubation on survival and neurological outcome: A controlled clinical trial. Jama 2000; 283: 783–790.

36. Stockinger ZT, McSwain NE, Jr. Prehospital endotracheal intubation for trauma does not improve survival over bag-valve-mask ventilation. J Trauma 2004; 56: 531–536.

37. Davis D, Ochs M, Hoyt D, Bailey D, Marshall L, Rosen P. Paramedic-administered neuromuscular blockade improves prehospital intubation success in severely head-injured patients. J Trauma 2003; 55: 713–719.

38. Bulger EM, Copass MK, Maier RV, Larsen J, Knowles J, Jurkovich GJ. An analysis of advanced pre-hospital airway management. J Emerg Med 2002; 23: 183–189.

39. Fisher DM. Neuromuscular blocking agents in paediatric anaesthesia. Br J Anaesth 1999; 83: 58–64.

40. Gronert GA. Cardiac arrest after succinylcholine: Mortality greater with rhabdomyolysis than receptor upregulation. Anesthesiology 2001; 94: 523–529.

41. Maree S. Succinylcholine: Friend or foe? Curr Rev Nurs Anesth 1994; 17: 89–100.

42. Mazze RI, Escue HM, Houston JB. Hyperkalemia and cardiovascular collapse following administration of succinylcholine to the traumatized patient. Anesthesiology 1969; 31: 540–547.

43. Wu CC, Tseng CS, Shen CH, Yang TC, Chi KP, Ho WM. Succinylcholine-induced cardiac arrest in unsuspected Becker muscular dystrophy—a case report. Acta Anaesthesiol Sin 1998; 36: 165–168.

44. U.S. Food & Drug Administration (Medwatch) http://www.fda.gov/medwatch/SAFETY/1997/safety97.htm#drugs

45. McDonald PF, Sainsbury DA, Laing RJ. Evaluation of the onset time and intubation conditions of rocuronium bromide in children. Anaesth Intensive Care 1997; 25: 260–261.

46. Sparr HJ. Choice of the muscle relaxant for rapid-sequence induction. Eur J Anaesthesiol Suppl 2001; 23: 71–76.

47. Gerardi MJ, Sacchetti AD, Cantor RM, Santamaria JP, Gausche M, Lucid W, Foltin GL. Rapid-sequence intubation of the pediatric patient. Pediatric Emergency Medicine Committee of the American College of Emergency Physicians. Ann Emerg Med 1996; 28: 55–74.

48. McAuliffe G, Bissonnette B, Boutin C. Should the routine use of atropine before succinylcholine in children be reconsidered? Can J Anaesth 1995; 42: 724–729.

49. Brain A. The laryngeal mask—a new concept in airway management. Brit J Anaes 1983; 55: 801–805.

50. Brimacombe J. The advantages of the LMA over the tracheal tube or facemask: A meta-analysis. Can J Anaesth 1995; 42: 1017–1023.

51. Davies P, Tigh S, Greenslade G, et al. Laryngeal mask airway and tracheal tube insertion by unskilled personnel. Lancet 1990; 336: 997–999.

52. Melissa W. Management strategies for the difficult pediatric airway. Anesthesiology Clinics of North America 1998; 16: 743–761.

53. Verghese C, Brimacombe JR. Survey of laryngeal mask airway usage in 11,910 patients: Safety and efficacy for conventional and nonconventional usage. Anesth Analg 1996; 82: 129–133.

54. Castresana MR, Stefansson S, Cancel AR, Hague KJ. Use of the laryngeal mask airway during thoracotomy in a pediatric patient with cri-du-chat syndrome. Anesth Analg 1994; 78: 817.

55. Denny NM, Desilva KD, Webber PA. Laryngeal mask airway for emergency tracheostomy in a neonate. Anaesthesia 1990; 45: 895.

56. Asai T, Vaughan RS. Misuse of the laryngeal mask airway. Anaesthesia 1994; 49: 467–469.

57. Smith I, White PF. Use of the laryngeal mask airway as an alternative to a face mask during outpatient arthroscopy. Anesthesiology 1992; 77: 850–855.

58. Paterson SJ, Byrne PJ, Molesky MG, Seal RF, Finucane BT. Neonatal resuscitation using the laryngeal mask airway. Anesthesiology 1994; 80: 1248–1253. Discussion, 27A.

59. Martin PD, Cyna AM, Hunter WA, Henry J, Ramayya GP. Training nursing staff in airway management for resuscitation. A clinical comparison of the facemask and laryngeal mask. Anaesthesia 1993; 48: 33–37.

60. Loh KS, Irish JC. Traumatic complications of intubation and other airway management procedures. Anesthesiol Clin North America 2002; 20: 953–969.

61. Neema PK, Sinha PK, S M, Rathod RC. Oversized endotracheal tube in pediatric anesthesia practice: Its objective detection. Anesth Analg 2003; 97: 1857–1858.

62. O'Connell JE, Stevenson DS, Stokes MA. Pathological changes associated with short-term nasal intubation. Anaesthesia 1996; 51: 347–350.

63. Weymuller EA, Jr., Bishop MJ, Santos PM. Problems associated with prolonged intubation in the geriatric patient. Otolaryngol Clin North Am 1990; 23: 1057–1074.

64. Eckenhoff JE. Some anatomic considerations of the infant larynx influencing endotracheal anesthesia. Anesthesiology 1951; 12: 401–410.

65. Cote C. Pediatric anesthesia, in *Anesthesia*. Edited by Miller R. Philadelphia, PA, Churchill-Livingstone, 2000, pp. 2088–2117.

66. Penlington GN. Letter: Endotracheal tube sizes for children. Anaesthesia 1974; 29: 494–495.

67. Fisher MM, Raper RF. The "cuff-leak" test for extubation. Anaesthesia 1992; 47: 10–12.

68. Mhanna MJ, Zamel YB, Tichy CM, Super DM. The "air leak" test around the endotracheal tube, as a predictor of postextubation stridor, is age dependent in children. Crit Care Med 2002; 30: 2639–2643.

69. Bishop MJ, Weymuller EA, Jr., Fink BR. Laryngeal effects of prolonged intubation. Anesth Analg 1984; 63: 335–342.

70. Nordin U, Lindholm CE, Wolgast M. Blood flow in the rabbit tracheal mucosa under normal conditions and under the influence of tracheal intubation. Acta Anaesthesiol Scand 1977; 21: 81–94.

Chapter 17

1. Ramsay M, Savege T, Simpson B, Goodwin R. Controlled sedation with alphaxalone-alphadolone. Br Med J 1974; 2: 656–659.

2. Kollef MH, Levy NT, Ahrens TS, Schaiff R, Prentice D, Sherman G. The use of continuous i.v. sedation is associated with prolongation of mechanical ventilation. Chest 1998; 114: 541–548.

3. Lewis KS, Whipple JK, Michael KA, Quebbeman EJ. Effect of analgesic treatment on the physiological consequences of acute pain. Am J Hosp Pharm 1994; 51: 1539–1554.

4. Shapiro BA, Warren J, Egol AB, Greenbaum DM, Jacobi J, Nasraway SA, Schein RM, Spevetz A, Stone JR. Practice parameters for intravenous analgesia and sedation for adult patients in the intensive care unit: An executive summary. Society of Critical Care Medicine. Crit Care Med 1995; 23: 1596–1600.

5. Abbuhl F, Reed D. Time to analgesia for patients with painful extremity injuries transported to the Emergency Department by ambulance. Prehosp Emerg Care 2003; 7: 445–447.

6. DeVellis P, Thomas S, Vinci R, Wedel S. Prehospital fentanyl analgesia in air-transported pediatric trauma patients. Pediatric Emergency Care 1998; 14: 321–323.

7. Dickinson E, Wurster F, Mechem C, Reyes J. Prehospital utilization and effectiveness of morphine (abstract). Prehosp Emerg Care 2004; 8: 103.

8. Frakes M, Lord W, Kocixzewski C, Wedel S. Efficacy of fentanyl for trauma analgesia in critical care transport. American Journal of Emergency Medicine 2006. May 24(3): 286–289.

9. Fullerton-Gleason L, Crandall C, Sklar D. Prehospital administration of morphine for isolated extremity injuries: A change in protocol reduces time to medication. Prehosp Emerg Care 2002; 6: 411–416.

10. McEachin C, McDermott J, Swore R. Few emergency medical services pateints with lower-extremeity fractures receive prehospital analgesia. Prehosp Emerg Care 2002; 6: 406–410.

11. Thomas S, Rago O, Harrison T, Biddinger P, Wedel S. Fentanyl trauma analgesia use in air medical scene transports. Journal of Emergency Medicine 2005; 29: 179–187.

12. White L, Cooper J, Chambers R, Gradisek R. Prehospital use of analgesia for suspected extremity fractures. Prehosp Emerg Care 2000; 4: 205–208.

13. DeVellis P, Thomas S, Wedel S. Prehospital and emergency department analgesia for air-transported patients with fractures. Prehosp Emerg Care 1998; 2: 293–296.

14. Murray MJ, DeRuyter ML, Harrison BA. Opioids and benzodiazepines. Crit Care Clin 1995; 11: 849–873.

15. Taylor N. *Plant Drugs That Changed the World*, First Edition. New York, Dodd, Mead & Company, 1965, p. 215.

16. Frakes M, Lord W, Kocixzewski C, Swedel. Efficacy of fentanyl for trauma analgesia in critical care transport. American Journal of Emergency Medicine 2006 May 24(3): 286–289.

17. Kanowitz A, Dunn T, Kanowitz E, Dunn WW, Vanbus K. Buskirk KV. Safety and effectiveness of fentanyl administration for prehospital pain management. Prehosp Emerg Care 2006; 10: 1–7.

18. Walls R. Airway management, in *Emergency Medicine Concepts and Clinical Practice*. Edited by Rosen P. St. Louis, Mosby, 1998, pp. 2–24.

19. Rodricks M. Emergent airway management. Indications and methods in the face of confounding conditions. Crit Care Clin 2000; 16: 389–409.

20. Vender J, Szokol J, Murphy G, Nitsun M. Sedation, analgesia, and neuromusclar blockade in sepsis: An evidence-based review. Crit Care Med 2004; 32: S554-S561.

21. Habibi S, Coursin DB. Assessment of sedation, analgesia, and neuromuscular blockade in the perioperative period. Int Anesthesiol Clin 1996; 34: 215–241.

22. Dowling J. Autonomic indices and reactive pain reports on the McGill Pain Questionnaire. Pain 1982; 14: 387–392.

23. Ellestad MH, Thomas LA, Bortolozzo TL, Abate JA, Greenberg PS. Autonomic responses in chest pain syndromes as compared to normal subjects. Cardiology 1987; 74: 35–42.

24. Simonnet G, Taquet H, Floras P, Caille JM, Legrand JC, Vincent JD, Cesselin F. Simultaneous determination of radio-immunoassayable methionine-enkephalin and radioreceptor-active opiate peptides in CSF of chronic pain suffering and non suffering patients. Neuropeptides 1986; 7: 229–240.

25. Ramsay M, Huddleston P, Henry C, Marcel R, Matter G. The patient state index as an indicator of inadequate pain management in unresponsive ICU Patients. Critical Care Medicine 2004; 32: A169.

26. Griffiths RD, Jones C. Recovery from intensive care. Brit Med J 1999; 319: 427–429.

27. Gerardi M. Rapid sequence induction of the pediatric patient. Ann Emerg Med 1996; 28: 55–74.

28. Lev R, Rosen P. Prophylactic lidocaine use preintubation: A review. J Emerg Med 1994; 12: 499–506.

29. Miller M, Levy P, Patel M. Procedural sedation and analgesia in the emergency department. Emerg Med Clin North Am 2005; 23: 551–572.

30. Murray K. The need for assessment of sedation in the critically ill. Nurs Crit Care 1997; 2: 297–302.

31. Shapiro BA. Bispectral Index: Better information for sedation in the intensive care unit? Crit Care Med 1999; 27: 1663–1664.

32. Practice guidelines for sedation and analgesia by non-anesthesiologists. A report by the American Society of Anesthesiologists Task Force on Sedation and Analgesia by Non-Anesthesiologists. Anesthesiology 1996; 84: 459–471.

33. Christensen BV, Thunedborg LP. Use of sedatives, analgesics and neuromuscular blocking agents in Danish ICUs 1996/97. A national survey. Intensive Care Med 1999; 25: 186–191.

34. Maze M. Sedation in the intensive care environment, in *Yearbook of Intensive Care and Emergency Medicine*. Edited by Vincent J-L. Berlin, Springer, 2000, pp. 405–413.

35. De Deyne C, Struys M, Decruyenaere J, Creupelandt J, Hoste E, Colardyn F. Use of continuous bispectral EEG monitoring to assess depth of sedation in ICU patients. Intensive Care Med 1998; 24: 1294–1298.

36. De Jonghe B, Cook D, Appere-De-Vecchi C, Guyatt G, Meade M, Outin H. Using and understanding sedation scoring systems: A systematic review. Intensive Care Med 2000; 26: 275–285.

37. Ely EW, Truman B, Shintani A, Thomason JW, Wheeler AP, Gordon S, Francis J, Speroff T, Gautam S, Margolin R, Sessler CN, Dittus RS, Bernard GR. Monitoring sedation status over time in ICU patients: Reliability and validity of the Richmond Agitation-Sedation Scale (RASS). Jama 2003; 289: 2983–2991.

38. Ostermann ME, Keenan SP, Seiferling RA, Sibbald WJ. Sedation in the intensive care unit: A systematic review. Jama 2000; 283: 1451–1459.

39. Riker RR, Picard JT, Fraser GL. Prospective evaluation of the Sedation-Agitation Scale for adult critically ill patients. Crit Care Med 1999; 27: 1325–1329.

40. Simmons LE, Riker RR, Prato BS, Fraser GL. Assessing sedation during intensive care unit mechanical ventilation with the Bispectral Index and the Sedation-Agitation Scale. Crit Care Med 1999; 27: 1499–1504.

41. Drover DR, Lemmens HJ, Pierce ET, Plourde G, Loyd G, Ornstein E, Prichep LS, Chabot RJ, Gugino L. Patient State Index: Titration of delivery and recovery from propofol, alfentanil, and nitrous oxide anesthesia. Anesthesiology 2002; 97: 82–89.

42. Ely EW, Truman B, Manzi DJ, Sigl JC, Shintani A, Bernard GR. Consciousness monitoring in ventilated patients: Bispectral EEG monitors arousal not delirium. Intensive Care Med 2004; 30: 1537–1543.

Chapter 18

1. Larson S, Jordan L. Preventable adverse patient outcomes: A closed claims analysis of respiratory incidents. AANA J 2001; 69: 386–392.

2. Huycke LI, Huycke MM. Characteristics of potential plaintiffs in malpractice litigation. Ann Intern Med 1994; 120: 792–798.

3. Merriam-Webster's Dictionary of Law 1996; 1996; Wikipedia contributors. **Misfeasance**. Wikipedia, The Free Encyclopedia. January 9, 2006, 20:26 UTC (available at http://en.wikipedia.org/w/index.php?title=Misfeasance&oldid=34526257). Accessed April 12, 2006.

4. Wikipedia contributors. **Proximate cause**. Wikipedia, The Free Encyclopedia. March 19, 2006, 02:33 UTC (available at http://en.wikipedia.org/w/index.php?title=Proximate_cause&oldid=44444671). (Accessed April 12, 2006. **Foreseeability**. Farlex. The Free Dictionary. April 12, 2006 (available at http://legal-dictionary.thefreedictionary.com/foreseeability). Accessed April 12, 2006.

5. Fla. Stat. 2002;766.102. Medical negligence; standards of recovery.

6. Florida Good Samaritan Act. Fla. Stat. 2002; 768.13. Reckless disregard standard in emergency room.

7. Circulation 2005; 112: IV-51–IV-57.

8. Scope and standards for nurse anesthesia practice. American Association of Nurse Anesthestists. 2002. (available at http://www.aana.com/resources.aspx? ucNavMenu_TSMenuTargetiD=51&ucNavMenu_TSMenuTargetType=48ucNavMenu_TSMenuID=6&id=783).

9. Standards for basic anesthetic monitoring, approved by American Society of Anesthesiologists House of Delegates on October 21, 1986, and last amended on October 27, 2004.

10. Kremer MJ, Faut-Callahan M, Hicks FD. A study of clinical decision making by certified registered nurse anesthetists. AANA J 2002; 70: 391–397.

11. Palsgraf v. Long Island R. Co., 248 N.Y. 339, 162 N.E. 99 (1928); Alegria v. Payon, 101 Idaho 617, 619 P.2d 135 (1980); Newton v. Davis Transport & Rentals, Inc., 312 So.2d 200 (Fla. App. 1975).

12. Federal Health Insurance Portability and Accountability Act of 1996. Public Law 104–191, 104th Congress.

13. Medical Experts & Establishing Standards of Care in Malpractice Cases. The 'Lectric Law Library. January 1998 (available at http://www.lectlaw.com/files/exp23.htm). Accessed April 12, 2006.

14. Caplan RA, Posner KL, Ward RJ, Cheney FW. Adverse respiratory events in anesthesia: A closed claims analysis. Anesthesiology. 1990; 72: 828–833.

15. Domino K, Posner K, Caplan R, Cheney F. Airway injury during anesthesia: A closed claims analysis. Anesthesiology 1999; 91: 1703–1711.

16. Jordan LM, Kremer M, Crawforth K, Shott S. Data-driven practice improvement: The AANA Foundation closed malpractice claims study. AANA J 2001; 69: 301–311.

17. Christy v. Salem, 366 N.J. Super. 535 (App. Div. 2004). 2004.

18. Payton v. New Jersey Turnpike Authority, 148 N.J. 524. 1977.

19. Public citizen, Inc. v. U. S. Department of Health and Human Services, 151 F.Supp.2d 64 (D.D.C. 2001) 2001.

20. Minnesota Statutes 2005. Sec. 145.64. Confidentiality of records of review organization.

21. 01–0438 Emmanuel E. Ubinas-Brache, M.D. v. Dallas County Medical Society and Texas Medical Association; from Dallas County; 5th district (05–97-00027-CV, ___ SW3d ___, 02–07-01).

22. Nicastro J. Court ruling suggests need to be clear about peer review. Vital Signs, Mass. Med. Soc, August 2002 (available at http://www.massmed.org/AM/Template.cfm?Section=August_2002TEMPLATE=/CM/ContentDisplay.cfm&CONTENTID=5697). Accessed April 12, 2006.

Chapter 19

1. Tait AR1, Tuttle DB. Preventing perioperative transmission of infection: A survey of anesthesiology practice. Anesth Analg 1995; 80: 764–769.

2. U.S. Department of Labor: Occupational Health and Safety Administration: Standards 29 Code of Federal Regulations: Bloodborne Pathogens 1910. 1030. Amended, April 03, 2006. www.osha.gov.

3. Bready L. Infectious disease and anesthesia. Advances in Anesthesia 1988; 5: 89–128.

4. Beck-Sague C, Jarvis WR, Martone WJ. Outbreak investigations. Infect Control Hosp Epidemiol 1997; 18: 138–145.

5. CDC. MRSA: Methicillin resistant Staphylococcus aureus fact sheet. Available from http://www.cdc.gov/ncidod/hip/Aresist/mrsafaq.htm.

6. Chrisco JA, DeVane G. A descriptive study of blood in the mouth following routine oral endotracheal intubation. AANA J 1992; 60: 379–383.

7. Kanefield J, Munro J, Eisele J. Are intubations bloody? Anesthesia and Analgesia 1989; 68: S124.

8. Recommendations for prevention of HIV transmission in health-care setting, in Morbidity and Mortality Weekly Report. 1987; 36:3S-18S .

9. Agerton T, Valway S, Gore B, Pozsik C, Plikaytis B, Woodley C, Onorato I. Transmission of a highly drug-resistant strain (strain W1) of Mycobacterium tuberculosis. Community outbreak and nosocomial transmission via a contaminated bronchoscope. Jama 1997; 278: 1073–1077.

10. Bond WW, Favero MS, Petersen NJ, Gravelle CR, Ebert JW, Maynard JE. Survival of hepatitis B virus after drying and storage for one week. Lancet 1981; 1: 550–551.

11. Michele TM, Cronin WA, Graham NM, Dwyer DM, Pope DS, Harrington S, Chaisson RE, Bishai WR. Transmission of Mycobacterium tuberculosis by a fiberoptic bronchoscope. Identification by DNA fingerprinting. Jama 1997; 278: 1093–1095.

12. Morell RC, Ririe D, James RL, Crews DA, Huffstetler K. A survey of laryngoscope contamination at a university and a community hospital. Anesthesiology 1994; 80: 960.

13. Nikkola R. Prevalence of visible and occult blood on airway management equipment used outside the perioperative setting. Annual meeting of the American Association of Nurse Anesthetists. Boston, MA, 1999.

14. Nolen M, Monaghan W. Presence of visible and occult blood on anesthesia airway equipment. American Association of Nurse Anesthetist Annual Meeting. Boston, MA, 2003.

15. Perry SM, Monaghan WP. The prevalence of visible and/or occult blood on anesthesia and monitoring equipment. AANA J 2001; 69: 44–48.

16. Phillips RA, Monaghan WP. Incidence of visible and occult blood on laryngoscope blades and handles. AANA J 1997; 65: 241–246.

17. Tobin MJ, Stevenson GW, Hall SC. A simple, cost-effective method of preventing laryngoscope handle contamination. Anesthesiology 1995; 82: 790.

18. HIV and its transmission, Divisions of HIV/Aids Prevention, Centers for Disease Control, 2003, http://www.cdc.gov/hiv/pubs/facts/transmission.htm.

19. Lowe, B. Staying Sharp in Phlebotomy, Advance for Medical Laboratory Professionals, 2004, 16(9), 25.

20. Llewelyn CA, Hewitt PE, Knight RS, Amar K, Cousens S, Mackenzie J, Will RG. Possible transmission of variant Creutzfeldt-Jakob disease by blood transfusion. Lancet 2004; 363: 417–421.

21. Peden AH, Head MW, Ritchie DL, Bell JE, Ironside JW. Preclinical vCJD after blood transfusion in a PRNP codon 129 heterozygous patient. Lancet 2004; 364: 527–529.

22. Gregori L, McCombie N, Palmer D, Birch P, Sowemimo-Coker SO, Giulivi A, Rohwer RG. Effectiveness of leucoreduction for removal of infectivity of transmissible spongiform encephalopathies from blood. Lancet 2004; 364: 529–531.

23. Miller D, Youkhana I, Karunaratne W, Pearce A. Presence of protein deposits on "cleaned" re-usable anaesthetic equipment. Anesthesia 2002; 57: 505–506.

24. Niedowski E. More to medical gloves than just rubber. The Miami Herald, (11 May, 2004), Section Health. Miami, FL, 2004.

25. Benkert N. Personnel protective equipment (PPE): Worth the effort, Advance for Medical Laboratory Professionals, 2003, pp. 27–28.

26. Rackl L. Doctors' neckties may be ailing patients. The Chicago Sun-Times. Chicago, Il, 2004, May 25, 2004.

27. Cyberspace: How Workplace Tech Can Make You Sick. USA, ABC News, 2005.

28. Leichman A. The average office is a breeding ground for germs. Northjersey.com, 2005.

Glossary

acromegaly   A condition caused by excessive secretion by the pituitary of growth hormone. It is characterized by enlargement of the bones of the extremities and the frontal bone and jaw, with enlargement of the nose and lips, tongue, and vocal cords, and thickening of facial tissues.

acute respiratory distress syndrome (ARDS)   Severe respiratory distress due to inflammatory damage that causes increased permeability of the alveolar capillary membranes, which in turn causes fluid leakage into the alveoli.

airway exchange catheter (AEC)   A long, thin, semirigid tube designed for use during endotracheal tube exchange. The tube is hollow and permits the flow of oxygen and carbon dioxide monitoring.

airway topicalization   Use of a topical agent, such as 4% lidocaine spray, to anesthetize the oropharynx in preparation for awake intubation.

ankylosing spondylitis   A form of chronic inflammation of the joints of the spine and sacroiliac joints, causing pain, stiffness and airway distortion.

anterior atlanto-axial dislocation   Displacement of the atlas from the axial spine.

antisialagogue agent   An agent that diminishes or prevents the flow of saliva (eg atropine, glycopyrrolate).

anxiolytic   A drug that relieves anxiety.

arthrogryposis   A condition in which a joint is fixed in the flexed position.

aryepiglottic folds   The aryepiglottic folds extend between the arytenoid cartilage and the lateral margin of the epiglottis on each side and constitute the lateral borders of the laryngeal inlet.

arytenoid cartilage   Either of two small cartilages at the posterior aspect of the larynx to which the vocal folds are attached.

arytenoid dislocation   Complete separation of the arytenoid cartilage from the cricoarytenoid joint. It usually results from severe laryngeal trauma and can be caused by attempts at intubation or removal of an ET tube with the cuff inflated.

atlanto-occipital dislocation   Dislocation of the base of the occiput and the arch of the atlas (C1), involving complete disruption of all ligaments between the occiput and the atlas. This injury usually causes immediate death from stretching of the brainstem, which causes respiratory arrest. Cervical traction is completely contraindicated in this injury because it can cause further stretching or dissection of the brainstem.

barotrauma   Injury from excess air pressure within the airways and lungs.

Beck airway airflow monitor   Also known as BAAM or Beck whistle. A device that fits on the 15-mm connector of the ET tube and makes a whistling sound as the patient breathes in and out. The sound gets louder when the proximal tip of the tube is closer to the glottis, rising to a maximum when the tube cuff is inflated within the trachea.

Becker dystrophy   A disease similar to Duchenne dystrophy but less serious. It affects mainly the pelvic girdle.

Beckwith-Wiedemann syndrome   A genetic disorder with some 30 manifestations, but the one that is pertinent to airway care is macroglossia, or enlarged tongue.

bilateral facet dislocation   An unstable flexion injury involving the articular joints between and posterior to adjacent vertebral bodies. The integrity of all the spinal ligaments as well as the intervertebral disc and facet joint capsules is lost. With complete dislocation, the inferior articular facets of the body above lie anterior to the superior facets of the body below.

bispectral index (BIS) monitor   A monitoring system that measures the effects of anesthetics and sedatives on the brain. Using a sensor placed on the patient's forehead, the device translates the patient's electroencephalogram (EEG) into a number from 0 to 100, indicating the patient's level of consciousness.

Bohr effect   The effect of a rise in blood acidity on oxyhemoglobin, increasing its ability to release oxygen.

Bougie-assisted tracheal intubation   A 60 cm to 70 cm long tracheal tube introducer with a 35 degree angled coude tip 2.5 cm from the distal end of the introducer. Facilitates tracheal intubation during poor laryngeal views when only the epiglottis or posterior arytenoids are visible during an optimal laryngoscopic attempt.

Bullard laryngoscope   One of several different types of rigid fiberoptic laryngoscopes.

BURP maneuver   Backward, upward, rightward pressure exerted on the thyroid cartilage to improve the laryngeal view.

capnography   A graphic recording or display of the capnometry reading over time.

capnometry   The measurement of expired carbon dioxide.

carboxyhemoglobin   The compound that results from carbon monoxide combining with hemoglobin.

Carpenter syndrome   A rare genetic disease with many manifestations, one of which is premature closure of the fontanelles, which causes a cone-shaped appearance of the head. The mandible and/or maxilla may be underdeveloped, contributing to a difficult airway situation.

cherubism   Painless mandibular enlargement, either with or without maxillary involvement.

cicatrical pemphigoid   An autoimmune disease characterized by blisters and scarring of the upper airway.

clay shoveler's fracture   A fracture of the spinous process (the posterior prominence that can be palpated on the back) resulting from abrupt flexion of the neck or a blow to the neck or the back of the head, causing forced flexion of the neck, usually occurring at C-7-T1.

commissure   The place where two structures meet.

Cormack and Lehane grading   A useful method for grading the laryngeal view of the airway as seen with the laryngoscope and estimating the difficulty of the intubation.

Cormack and Lehane laryngoscopic grades   A system of grading the view seen with the laryngoscope, with Grade 1 being the visualization of the entire vocal cords and Grade 4 being an inability to see any laryngeal anatomy, either the epiglottis or the cords. Grade 3 defines the difficult airway and is present when only the epiglottis is visible. Grade 2 is a partial view of the vocal cords.

crash airway   A patient with a Glasgow Coma Scale (GCS) score of 9 or less on an AVPU score of "P" or "U", an oxygen saturation of less than or equal to 92%, a respiratory rate of less than 10 or greater than 30 breaths per minute, and who has not responded to basic methods of ventilation. He/she requires immediate rescue ventilation to survive.

Cribriform plate   The sievelike bone that forms part of the braincase at the roof of the nasal cavity. The sievelike holes allow axons of the olfactory nerves to connect with the neurons of the olfactory bulbs.

cricothyroidotomy   Creation of access to the airway through the cricothyroid membrane.

critical airway event   Any cannot-mask-ventilate/cannot-intubate situation, three or more failed intubation attempts or attempting intubation for longer than 10 minutes (by an experienced practitioner), or sustained hypoxemia that is refractory to positive pressure ventilation with 100% oxygen.

Crouzon syndrome   A genetic disease involving premature closure of the cranial suture, causing (among other things) a beaked nose, short upper lip, underdeveloped maxilla, and a relatively small mandible.

depolarizing muscle relaxant   A muscle relaxant that causes muscle depolarization at the postsynaptic neuromuscular cleft. Succinylcholine is the only depolarizing agent available today.

difficult intubation   Multiple laryngoscopies, maneuvers, and/or blades are needed by an experienced practitioner to perform an intubation.

difficult laryngoscopy   No portion of the glottic opening can be seen during an optimal laryngoscopic attempt.

Down syndrome   Also known as trisomy 21. A congenital defect characterized by extra chromosome 21 material, leading to physical abnormalities and mild to moderate mental retardation. The Down patient may have a flat face and nose, a small mouth from which the relatively large tongue sometimes protrudes, and a short neck, all making airway management difficult.

Duchenne dystrophy   A progressive disease with childhood onset that is transmitted as a sex-linked recessive trait and that causes weakness in muscles, particularly the pelvic and shoulder muscles. Most patients die before age 20.

ELM   External laryngeal manipulation on the thyroid cartilage to improve the laryngeal view.

end-tidal carbon dioxide (ETCO$_2$)   The measurement of the CO$_2$ concentration at the end of expiration.

esophageal detector device (EDD)   Either a syringe with an adapter that fits on an ET tube, or a bulb syringe designed to attach to the ET tube. When the plunger on the syringe is drawn back, and if the tube is properly placed, the syringe should immediately and easily fill with air. The bulb syringe is depressed and the air is forced out of it; then it is attached to the ET tube. If the tube is correctly placed, the bulb syringe should fill rapidly.

failed intubation   Intubation that cannot be achieved by an experienced operator after three attempts, or the attempts have lasted for more than 10 minutes.

flexion teardrop fracture   The most severe fracture of the cervical spine, usually occurring at C5–C6, often caused by a dive into shallow water. Characterized by complete instability of the cervical spine, often resulting in quadriplegia. On x-ray, identified by a teardrop-shaped bone fragment that is separated from the vertebral body.

Freeman-Sheldon syndrome   A very rare genetic condition manifested by a small mouth that makes a person look like she or he is whistling, a flat face, club feet, contracted muscles of the joints of the fingers and hands, and underdeveloped nose cartilage.

friable lesion   An injury, wound, or other disruption of local tissue that might easily be punctured.

GABA agonist   An amino acid derivative, g-aminobutyrate (GABA) is a well-known inhibitor of presynaptic transmission in the central nervous system. Benzodiazepines exert their soothing effects by potentiating the responses of GABA-A receptors to GABA binding.

glycopyrrolate   Also known as Robinol. An anticholinergic drug that may occasionally be used as an alternative to atropine and does not cross the blood–brain barrier.

Goldenhar syndrome   A genetic defect that involves deformities of the face, usually affecting one side of the face only. Characteristics include a partially formed or absent ear, one corner of the mouth may be higher than the other, the chin may be closer to the affected ear, and sometimes an eye is missing.

gross negligence   Negligence committed with an element of reckless or wanton disregard for the person affected.

gum-elastic bougie   A long flexible "stylet" that is placed in the trachea as a guide for the ET tube. It is useful when a good view of the cords is impossible, but the epiglottis or posterior arytenoids is identifiable.

hangman's fracture of C2   Named for the fracture that occurs with hanging, now it usually results from hyperextension in trauma such as motor-vehicle collisions. May be stable or unstable, depending on whether the fracture extends through the pedicles and results in facet dislocation.

HELP   Head-elevated laryngoscopy position.

hemangioma   A tumor composed of dilated blood vessels.

hematocrit   Percentage of blood volume occupied by red cells, or erythrocytes, when they are packed together. In adult males, this is normally between 41% and 50%; in adult females, it is normally between 36% to 44%.

hemoglobin   The oxygen-carrying, iron-containing compound of the blood. It is measured by weight per unit volume, such as 14.5 grams per deciliter, or 14.5 g/dl.

Hering-Breuer reflex   A reflex, initiated by stretch receptors in the airways and lungs, that causes inspiration to stop and thus prevents overinflation of the lungs.

hypotonia   Diminished muscle tone.

imidazole   An organic crystalline base that is an inhibitor of histamine. Many drugs contain an imidazole ring (e.g., etomidate, ketoconazole, and miconazole).

inadequate ventilation   An inability to prevent or reverse hypoxemia using one- or two-person positive-pressure bag-valve-mask (BVM) ventilation in conjunction with an oropharyngeal and/or two nasopharyngeal airways and 100% oxygen.

inspissated secretions   Thickened secretions.

intercostal retractions   Inward movements of the muscles between the ribs. A sign of severe airway restriction and respiratory distress.

interincisor gap   The distance between the incisors.

Jefferson fracture   A burst fracture of the ring of C1. A fracture of the atlas caused by a downward compression. The anterior and posterior arches, and possibly the transverse processes and ligaments, are fractured.

Klippel-Feil syndrome   A rare disorder characterized by the congenital fusion of any two of the seven cervical vertebrae. This may result in restricted neck movement.

laryngocele   An abnormal dilation of the larynx.

Le Fort's fracture   Réné Le Fort, a French physician, described three different types of facial fractures: Le Fort I, a transverse fracture of the body of the maxilla just under the nasal septum; Le Fort II, a fracture of the central maxilla and palate, wherein the nose and its structures are displaced; and Le Fort III, a fracture in which the whole facial skeleton separates from the skull. Le Fort IV, not one of Le Fort's original classifications, involves the frontal bone as well as the facial skeleton. These serious injuries usually require aggressive airway management.

lymphangioma   A tumor composed of lymphatic vessels.

macroglossia   Literally, large tongue.

malfeasance   Doing a wrongful act, sometimes intentionally.

Mallampati view   The Mallampati classification system of airway views, which is different from Cormack and Lehane. The Cormack and Lehane system grades the laryngoscopic view, whereas the Mallampati system grades the view seen within the oral cavity when the patient sits upright, opens his or her mouth, and maximally protrudes the tongue.

Mason's PU-92 concept   A simple scheme to identify patients requiring immediate or rescue ventilation.

masseter muscle   The muscle involved in chewing and clenching the jaw.

methicillin-resistant S. aureus (MRSA)   A type of bacteria that is resistant to certain antibiotics, such as methicillin and other more common antibiotics, such as oxacillin, penicillin, and amoxicillin.

microatelectasis   Microscopic collapse of alveoli.

micrognathia   Abnormal smallness of the jaw.

misfeasance   Doing a lawfully required act in an improper manner.

Morquio syndrome   An inherited disease characterized by, among other things, a large head and coarse facial features, widely spaced teeth, and abnormal development of the spine. It can cause difficulty in intubation because of deformity, redundant pharyngeal mucosa, and contraindicated manipulation of the spine.

mucopolysaccharidosis (MPS)   There are seven different varieties of MPS, with many different manifestations; however, the implications for airway management are short neck, macrocephaly (large head), spinal malformations, poor development of facial bones, cardiac valvular disease, and frequent respiratory infections.

myoclonus   Twitching of muscles.

negligence   Failure to act as a reasonable and prudent person would have acted under the same or similar circumstances.

neoplasm   A growth or tumor. It may be benign or malignant.

neurofibroma   A tumor composed of the cells that form the myelin sheath of nerve fibers, the nerve fibers themselves, and connective tissue.

nondepolarizing relaxant   A muscle relaxant that inhibits neuromuscular transmission by competitively blocking (as opposed to depolarizing) nicotinic sites on the postsynaptic cleft. Nondepolarizing relaxants do not cause hyperkalemia.

nonfeasance   Failure to do what was required.

nosocomial infection   An infection acquired in a hospital.

nystagmus   Involuntary movement of the eyeballs in any direction. Often occurs with drug or ETOH ingestion but may be congenital or caused by neurological conditions. There are many types of nystagmus, but all are constant and involuntary.

odontoid fracture with lateral displacement   The odontoid, also called the dens, is a toothlike bony process extending upward from the atlas. This fracture is usually stable but may become unstable.

ovassapian airway   The fiberoptic intubating airway.

oxyhemoglobin   The compound that results from oxygen combining with hemoglobin.

oxymetazoline   A spray-type vasoconstrictor commonly available over-the-counter under a variety of trade names that can assist in both dilating the nores preventing nosebleeds during instrumentation of the nares.

peak inspiratory pressure (PIP)   The greatest air pressure within an inspiratory cycle, no matter the source of ventilation.

percussion   A tapping on the chest by placing one middle finger against the chest wall and tapping it with the tip of the other middle finger.

Pierre-Robin sequence   A syndrome characterized by unusual smallness of the jaw with cleft palate, downward displacement of the tongue, and absent gag reflex.

pneumocyst   A pocket of air in the tissues.

pneumomediastinum   Air in the mediastinum.

posterior atlanto-axial dislocation   A rare injury in which the posterior atlas is dislocated onto the axis without fracture of the odontoid process.

posterior neural arch fracture   A hyperextension injury wherein the posterior neural arch of C1 is compressed between the occiput and the spinous process of C2. The posterior arch of C1 is thin, and this compression causes it to break.

prion   A proteinaceous infectious particle; an infectious particle made entirely of protein.

proximate cause   An event that sets off a continuous and unbroken chain of events that results, in law, in injury.

pulmonary toilet   Endotracheal suctioning of secretions.

Quinsy and retropharyngeal abscess   Abscess of the area between the tonsils and the pharyngeal wall.

rales   Also called crepitations. Tiny crackling, bubbling, or rattling noises within the lungs that sound like hair being twisted together or salt being poured on a piece of paper.

Ramsay sedation scale (RSS)   A way of measuring a patient's response to sedation involving six levels of sedation.

retrograde intubation   A method by which a wire is inserted into the cricothyroid membrane through a catheter and threaded upward into the oral cavity, where it is used as a guide wire for a hollow stylet over which an endotracheal tube is advanced into the trachea.

rhabdomyolysis   Breakdown of muscle fibers leading to release of particles of muscle fiber into the circulatory system. It may be the result of crushing injury, burns, stress of muscle fibers, and other causes and can lead to kidney failure.

rhonchi   Coarse sounds resembling soft snoring that come from the larger airways.

Seldinger technique   Used in both antegrade and retrograde cricothyrotomy techniques, this is a method in which a wire is inserted through a catheter into a blood vessel or the airway and a catheter or guide is advanced over it. The wire is removed once the catheter or airway device is in place.

Sellick's maneuver   The application of pressure on the cricoid cartilage to occlude the esophagus and prevent silent regurgitation of gastric contents.

Shikani seeing stylet   A device for endotracheal intubation consisting of a high resolution (30,000 pixels) endoscope within a bendable stylet that is inserted through an endotracheal tube to allow placement under direct vision.

shunting   A condition that occurs when deoxygenated blood passes straight through unventilated sections of the lung without picking up oxygen or shedding carbon dioxide. This can happen when alveoli collapse (atelectasis) or pulmonary edema replaces the air in the alveoli.

6-D Method   Method of assessing the airway for distortion, disproportion, decreased thyromental distance, decreased interincisor gap, decreased range of motion, and dental overbite (all signs begin with "D" like the word "difficult").

SLAM concept   The idea that most airway techniques used in anesthesiology can be applied from the prehospital environment through all areas of the hospital.

sniffing position   The position when the patient's neck is slightly flexed and the head is extended, which brings the oral, pharyngeal, and laryngeal axes into alignment.

standard of care   Care that is recognized as acceptable and appropriate by reasonably prudent health care providers.

Stickler's syndrome   A genetic disease of the connective tissue. It is expressed in many ways, including cleft palate, cataracts, retinal detachments, blindness, flat face with a small jaw, and hyperextensible joints.

stomal granulation   Granular tissue that develops around the stoma, or opening, created by a surgical procedure.

stridor   A harsh, vibrating noise caused by an obstruction high in the airway.

SUAAF   SLAM Universal Adult Airway Flowchart.

subglottic web   A membrane, tissue, or tissues that extend across the lumen of the trachea.

subluxation   Dislocation of vertebrae.

thalassanemia   A group of inherited anemias that occur in Mediterranean and Southeast Asian populations.

thyromental distance   The distance from the tip of the chin to the superior aspect of the thyroid cartilage (the upper prominence of the larynx).

tortfeasor   One who commits an act of negligence that is actionable under the law of torts.

tracheo-esophageal malacia   A softening of the tissues, leading to tissue structural collapse.

tracheo-innominate fistula   An abnormal passageway or "tube" between the trachea and the innominate artery, resulting in hemorrhage into the trachea or into the surrounding tissues.

tracheopathia osteochondroplastica   Benign dysplasia (abnormal growth) of the trachea and large bronchi, which gradually causes narrowing of the tracheal lumen.

tracheotomy   A surgical procedure in which a portion of the anterior trachea below the cricoid cartilage is dissected and an airway device is inserted.

transillumination   The light from a lighted stylet that can be seen externally through the tissues. If the stylet is properly placed, a bright light can be seen in the anterior neck.

transtracheal anesthesia   Puncture of the cricothyroid membrane and injection of lidocaine at the end of inspiration to produce anesthesia below the vocal chords and upper trachea.

transtracheal jet ventilation   Ventilation through the cricothyroid membrane with a needle or catheter connected to a special controlled-pressure oxygen system.

transverse process fracture   A fracture of the bony protrusions extending out from each side of the vertebral column at about a 45° angle. It is usually stable. The most common transverse process fractures are in the lower thoracic and lumbar spine.

Treacher-Collins syndrome   Also called mandibulofacial dysostosis. Characterized by down-slanted eyes; notched lower eyelids; underdevelopment or absence of cheekbones and the side wall and floor of the eye socket; an often small and slanting lower jaw; underdeveloped, malformed ears; and a fish-face appearance often causing difficult laryngoscopy.

trismus   Restriction of the mouth opening. Also a contraction of the muscles in the jaw.

velocardiofacial syndrome   A genetic condition characterized by structural or functional abnormalities of the palate, cardiac defects, and many other manifestations.

ventilation/perfusion mismatch   A condition that occurs when some alveoli are over-ventilated and underperfused, and others are underventilated and overperfused, resulting in suboptimal oxygenation of the blood. This is also known as pulmonary shunting.

vesicular breath sounds   Normal breath sounds.

wedge fracture   A vertebral compression fracture occurring anteriorly (front) or laterally (side).

xeroderma pigmentosum   A rare genetic disease provoked by sunlight.

INDEX

Endotracheal intubation, 57, 66, 144*t*
   anesthesia for, 128–35
   cervical-spine injuries and, 254*t*
   lighted stylet, 206, 208*f*, 209
Endotracheal tubes, 38, 49, 58–59, 63, 81*f*, 87*f*, 114, 122,
     167*f*, 174–75
   cuffed. *See* Cuffed endotracheal tubes
   guide for, 106
   obstruction, 122*f*
   selecting according to age, 285*t*
ENK cricothyrotomy needle, 221*f*
ENK oxygen flow modulator, 223*f*
Epiglottis, 2, 24–25, 24*f*, 27, 59, 91, 274*t*
   cartilage, 20, 23
   vallecula, 25
ERC (European Resuscitation Council), 67
ERV (expiratory reserve volume), 42*f*
Eschmann introducer, 102, 105–6, 119–20
Esmolol, 143*t*, 144*t*
Esophageal detector device, 80, 88, 112–15, 119, 120, 162
   self-inflating bulb, 14, 114, 115*f*, 119, 158
   syringe, 114
Esophageal gastric tube airway, 166
Esophageal intubation, 4, 80, 112, 119
Esophageal tracheal combitube, 9*t*, 149, 158–71,
     160*t*, 165*f*
   advantages, 164–66, 165*t*
   and airway management, 168*f*
   closed space rescue and, 168*f*
   complications, 169
   insertion, 160–62
   and laryngeal mask airway, 171*t*
   limitations and contraindications, 169, 169*t*
   lung ventilation and, 162
   manikin training with, 163–64
   patient positioning for, 161
   placement, 163, 164
   replacement for definitive airway, 166–67, 167*f*
Esophageal ventilation, 114
Esophagus, 24–27, 26*f*, 49
ETC. *See* Esophageal tracheal combitube
ETCO$_2$. *See* End-tidal carbon dioxide
Etomidate, 129*t*, 130, 140, 140*t*, 141*t*, 143*t*, 144*t*, 150
ETT. *See* Endotracheal tubes
Euromedical tracheal tube, 182*f*, 185
Exaggerated hyperkalemia, 141*t*
Exhalation, 41*f*
Expiration, 39–40, 42*f*, 52
   forced, 41*f*, 42

   obstruction, 122
   passive, 40
Expiratory reserve volume, 42*f*
External laryngeal manipulation. *See* ELM (external
     laryngeal manipulation)

F

Face tents, 53
Face-to-face patient positioning, 209
Facial trauma, 62, 238–41, 240*f*
Failed intubation, 80, 99–109, 112, 149, 176, 178
   contingency plans for, 108–9
   fiberoptic bronchoscope and, 191
   orotracheal, 148
Failed laryngoscopy, 99
Failed orotracheal intubation, 148
False vocal cords, 27
FDA (Food and Drug Administration), 218, 280
Fentanyl, 129*t*, 134, 142*t*, 143*t*, 144*t*, 289
Fiberoptic intubation. *See* Fiberscopic and video-assisted
     intubation
Fiberscopic and video-assisted intubation, 166, 167*f*,
     186, 189–204
   case study, 189
   in cervical spine injuries, 103
   and lightwand intubation, 210
Fibrocartilage, 24
Fistula, tracheo-innominate, 234
Flexible fiberoptic bronchoscope, 190–94
Flexion teardrop fracture, 250
Flip test, 153*f*
Flow meters, 81
FOB (flexible fiberoptic bronchoscope), 190–94
Foley Airway Stylet Tool, 198
Foreign body, 43, 55, 83, 270
   and cricothyrotomy, 218–19
   removal, 83*f*, 108
Fractures, 238, 241, 250–53, 250*t*
FRC (functional residual capacity), 42*f*, 57, 88–89, 276
Freeman-Sheldon syndrome, 273*t*, 274
Friable lesion, 210
Frova Intubating Introducer, 106
Functional residual capacity, 42*f*, 57, 88–89, 276

G

GABA agonists, 290
Gas diffusion, 38
Gas exchange, 46–47, 57, 139
Gas transport, 38, 39

CPSIA information can be obtained at www.ICGtesting.com
Printed in the USA
LVOW02s1939220515

439531LV00005B/7/P